T0198176

CLINICAL CARDIAC ELECTROPHYSIOLOGY

A PRACTICAL GUIDE

CLINICAL CARDIAC ELECTROPHYSIOLOGY

A PRACTICAL GUIDE

Demosthenes G Katritsis, MD, PhD, FRCP, FESC, FACC

Director, Department of Cardiology
Hygeia Hospital
Athens, Greece
Honorary Consultant Cardiologist
St Thomas' Hospital
London, UK
Adjunct Assistant Professor of Cardiology,
Johns Hopkins University School of Medicine,
Baltimore, Maryland, USA

Fred Morady, MD, FACC

McKay Professor of Cardiovascular Diseases
Professor of Internal Medicine
University of Michigan Medical School
Ann Arbor, Michigan
USA

ELSEVIER

Elsevier
1600 John F. Kennedy Blvd.
Ste 1600
Philadelphia, PA 19103-2899

CLINICAL CARDIAC ELECTROPHYSIOLOGY: ISBN: 9780323793384
A PRACTICAL GUIDE

Notice

Practitioners and researchers must always rely on their own experience and
knowledge in evaluating and using any information, methods, compounds
or experiments described herein. Because of rapid advances in the medical
sciences, in particular, independent verification of diagnoses and drug
dosages should be made. To the fullest extent of the law, no responsibility is
assumed by Elsevier, authors, editors or contributors for any injury and/or
damage to persons or property as a matter of products liability, negligence
or otherwise, or from any use or operation of any methods, products,
instructions, or ideas contained in the material herein.

**Front cover image from Katritsis DG. A unified theory for the circuit of
atrioventricular nodal reentrant tachycardia. Europace 2020 Sep 26:euaa196.**

Library of Congress Control Number: 2020943677

Director, Content Development: Ellen Wurm-Cutter
Content Strategist: Robin Carter
Content Development Specialist: Dominque McPherson
Publishing Services Manager: Shereen Jameel
Senior Project Manager: Kamatchi Madhavan
Design: Amy Buxton

Printed in China

Last digit is the print number: 9 8 7 6 5 4 3 2 1

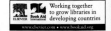

If one asks me where we go from here, I would respond, "back to basics—learn electrophysiology."

Mark E. Josephson

Preface

The *term electrophysiology study (EPS)* denotes an invasive procedure for the examination of the conducting system of the heart and cardiac arrhythmias. In contemporary practice, an EPS often includes catheter ablation. A standardized approach in every laboratory is helpful for obtaining reproducible results that ensure an accurate diagnosis, and effective therapy. This book presents the fundamental steps that comprise the framework for EPS in contemporary EP laboratories, as well as an overview of all clinical arrhythmias. It is not a reference textbook of basic or clinical cardiac electrophysiology. It is aimed at succinctly presenting the methodology of when and how to perform an EPS and catheter ablation, in the context of a practical guide on how to manage patients with arrhythmia problems. It is, therefore, aimed both at cardiology and EP fellows and trainees who wish to learn electrophysiology, and study the diagnosis and invasive therapy of arrhythmia disorders.

The fundamentals of mechanisms of arrhythmogenesis, anatomy of cardiac structures, and hardware needed for an EPS that the electrophysiologist must be aware of are presented in the first section of the book. The following chapters deal with the clinical indications for an EPS, the tools and techniques used to perform an EPS, and the potential problems encountered during the study of specific arrhythmias in clinical practice.

We both have been attracted to clinical cardiac electrophysiology by the cognitive challenges it presents, and the satisfaction derived from identifying the mechanism of a challenging arrhythmia using an analytical approach. In the era of computerized, video-game-style approaches that are now available for atrial fibrillation, supraventricular tachycardia, and ventricular tachycardia ablation, in-depth knowledge of electrophysiologic principles and deductive reasoning for arrhythmia diagnosis remain essential for the clinical cardiac electrophysiologist, as well as the cardiologist who takes care of patients with arrhythmic disorders.

For the sake of consistency and to avoid the redundancy often present in books with multiple contributors, we decided to undertake the writing of the book ourselves. Of course, several colleagues, senior and junior, have reviewed and commented on our manuscript—our sincerest thanks to them all. We are particularly grateful to Yannis Pantos, PhD, George Katritsis, BSc, MRCP, Vishal Luther, PhD, MRCP, and Theodore Xenos, MSc, who kindly provided their expertise and help on the issues of physics of ablation and electroanatomic mapping. We are also grateful to Kamatchi Madhavan, Dominque McPherson, and involved staff at Elsevier for their incredible help and efficiency. Finally, our appreciation and thanks to Robin Carter, our editor at Elsevier, for her professionalism, wholehearted support, and commitment to our purpose.

Demos Katritsis
Fred Morady

Contents

1

Classification of Arrhythmias

Bradyarrhythmias are due to ***sinus nodal disease*** (Box 1.1) or ***atrioventricular conduction block*** (Box 1.2).

Tachyarrhythmias are classified as **ventricular** or **supraventricular**. The term *supraventricular* literally indicates tachycardias (atrial rates > 100 beats per minute [bpm] at rest) arising from the His bundle or above.[1-3] Traditionally, the term *supraventricular tachycardia* (SVT) has been used to describe all tachycardias that are not solely infra-Hisian in origin, including atrial fibrillation and tachycardias such as atrioventricular reentry as a result of an accessory connection that involves both the atrium and ventricle (Box 1.3). The term *narrow QRS tachycardia* indicates tachycardia with a QRS duration ≤ 120 milliseconds (ms). A *wide QRS tachycardia* refers to one with a QRS duration > 120 ms.

Box 1.1 Sinus Node Dysfunction (with accompanying symptoms)

Sinus bradycardia
Sinoatrial exit block
Sinus pauses (>3 s)
Sinus node arrest
Tachycardia-bradycardia syndrome
Chronotropic incompetence*

---

*Maximum predicted heart rate is calculated as 220 – age (y).

Box 1.2 Atrioventricular Block

First-degree AV block
Second-degree AV block
    Type I AV block (Mobitz I or Wenckebach)
    Type II AV block (Mobitz II)
Third-degree (complete) AV block.

AV, Atrioventricular.

Box 1.3 Classification of Tachyarrhythmias

ATRIAL TACHYCARDIAS

Sinus tachycardia
- Physiologic sinus tachycardia
- Inappropriate sinus tachycardia
- Sinus nodal reentrant tachycardia

Focal atrial tachycardia
- Microreentry
- Automatic

Multifocal atrial tachycardia

Macroreentrant atrial tachycardia
- Cavotricuspid isthmus dependent
  - Typical atrial flutter, counterclockwise (common) or clockwise (reverse)
  - Other cavotricuspid isthmus dependent
- Noncavotricuspid isthmus dependent
  - Right atrial
  - Left atrial

Atrial fibrillation

ATRIOVENTRICULAR JUNCTIONAL TACHYCARDIAS

Atrioventricular nodal reentrant tachycardia
- Typical
- Atypical

Nonreentrant junctional tachycardia
- Junctional ectopic tachycardia (focal or automatic junctional tachycardia)
- Other nonreentrant variants

Box 1.3 Classification of Tachyarrhythmias—cont'd

ATRIOVENTRICULAR TACHYCARDIAS
- Orthodromic
  - Concealed or manifest atrioventricular accessory pathway conducting in retrograde direction, with anterograde conduction through the atrioventricular node node/His-Purkinje system
  - Nodofascicular or nodoventricular bypass tract conducting in retrograde direction, with anterograde conduction through the atrioventricular node/His-Purkinje system
- Antidromic
  - Atrioventricular accessory pathway conducting anterograde with retrograde conduction through the AV node or, rarely, over another pathway
  - Atriofascicular, atrioventricular, nodofascicular, or nodoventricular bypass tract conducting in the anterograde direction, with retrograde conduction through the AV node or rarely through another pathway

VENTRICULAR TACHYCARDIAS
- Monomorphic ventricular tachycardia
  - Scar-related reentry
  - Bundle branch reentry
  - Idiopathic (automatic, reentrant, interfascicular)
- Accelerated idioventricular rhythm
- Polymorphic ventricular tachycardia
- Pleomorphic ventricular tachycardia
- Bidirectional ventricular tachycardia
- Torsades de pointes
- Ventricular flutter
- Ventricular fibrillation

AV, Atrioventricular.

References

1. Page RL, Joglar JA, Caldwell MA, et al. 2015 ACC/AHA/HRS guideline for the management of adult patients with supraventricular tachycardia. *J Am Coll Cardiol.* 2016;67(13):1575-1623.
2. Katritsis DG, Boriani G, Cosio FG, et al. European Heart Rhythm Association (EHRA) consensus document on the management of supraventricular arrhythmias, endorsed by Heart Rhythm Society (HRS), Asia-Pacific Heart Rhythm Society (APHRS), and Sociedad Latinoamericana de Estimulación Cardiaca y Electrofisiologia (SOLAECE). *Eur Heart J.* 2018;39(16):1442-1445.
3. Brugada J, Katritsis DG, Arbelo E, et al. 2019 ESC Guidelines for the management of patients with supraventricular tachycardia. *Eur Heart J.* 2020;41(5):655-720.

2

Electrophysiologic Mechanisms of Arrhythmogenesis

NORMAL EXCITATION OF THE HEART

Cardiac electrical activity starts by the spontaneous excitation of "pacemaker" cells in the sinoatrial node in the right atrium. Pacemaker automaticity is due to spontaneous diastolic repolarization of phase 4 that generates rhythmic action potentials and determines the heart rate through various currents, including the If current.[1] There are no histologically specialized conduction tissues between the sinus and AV node, and the sinus impulse is transmitted via several exit pathways which electrically bridge the nodal tissue and atrial myocardium,[2] and then preferentially toward the AV node via muscle bundles with well aligned arrangement of cardiomyocytes.[3] By traveling through intercellular gap junctions (cell-to-cell connections), the excitation wave depolarizes adjacent atrial myocytes, ultimately resulting in excitation of the atria. The excitation wave then propagates via the atrioventricular node and the Purkinje fibers to the ventricles, where ventricular myocytes are depolarized, resulting in excitation of the ventricles. Depolarization of each atrial or ventricular myocyte is represented by the initial action potential (AP) upstroke (phase 0), where the negative resting membrane potential (approximately −85 mV) depolarizes to positive voltages (Figs. 2.1 and 2.2 and Table 2.1).[4] The action potential is produced by transmembrane flow of ions (inward depolarizing currents mainly through Na^+ and Ca^{2+} channels, and outward repolarizing currents mainly through K^+ channels).[5,6] The resting potential of atrial and ventricular myocytes during AP phase 4 (resting phase) is stable and negative (–85 mV) because of the high conductance of the potassium channels. Excitation by electrical impulses from adjacent cells activates the inward Na^+ current that depolarizes myocytes rapidly (phase 0). Transient outward K^+ current (phase 1) creates a notch during the early phase of repolarization (I_{to}). Balance of the inward depolarizing L-type Ca^{2+} current (I_{Ca-L}) and outward rectifier K^+ currents (slow I_{Ks}, rapid I_{Kr}, and ultra-rapid I_{Kur}) forms a plateau phase (phase 2). Deactivation (closing) of the inward current I_{Ca-L} and increase of the outward currents creates phase 3 with final repolarization mainly because of potassium efflux through the inward rectifier I_{K1} channels, and the membrane potential returns to its resting potential (phase 4). The pacemaker current (I_f) contributes to action potential generation in the sinus node and significantly determines heart rate.[7] I_f is an inward current activated on hyperpolarization. It is called the funny current because despite being an inward current, it behaves like a pure K^+ current (as a result of superimposition of I_{k1}).[8] In Purkinje fibers, a similar behavior is expressed by current I_{k2}. I_f activation is accelerated by intracellular cyclic adenosine monophosphate (cAMP) levels and thus regulated by sympathetic and parasympathetic activity, which controls synthesis and degradation of intracellular cAMP, respectively.

Opening and closing (gating) of ion channels enable transmembrane ion currents that consist of proteins called pore-forming alpha (α) subunits and accessory beta (β) subunits. Terminology of genes encoding for these proteins describes their function. For example, the gene encoding the α subunit of the cardiac sodium channel is called *SCN5A*: sodium channel, type 5, α subunit. The α subunit is termed Nav 1.5: Na^+ channel family, subfamily 1, member 5; *V* means that channel gating is regulated by transmembrane voltage changes (voltage dependent).[4] Polymorphisms and mutations in genes encoding for ion channels are associated with slow conduction and QRS prolongation and, consequently, future development of cardiac arrhythmias.[9,10]

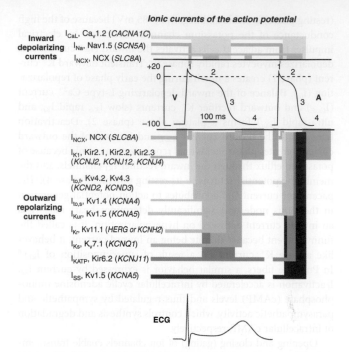

FIG. 2.1. The Ionic currents of the action potential (AP). Activation and inactivation of ion channels, currents, underlying proteins, and encoding genes and their contributions to inward depolarizing and outward repolarizing currents. Ventricular *(V)* and atrial *(A)* APs comprise rapid depolarizing (phase 0), early repolarizing (phase 1), brief (atrial) or prolonged (ventricular) phase 2 plateaus (phase 2), phase 3 repolarization, and phase 4 electric diastole. In these, inward Na^+ or Ca^{2+} currents drive phase 0 depolarization and Ca^{2+} current maintains the phase 2 plateau, and a range of outward K^+ currents drive phase 1 and phase 3 repolarization. Phase 4 resting potential restoration is accompanied by a refractory period required for Na^+ channel recovery. Abbreviation of ionic currents are presented in Table 2.1.

ECG, Electrocardiogram. (Adapted from Huang CL. Murine electrophysiological models of cardiac arrhythmogenesis. *Physiol Rev.* 2017;97(1):283-409. © 2017 the American Physiological Society.)

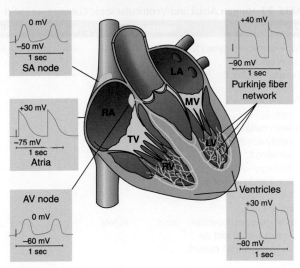

FIG. 2.2. Functional anatomy of the cardiac conduction system. The cardiac impulse is initiated in the sinoatrial node and propagates through the atria. The electric impulse is then delayed in the AVN before rapid conduction through the right and left bundle branches before terminating in the Purkinje fiber network, which directly interfaces with ventricular cardiomyocytes. Distinct time-voltage relationships are noted in the sinoatrial node, atria, AVN, Purkinje fibers, and ventricles.

AV, Atrioventricular; *AVN,* atrioventricular node; *LA,* left atrium; *LV,* left ventricle; *MV,* mitral valve; *RA,* right atrium; *RV,* right ventricle; *SA,* sinoatrial node; *TV,* tricuspid valve. (Munshi NV. Gene regulatory networks in cardiac conduction system development. *Circ Res.* 2012; 110(11):1525-1537. © 2012 American Heart Association, Inc.)

TABLE 2.1 Human Atrial and Ventricular Ionic Currents

CURRENT/SYMBOL	PROTEIN	GENE	VENTRICLE	ATRIUM
Voltage-Gated Inward Currents				
Fast Na⁺ current, I_{Na}	Na$_V$1.5	*SCN5A*	+++	+++
L-type Ca²⁺ current, I_{CaL} (dihydropyridine receptor: DHPR)	Ca$_V$1.2	*CACNA1C*	+++	++
Voltage-Gated Outward Currents				
Fast transient outward K⁺ current, $I_{to,f}$	Kv4.2	*KCND2*	++	+++
	Kv4.3	*KCND3*		

Continued

TABLE 2.1 Human Atrial and Ventricular Ionic Currents—cont'd

CURRENT/SYMBOL	PROTEIN	GENE	VENTRICLE	ATRIUM
Slow transient outward K$^+$ current, $I_{to,s}$	KV1.4	KCNA4	++	+++
Delayed rectifier K$^+$ current, I_{Kr}	Kv11.1	KCNH2 (HERG)	+++	+
Delayed rectifier K$^+$ current, I_{Ks}	Kv7.1	KCNQ1	+++	+
4-Aminopyridine-sensitive, rapidly activating, slowly inactivating K$^+$ current, I_{Kslow}	Kv1.5	KCNA5	−	−
4-Aminopyridine-insensitive, rapidly activating, slowly inactivating K$^+$ current, I_{Kslow2}	Kv2.1	KCNB1	−	−
Sustained 4-aminopyride-sensitive ultrarapid delayed rectifier K$^+$ current, I_{Kur}	Kv1.5	KCNA5	−	++
Inward Rectifiers				
Inwardly rectifying current I_{K1}	Kir2.1	KCNJ2	+++	++
	Kir2.2	KCNJ12		
Acetylcholine-activated, K$^+$ current, I_{KACh}	Kir3.1	KCNJ3	−	+++
	Kir3.4,	KCNJ5		
ATP-sensitive potassium channel, $I_{k2}p$	Kir6.2	KCNJ11	++	++
Leak Currents				
Two-pore domain K$^+$ leak current, $I_{k2}p$	K2p3.1	KCNK3	+++	++
Ca^{2+}-activated K$^+$ current, I_{KCa}	KC$_a$2.x-	KCNNx	−	+++
Exchange Currents				
Transient, inward, Na$^+$-Ca^{2+} exchange current, I_{ti}	NCX	SLC8A1	++	++

ATP, Adenosine triphosphate.
From Huang CL. Murine electrophysiological models of cardiac arrhythmogenesis. *Physiol Rev.* 2017;97(1):283-409.

MECHANISMS OF ARRHYTHMIAS

Although the initiation of tachycardias is a complex process depending on the interaction of several factors, the main mechanisms responsible for the initiation of tachycardias are thought to be cell membrane hyperexcitability (i.e., enhanced automaticity or triggered activity) and reduction in cell-to-cell electrical coupling resulting in conduction block and reentry.[11]

Abnormal or Enhanced Automaticity

Abnormal or enhanced automaticity is due to the maximum diastolic potential spontaneously becoming less negative (−40 to −60 mV; phase 4 of the AP). In nonpacemaker myocytes, an imbalance between hyperpolarizing and depolarizing diastolic currents can occur under pathologic conditions and lead to enhanced automaticity.[12] This is facilitated by factors including ischemia, hypokalemia, and sympathetic activation.

Triggered Activity

Triggered activity is caused by early after-depolarizations or delayed after-depolarizations (i.e., depolarizing oscillations in membrane voltage usually mediated by increases in intracellular calcium. **Early after-depolarizations** occur during phase 3 of the action potential and may be due to electrolyte disturbances such as hypokalemia, hypomagnesemia, antiarrhythmic drugs (classes Ia and III), hypoxia, or hypercapnia. Although promoted by bradycardia, early after-depolarizations are enhanced by adrenergic stimulation. Typically they occur in long QT syndrome. Moderate hypokalemia is a potent inducer of ventricular arrhythmias mediated by early after-depolarizations.[13] **Delayed after-depolarizations** occur after complete repolarization of the action potential and may be due to calcium overload, digoxin, and artificial pacing. They are facilitated by tachycardia and adrenergic stimulation. Typically they occur in idiopathic outflow tract tachycardia. Delayed after-depolarizations are generated by diastolic Ca^{2+} release from the sarcoplasmic reticulum to form intracellular "Ca^{2+} waves."[12,14]

Reentry

Reentry denotes circulation of a wave of depolarization that is initiated when the following occur:

- Two functionally distinct pathways are present.
- Unidirectional block is induced in one pathway—for example, by a premature depolarization or by a physiologic tachycardia.
- Sufficiently slow conduction exists to allow recovery of excitability in the blocked pathway and permit retrograde conduction over that pathway and completion of the circuit.

The activation wave front travels around the obstacle (anatomic or functional). For reentry to continue, the circuit length (set by anatomic obstacle size or functional tissue properties) must be larger than the "wavelength" (WL) (Fig. 2.3). The WL concept is based to the mode of reentry first described and named "*leading circle.*"[12] The minimum circuit length theoretically achievable depends on myocardial properties as follows: WL = CV × RP, where *CV* is conduction velocity and *RP* is the refractory period. The smaller the WL, the more likely is reentry; accordingly, either conduction slowing or decreased refractoriness facilitates reentry. An excitable gap (EG = circuit length − WL) separates the circuit head from the tail. If the circuit length is smaller than the WL, the circuit head collides with the tail and propagation is extinguished.

Reentrant mechanisms conventionally are classified as follows:

- *Anatomic,* caused by a defined loop. There is a large excitable gap between the crest and tail of impulse, such that properly timed stimuli can capture the circuit and reset the tachycardia. A typical example of this is atrioventricular reentrant tachycardia using an accessory atrioventricular connection.
- *Functional,* caused by altered cellular electrophysiologic properties of myocardial tissue such as functional barriers of conduction block or decremental conduction leading to propagation failure. Functional reentry is exemplified by the "leading circle" hypothesis, which may be important in atrial fibrillation.[15] In this model the reentrant pathway is the shortest possible one and is determined on an instantaneous basis by refractoriness ahead of the activation wave front. The cycle length therefore is determined only by refractoriness, and the excitable gap is as short as possible, independent of the cycle

length. Functional reentry may also take the form of a "spiral wave," which has been implicated in both atrial and ventricular fibrillation.[16,17]

- *Anisotropic,* caused by changes in microanatomic structures such as cellular coupling and fiber disarray, which lead to anisotropic conduction or spatial inhomogeneity of refractoriness.[18] The length of the circular pathway is determined by electrophysiologic-anatomic changes, and there may be an excitable gap. This kind of reentry can be seen after myocardial infarctions.

There is evidence that more than 90% of clinical tachycardias are due to reentrant mechanisms.[19] Typical examples of reentry are tachycardias associated with Wolff-Parkinson-White syndrome, the atrioventricular junctional reentry tachycardias, atrial flutter, and most probably (at least in part) atrial fibrillation. In addition, certain forms of sustained monomorphic ventricular tachycardia (VT) such as VT in patients with coronary artery disease and bundle branch reentry in cases of dilated cardiomyopathy demonstrate a reentrant circuit with a fully excitable gap. Anisotropic reentry appears to play an important role in ventricular tachycardias occurring in the setting of chronic healed myocardial infarcts. Torsades de pointes and some forms of ventricular tachycardia complicating coronary artery disease are due to after-depolarization–induced triggered activity.

Reentrant mechanisms are postulated when programmed stimulation demonstrates that the tachycardia behaves in a manner similar to that of reentry. Inducibility and termination by programmed stimulation and entrainment of the tachycardia indicate a reentrant mechanism. Tachycardias as a result of triggered activity may also be initiated and terminated by pacing and may be distinguished from reentrant ones because progressively more premature stimulation may cause progressively faster triggered activity. VT caused by triggered activity is distinguished from reentrant VT by the inability to entrain this type of tachycardia. Distinction of supraventricular tachycardias caused by triggered activity from reentry may be more difficult. Arrhythmias caused by abnormal automaticity occur spontaneously or in response to isoprenaline and are not induced by programmed stimulation.

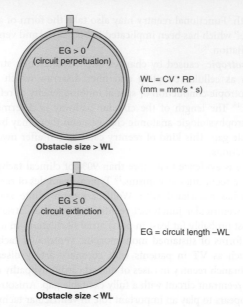

FIG. 2.3. Reentry "wavelength." The activation front travels around the obstacle (anatomic or functional). For reentry to continue, the circuit length (set by anatomic obstacle size or tissue functional properties) must be larger than the "wavelength" *(WL)*. In this case an excitable gap *(EG)* separates the circuit head from the tail. If the circuit length is smaller than the WL, the circuit head collides with the tail (no EG) and propagation is extinguished.

CV, Conduction velocity; *RP,* absolute refractory period. (Brugada J, Katritsis D, Arbelo E, et al. 2019 ESC Guidelines for the management of supraventricular tachycardias. *Eur Heart J.* 2019;40[47]:3812-3813.)

References

1. Park DS, Fishman GI. The cardiac conduction system. *Circulation.* 2011;123(8):904-915.
2. Fedorov VV, Glukhov AV, Chang R, et al. Optical mapping of the isolated coronary-perfused human sinus node. *J Am Coll Cardiol.* 2010;56(17):1386-1394.
3. Ho SY, Anderson RH, Sánchez-Quintana D. Atrial structure and fibres: morphologic bases of atrial conduction. *Cardiovascular Research.* 2002;54(2):325-336.
4. Amin AS, Tan HL, Wilde AA. Cardiac ion channels in health and disease. *Heart Rhythm.* 2010;7(1):117-126.
5. Huang CL. Murine electrophysiological models of cardiac arrhythmogenesis. *Physiol Rev.* 2017;97(1):283-409.

6. Lei M, Wu L, Terrar DA, Huang CL. Modernized classification of cardiac antiarrhythmic drugs. *Circulation.* 2018;138(17):1879-1896.

7. Verkerk AO, Wilders R, van Borren MM, et al. Pacemaker current (I(f)) in the human sinoatrial node. *Eur Heart J.* 2007;28(20):2472-2478.

8. DiFrancesco D. The role of the funny current in pacemaker activity. *Circ Res.* 2010;106(3):434-446.

9. Ritchie MD, Denny JC, Zuvich RL, et al. Genome- and phenome-wide analyses of cardiac conduction identifies markers of arrhythmia risk. *Circulation.* 2013;127(13):1377-1385.

10. Obeyesekere MN, Antzelevitch C, Krahn AD. Management of ventricular arrhythmias in suspected channelopathies. *Circ Arrhythm Electrophysiol.* 2015;8(1):221-231.

11. Zipes DP. Mechanisms of clinical arrhythmias. *Heart Rhythm.* 2004;1(suppl 5): 4C-18C.

12. Wit AL, Wellens HJ, Josephson ME. *Electrophysiological Foundations of Cardiac Arrhythmias.* 1st ed. Minneapolis: Cardiotext Publishing; 2017.

13. Pezhouman A, Singh N, Song Z, et al. Molecular basis of hypokalemia-induced ventricular fibrillation. *Circulation.* 2015;132(16):1528-1537.

14. Zaza A, Rocchetti M. Calcium store stability as an antiarrhythmic endpoint. *Curr Pharm Des.* 2015;21(8):1053-1061.

15. Comtois P, Kneller J, Nattel S. Of circles and spirals: bridging the gap between the leading circle and spiral wave concepts of cardiac reentry. *Europace.* 2005;7(suppl 2):10-20.

16. Vaquero M, Calvo D, Jalife J. Cardiac fibrillation: from ion channels to rotors in the human heart. *Heart Rhythm.* 2008;5(6):872-879.

17. Grace AA, Roden DM. Systems biology and cardiac arrhythmias. *Lancet.* 2012;380(9852):1498-1508.

18. Valderrabano M. Influence of anisotropic conduction properties in the propagation of the cardiac action potential. *Prog Biophys Mol Biol.* 2007;94(1-2):144-168.

19. Brugada J, Katritsis DG, Arbelo E, et al. 2019 ESC Guidelines for the management of patients with supraventricular tachycardia: The Task Force for the management of patients with supraventricular tachycardia of the European Society of Cardiology (ESC). *Eur Heart J.* 2020;41(5):655-720.

3

Cardiac Anatomy for the Electrophysiologist

Some of the descriptive terms conventionally used for cardiac structures are inaccurate. Conventionally the heart and its associated structures have been described in accordance with their position when the heart has been removed from the body and positioned with the apex down, rather than according to their in vivo positions.[1,2] For example, when defining positions along the mitral and tricuspid valve annuli and the triangle of Koch, the superior aspect of the heart has been described as being anterior, whereas the anterior and posterior aspects have been described as right and left lateral.[2]

When entering the chest through a sternotomy, the most anterior chamber of the heart is the right ventricle (RV). A small portion of the left ventricle (LV) can be seen along the left border of the RV, and the remainder of the LV lies posterior to the RV (Fig. 3.1).[1,2] The apex of the heart (point of maximal impulse) is formed by the left ventricular apex, which is slightly superior to its right ventricular counterpart. To the right of the RV is the right atrium (RA), the only appropriately named cardiac chamber with respect to its position. Posteriorly and just anterior to the vertebral column is the left atrium (LA). Therefore, in view of the in vivo position of the heart, the ventricles are anterior to their respective atria and the right-sided chambers are anterior to the left-sided chambers. The LA is the most posterior cardiac chamber and the RV is the most anterior cardiac chamber.[1,2]

Fig. 3.2 presents the inaccurate nomenclature that has been conventionally used for the locations of accessory pathways and the anatomically correct terminology.

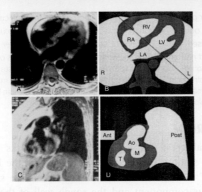

FIG. 3.1. (A) View of the heart through the mitral and tricuspid planes, atria, and ventricles using horizontal magnetic resonance imaging (MRI). (B) Schematic reproduction of (A) with appropriate labels. The main direction of the valvar planes, marked by the *dotted line* in (B), is from the anterior *(right)* to the posterior *(left)*. (C) Oblique sagittal MR image of the heart, parallel to the plane of the atrioventricular valves *(dotted line* in [B]), showing the position of the mitral and tricuspid valvar orifices and the aortic root in the left anterior oblique view. (D) schematic reproduction of (C) with appropriate labels.

Ant, Anterior; *Ao,* aortic root; *L,* left; *LA,* left atrium; *LV,* left ventricle; *M,* mitral valve; *Post,* posterior; *R,* right; *RA,* right atrium; *RV,* right ventricle; *T,* tricuspid valve. (Cosio FG, Anderson RH, Kuck KH, et al. ESCWGA/NASPE/P experts consensus statement: living anatomy of the atrioventricular junctions. *J Cardiovasc Electrophysiol* 1999;10(8):1162-1170.)

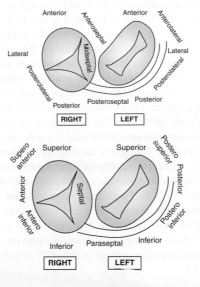

FIG. 3.2. *Upper panel:* Schematic representation of the atrioventricular junctions in the left anterior oblique projection, showing the anatomically inaccurate nomenclature currently used for the locations of accessory pathways. *Lower panel:* An anatomically correct nomenclature is shown for the different segments of the junctions. (Cosio FG, Anderson RH, Kuck KH, et al. ESCWGA/NASPE/P experts consensus statement: living anatomy of the atrioventricular junctions. A guide to electrophysiologic mapping. Working Group of Arrhythmias of the European Society of Cardiology. North American Society of Pacing and Electrophysiology. *J Cardiovasc Electrophysiol.* 1999;10(8):1162-1170.)

RIGHT ATRIUM

The **terminal crest** (or **crista terminalis**) marks the border between the smooth intercaval posterior wall of the RA and the appendage.[3,4] It delineates the border between the smooth wall of the venous component and the rough wall of the appendage (Fig. 3.3). A series of muscle bundles known as pectinate muscles arise from the lateral margin of the terminal crest with branches between the crest and the smooth vestibule that surrounds the tricuspid valve orifice. The vestibule itself is composed mainly of a circumferential arrangement of myofibers. The nonuniform arrangement of the terminal ramifications of the terminal crest may account for delay and discontinuity in the spread of an excitatory wave front, leading to reentry that uses the cavotricuspid isthmus (CTI), a critical component of the typical atrial flutter reentry circuit. Surgical scars in the right atrium after open heart surgery can also create the substrate for non–CTI-dependent, macroreentrant atrial tachycardias.[5]

The **triangle of Koch** (Fig. 3.4), which is the anatomic landmark for the location of the atrioventricular node, is the portion of the vestibule that is located anterosuperior to the orifice of the coronary sinus.[6] Its posterior border is the **tendon of Todaro** (the hypotenuse of the triangle) within the **Eustachian ridge,** whereas its anterior border is the annulus of the septal leaflet of the tricuspid valve, and the orifice of the coronary sinus marks its base. The atrioventricular node (AVN) and His bundle lie at its apex, and the orifice of the coronary sinus marks its base. The inferior extensions of the compact AVN are thought to account for the slow pathway in nodal reentry tachycardia, although the arrangement of the cardiomyocytes in this area may also play a role.[7] The valve of the inferior vena cava (IVC) or **Eustachian valve** is derived embryologically from the right venous valve and can be absent or extremely prominent (in which case it is referred to as a **Chiari network**). The Chiari network is a complex remnant of a large valve of the Eustachian ridge present in about 2% of individuals. It can be mistaken for a thrombus on cardiac imaging and occasionally can produce a nearly complete partitioning of the RA (cor triatriatum dexter). The extension of the Eustachian valve continues as the tendon of Todaro medially along the Eustachian ridge.

The **coronary sinus** (CS) is the cardiac venous system that begins at its ostium in the right atrium and ends at the origin of the great cardiac vein. The major tributaries of the CS include the great cardiac vein (anterior cardiac vein), the left obtuse marginal vein, the posterior (or inferior) left ventricular vein, the middle cardiac vein, and the right coronary vein. In addition, atrial veins and, notably, the **vein** (or **ligament**) **of Marshall** (or oblique left atrial vein) also enter the coronary sinus vein.[8] From the perspective of electrophysiologists, the CS represents an anatomic structure of particular interest. First, it provides access to epicardial accessory AV connections and to both atria and ventricular arrhythmias. Second, the muscle that wraps around the CS can be a source of atrial arrhythmias.[9]

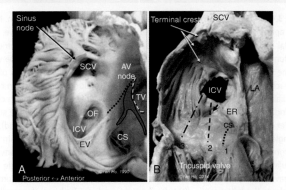

FIG. 3.3. (A) This display of the inside of the right atrium with the lateral wall of the appendage deflected posteriorly shows the atrial septum enface and the terminal crest with its array of pectinate muscles. The sinus and atrioventricular nodes are superimposed. The *dotted line* marks the position of the tendon of Todaro and the *white broken line* marks the annulus of the septal leaflet of the tricuspid valve, the borders of the triangle of Koch. (B) This four-chamber section shows three lines in the cavotricuspid isthmus corresponding to the paraseptal isthmus *(1)*, inferior/central isthmus *(2)*, and inferolateral isthmus *(3)*. The *short arrow* indicates a pouchlike depression crossed by line 2.

AV, Atrioventricular; *CS,* coronary sinus; *ER,* Eustachian ridge; *EV,* Eustachian valve; *ICV,* inferior caval vein; *LA,* left atrium; *OF,* oval fossa; *SCV,* superior caval vein; *TV,* tricuspid valve. (Brugada J, Katritsis D, Arbelo E, et al. 2019 ESC Guidelines for the management of supraventricular tachycardias. *Eur Heart J.* 2019;40(47):3812-3813.)

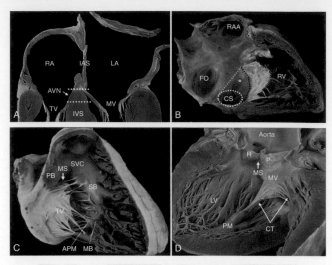

FIG. 3.4. (A) The right and left atria are separated by the interatrial septum. Note the apical displacement of the tricuspid valve relative to the mitral valve. The septal tissue in between these two valves *(dashed lines)* is the atrioventricular septum, which houses the atrioventricular node. (B) Right anterior oblique view of the septal aspect of the right atrium and right ventricle. The extension of the Eustachian valve continues as the tendon of Todaro along the Eustachian ridge medially *(blue line)*. It forms the hypotenuse of the triangle of Koch with other boundaries supplied by the coronary sinus ostium *(dashed oval)* and the septal leaflet of the tricuspid valve *(black line)*. Toward its apex (superiorly located), the triangle of Koch houses the atrioventricular node *(asterisk)*. (C) Right ventricular anatomy is shown (free wall has been removed) demonstrating the many trabeculations (trabeculae carneae), moderator band, anterior papillary muscle, and supraventricular crest. The membranous septum can be seen with transillumination from the left ventricle. (D) Left ventricular anatomy is shown (free wall has been displaced laterally) demonstrating the inferior papillary muscle, aortomitral continuity, and left ventricular outflow tract. The membranous septum is seen from the left ventricular aspect, located at the junction of the right and posterior aortic sinuses of Valsalva.

APM, Anterior papillary muscle; *AVN,* atrioventricular node; *CS,* coronary sinus; *CT,* chordae tendineae; *FO,* fossa ovalis; *IAS,* interatrial septum; *IVS,* interventricular septum; *LA,* left atrium; *LV,* left ventricle; *MB,* moderator band; *MS,* membranous septum; *MV,* mitral valve; *P,* posterior aortic valve cusp; *PB,* parietal band; *PM,* papillary muscle; *R,* right aortic valve cusp; *RA,* right atrium; *RV,* right ventricle; *SB,* septal band; *SOV,* sinus of Valsalva; *SVC,* supraventricular crest; *TV,* tricuspid valve. (Killu AM, Asirvatham SJ. Cardiac anatomy in the interventional era: an overview. In Camm AJ, Lüscher TF, Maurer G, Serruys SW, eds. *ESC Textbook of Cardiovascular Medicine.* 3rd ed. Oxford, UK: Oxford University Press; 2018.)

LEFT ATRIUM

The **interatrial septum** is located posteromedially and is slightly angu lated given the cephalad position of the LA (Fig. 3.4 and 3.5). It consists of a thin, fibrous portion centrally (fossa ovalis, the remnant of the foramen ovale/septum primum) that is surrounded by a thicker muscular portion (the limbus of the fossa ovalis, the remnant of the septum secundum). The wall of the LA is generally thicker than the wall of the RA. Apart from muscular continuity at the margins and the floor of the oval fossa, there are muscle bundles that allow conduction between the atria. In the majority of hearts, the most obvious muscular interatrial bridge is **Bachmann's bundle,** which has a parallel alignment of myofibers in the subepicardium, crossing over the interatrial groove, in parallel fashion to the plane of the atrioventricular junction.[1] The change in fiber orientation and wall thickness at the boundary of these bundles may lead to conduction block during sinus rhythm propagation or may become the substrate for atrial fibrillation.

The **LA appendage** is a flattened tubular structure with considerable variability in shape and size. The tip of the appendage is commonly directed anteriorly, overlying the pulmonary trunk or the LV summit, where its floor sits on the early branches of the left coronary artery and the interventricular vein.[10] In the LA, depressions ("pits") are often seen in the region of the LA appendage ostium. The atrial wall inside these depressions is thin, thus care is needed when manipulating catheters and sheaths in this region to minimize the risk of atrial perforation.

Inside the atrium, a prominent ridge lies between the orifices of the left PVs and the ostium of the appendage. Epicardially the ridge is a fold containing the remnant of the **vein of Marshall** with its accompanying autonomic nerves and can be the source of atrial arrhythmia. It can be approached and ablated through the distal coronary sinus.[11]

Although there are usually four **pulmonary venous** orifices, two on each side of the venous component, variations in number of orifices, length of conjoined veins, and atypical locations are common.[12,13] The superior pulmonary venous orifices are larger and have a longer trunk (up to 20 mm). Complex muscular architecture is found at the venoatrial junctions where the LA wall extends over the outer surface of the venous wall, creating muscular sleeves, longest along the upper veins.[13] The sleeves are thicker and circumferential at the venoatrial junctions, especially around the superior pulmonary veins (PVs), and thinner and more irregular toward the lung hilum. The areas of the oatrial junctions and adjoining PVs are also highly innervated by ganglionated nerves originating from the cardiac neural plexus.[14] They may play a role in initiating an sustaining atrial arrhythmias.[15,16]

The **phrenic nerves** track along the lateral mediastinum coursing along the outer surface of the fibrous pericardium. The right phrenic nerve has a close relationship with the superior vena cava and the anterior border of the orifice of the right superior PV. In the majority of individuals the left phrenic nerve passes over the LA appendage.[17] The esophagus is located in close proximity to the posterior wall and the vagal plexus descends on its anterior surface.[12]

LA fibrosis can be assessed with tissue echocardiography techniques and late gadolinium contrast–enhanced cardiovascular magnetic resonance (CMR) imaging and has been related to atrial tachycardia and fibrillation.[18,19]

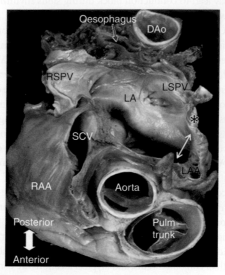

FIG. 3.5. The LA of this heart has been cut in a plane along the short axis of the thorax through the orifices of the right and left superior pulmonary veins. The *double-headed arrow* marks the ostium of the LAA, and the *asterisk* marks the ridge. The esophagus and DAo pass behind the left atrium.

DAo, Descending aorta; *LA,* left atrium; *LAA,* left atrial appendage; *LSPV,* left superior pulmonary vein; *RAA,* right atrial appendage; *RSPV,* right superior pulmonary vein; *SCV,* superior caval vein. (Brugada J, Katritsis D, Arbelo E, et al. 2019 ESC Guidelines for the management of supraventricular tachycardias. *Eur Heart J.* 2019;40(47):3812-3813.)

RIGHT AND LEFT VENTRICLES

The RV is a complex structure containing many t. (trabeculae carneae) that extend from the inflow of the apex, whereas the infundibulum (right ventricular outfr contains only a few (see Fig. 3.4). However, the LV also po trabeculations, albeit more diminutive, especially in the apex RV is anterior to the LV in a way that the septum is directly pos rior to the RV outflow tract, and to the left and posterior to the R in the inflow portion.[1,20] The RV wall is thinner than the LV (unless there is pressure overload against the RV).

The **interventricular septum** is a complicated structure that has a spiral course and exhibits both membranous and muscular portions. The membranous portion of the interventricular septum is an important landmark that contains the bundle of His. It consists of both interventricular and atrioventricular segments (the latter arising because of the apical displacement of the tricuspid valve relative to the mitral valve). In the inflow portion, the septum is to the left and posterior to the RV. However, in the outflow tract, the septum is directly posterior to the RV outflow tract. The outflow tract of the RV is completely encircled by muscular tissue, whereas that of the LV has nonmuscular parts formed by the aortomitral continuity/intervalvular fibrosa (Fig. 3.6). Of note, the distal part of the RV outflow tract actually lies toward the left of the body, whereas the distal part of the LV outflow tract lies toward the right of the body.[1] The RVOT is an important substrate for ventricular arrhythmia in patients with Brugada syndrome.[21,22]

Both ventricles have **papillary muscles.** The RV typically has three papillary muscles: septal, anterior, and inferior (see Fig. 3.4). The LV typically has two that are usually described as being posteromedial and anterolateral (or, more correctly, inferior and lateral). In addition, both ventricles may contain **false tendons.** These are chordlike structures that traverse the ventricular cavity and may variably attach to the septum, papillary muscles, or free wall, without being attached to the atrioventricular valve. At autopsy, they may be found in more than 50% of individuals and may be more common in men. They have also been implicated as the site of some arrhythmias.[7] The RV also contains a moderator band that is not found in the LV and that is the extension of the septoparietal band that carries right bundle branch conduction tissue to the free wall of the RV.

...les, the myocytes are aggregated together as a ...nal mesh within a supporting matrix of fibrous ...e are three interconnecting "layers" described as ... (subepicardial), middle, and deep (subendocardial) ...g to the longitudinal alignment of the myocardial myo- ...hese "layers" represent changes in orientation of the ...bers transmurally, without being separated by cleavage ...es or sheets of fibrous tissue. Myofibers of one layer intercon-...ect with those of the next layer and so forth in a continuum. In the right ventricle the myofibers in the superficial layer are arranged more circumferentially than in the left ventricle, and a distinct middle layer is not present in the RV, as occurs in the LV.[24] The QT interval on the electrocardiogram (ECG) represents the longest repolarization in the mid-myocardial M-cell region—that is, a physiologic transmural dispersion of repolarization. Gene mutations or medications that cause selective action potential prolongation in the M-cell region can lead to increased transmural repolarization gradients and thus create the conditions for functional reentry and subsequent torsades, as probably happens in patients with the long QT syndrome.[25,26]

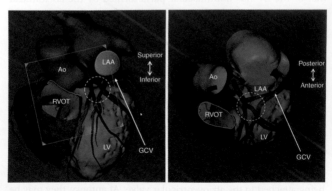

FIG. 3.6. Three-dimensional computed tomography reconstruction of cardiac anatomy illustrating the complex anatomy of the ventricular outflow tract. The left anterior oblique (left) and superior (right) views show the anatomic proximity of the RVOT, LV outflow tract, Ao, GCV, and LAA to the summit (yellow circle). The distal RVOT and pulmonary artery are not seen in the images, but these structures are also in close proximity to the summit. Outflow tract premature ventricular contractions and ventricular tachycardia have been reported to be successfully ablated from each of these structures.

FIG. 3.6, cont'd The proximity of the coronary arteries is also shown, and their course must be appreciated to avoid collateral damage during ablation.
Ao, Aorta; GCV, great cardiac vein; LAA, left atrial appendage; LV, left ventricular; RVOT, right ventricular outflow tract. (Dukkipati SR, Koruth JS, Choudry S, et al. Catheter ablation of ventricular tachycardia in structural heart disease: indications, strategies, and outcomes—part II. J Am Coll Cardiol. 2017;70(23):2924-2941.)

CARDIAC VALVES

The **atrioventricular valves** arise from the fibrous ring of the atrioventricular septum in distinction to the semilunar valves, which can be regarded as arising from the arterial wall of the respective major artery. The tricuspid valve is apically displaced relative to the mitral valve and contains three leaflets—septal, anterior, and inferior (the latter often incorrectly referred to as posterior, the position actually occupied by the septal leaflet).[1] The mitral valve contains two leaflets (anterior and posterior), although there are also two smaller commissural cusps. In contrast to the right-sided cardiac valves, which are distinctly located from one another, the anterior leaflet of the mitral valve forms part of the aortomitral continuity with the left and posterior cusps of the aortic valve. The anterior leaflet corresponds to one-third of the circumference and is deep. The posterior corresponds to two-thirds of the circumference but is much shallower and consists of three subunits (scallops). In between each leaflet are the valve commissures, which extend a variable distance to the annulus.[1] The **chordae tendineae** are strong cords and may be referred to as *primary, secondary,* or *tertiary* depending on their insertion site into the valve leaflets or their origination. Primary cords are thin, high in number, and arise from the papillary muscle to attach to the free margin of the leaflets. Secondary cords are thicker, fewer in number, and also arise from the papillary muscle yet attach a few millimeters in from the valve margin on the ventricular aspect of the leaflet at the level of the noduli Albini (white nodules found on the atrial surface of the valve). These may be referred to as valve struts.

Semilunar valves, the pulmonary and aortic trileaflet valves, demarcate the ventriculoarterial junction. The pulmonary valve is the most superiorly and anteriorly located cardiac valve. The aortic valve is the central valve of the heart posterior to the RV outflow tract and pulmonic valve and between the tricuspid and mitral

annulus with the interatrial septum located posteriorly. At the tip
of each cusp are small fibrous nodes (of *Morgagni* for the pulmonary valve and of *Arantius* for the aortic valve). These represent
thickening of the tunica intima layer and arise at the points of
leaflet coaptation. In the aorta, each cusp is associated with a corresponding outpouching (**sinus of Valsalva**) that is bounded inferiorly by the leaflet attachment and superiorly by the sinotubular
junction. The right cusp is associated with the right sinus of
Valsalva, from which the right coronary artery usually arises. The
left cusp is associated with the left sinus of Valsalva, from which
the left coronary artery usually arises. The posterior cusp (adjacent
to the interatrial septum) and its related sinus do not normally
have a coronary artery associated with them (also called *noncoronary sinus/cusp*).[1]

THE CONDUCTION SYSTEM

At the RA–SVC junction, the **sinus node** lies in a subepicardial
position, although this structure has extensions that approach
the endocardial surface (see Fig. 3.3). The **sinus node** is a
crescent-like, 2.5 mm long subepicardial structure with irregular margins and is not insulated by a sheath of fibrous tissue.[27]
Impulses arrive at the non-insulated **AV node** of average length
of 5 mm and width 3 mm, that functions as a filter for ventricular
protection from fast atrial rates as well as a backup pacemaker in
case of sinus node dysfunction.[28,29] The inferior extensions of
the AV node most probably represent the anatomic substrate
of the slow pathway.[30] Conduction to the ventricles is then
through the insulated **bundle of His,** which passes via the annulus fibrosus and penetrates the membranous intraventricular
septum before separating into the left and right bundle branches
at the superior margin of the muscular septum (Fig. 3.7).[31] The
right bundle crosses the anterior part of the intraventricular
septum and reaches the apex of the ventricle and the base of the
anterior papillary muscle. The **left bundle** is anatomically less
discrete and subdivides into the **anterior (superior)** and **posterior (inferior) fascicle.** Finally, the bundle branches ramify to
produce the endocardial **Purkinje fibers,** which activate the
ventricles. Dense innervation of the sinus node and the conduction system by postganglionic adrenergic and cholinergic nerve
terminals determine sinus rate and AV conduction.

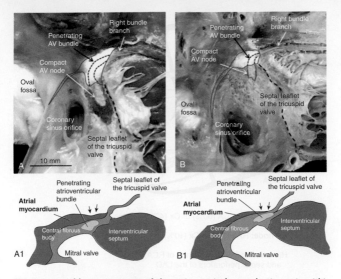

FIG. 3.7. Variable arrangement of the atrioventricular conduction axis within the triangle of Koch. (A, B) Gross dissections of the human atrioventricular (AV) conduction axis relative to the triangle of Koch and subsequent transillumination of the membranous septum are shown. The compact node becomes the penetrating AV bundle as the axis itself enters the AV component of the membranous septum (transillumination), thus becoming encircled by the fibrous tissue of the central fibrous body (CFB). In almost three-fifths of specimens, this site of penetration was found superiorly within the triangle of Koch, with an inferior transition found in the remaining two-fifths. (A) An inferior origin of the penetrating AV bundle, which is surrounded in the AV component of the membranous septum by a thick layer of atrial muscle fibers, is represented in the schematic drawing (A1). (B) A superior origin of the penetrating AV bundle, which is surrounded by the connective tissue of the CFB and a thin layer of atrial muscle fibers, is represented in schematic drawing (B1).

(Cabrera JA, Anderson RH, Macias Y, et al. Variable arrangement of the atrioventricular conduction axis within the triangle of Koch: implications for permanent his bundle pacing. JACC Clin Electrophysiol. 2020;6:362-377.)

The sinus nodal branch of the right coronary artery (sinus nodal branch may also originate from the proximal circumflex artery in up to 40% of cases) provides blood supply to sinus node (Fig. 3.8). In 85% to 90% of human hearts, blood supply to the AV node (AV nodal artery) is provided by the distal right

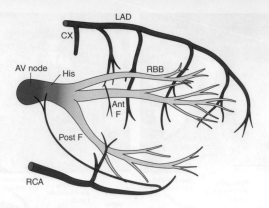

Sinus Node: RCA (60%) or Cx (40%)

AV node: RA (90%) or Cx (10%)

His bundle: AV nodal branch of RCA, and septal perforators of the LAD

RBB: septal perforators of the LAD

LBB: septal perforators from LAD, and AV nodal branch of RCA

FIG. 3.8. Vascular supply to the conducting system. *Ant F,* Anterior fascicle; *AV,* atrioventricular; *Cx,* left circumflex artery; *LAD,* left anterior descending; *LBBB,* left bundle branch block; *Post F,* posterior fascicle; *RBB,* right bundle branch; *RBBB,* RBB block; *RCA,* right coronary artery.

coronary artery; it is provided by the left circumflex in the remainder. Septal branches of the left anterior descending artery also provide blood to the upper muscular interventricular septum and the conduction system. The specialized cells of the cardiac conduction system have relatively poor contractility and express specialized ion channels and gap-junction proteins, such as connexins, that mediate electrical coupling with neighboring cells.

References

1. Killu AM, Asirvatham SJ. Cardiac anatomy in the interventional era: an overview. In: Camm AJ, Lüscher TF, Maurer G, Serruys SW, eds. *ESC Textbook of Cardiovascular Medicine*. 3rd ed. 2018. Oxford University Press. Oxford, United Kingdom.
2. Cosio FG, Anderson RH, Kuck KH, et al. ESCWGA/NASPE/P experts consensus statement: living anatomy of the atrioventricular junctions. A guide to electrophysiologic mapping. Working Group of Arrhythmias of the European Society of Cardiology. North American Society of Pacing and Electrophysiology. *J Cardiovasc Electrophysiol*. 1999;10(8):1162-1170.
3. Ho SY, Anderson RH, Sánchez-Quintana D. Atrial structure and fibres: morphologic bases of atrial conduction. *Cardiovasc Res*. 2002;54(2):325-336.
4. Ueda A, McCarthy KP, Sánchez-Quintana D, Ho SY. Right atrial appendage and vestibule: further anatomical insights with implications for invasive electrophysiology. *Europace*. 2013;15(5):728-734.
5. Katritsis DG, Boriani G, Cosio FG, et al. European Heart Rhythm Association (EHRA) consensus document on the management of supraventricular arrhythmias, endorsed by Heart Rhythm Society (HRS), Asia-Pacific Heart Rhythm Society (APHRS), and Sociedad Latinoamericana de Estimulacion Cardiaca y Electrofisiologia (SOLAECE). *Europace*. 2017;19(3):465-511.
6. Sanchez-Quintana D, Davies DW, Ho SY, Oslizlok P, Anderson RH. Architecture of the atrial musculature in and around the triangle of Koch: its potential relevance to atrioventricular nodal reentry. *J Cardiovasc Electrophysiol*. 1997;8(12):1396-1407.
7. Katritsis DG, Becker A. The atrioventricular nodal reentrant tachycardia circuit: a proposal. *Heart Rhythm*. 2007;4(10):1354-1360.
8. Katritsis DG. Arrhythmogenicity of the coronary sinus. *Indian Pacing Electrophysiol J*. 2004;4(4):176-184.
9. Katritsis DG. The coronary sinus: passive bystander or source of arrhythmia? *Heart Rhythm*. 2004;1(1):113-116.
10. Su P, McCarthy KP, Ho SY. Occluding the left atrial appendage: anatomical considerations. *Heart*. 2008;94(9):1166-1170.
11. Katritsis D, Ioannidis JP, Anagnostopoulos CE, et al. Identification and catheter ablation of extracardiac and intracardiac components of ligament of Marshall tissue for treatment of paroxysmal atrial fibrillation. *J Cardiovasc Electrophysiol*. 2001;12(7):750-758.
12. Ho SY, Cabrera JA, Sanchez-Quintana D. Left atrial anatomy revisited. *Circ Arrhythm Electrophysiol*. 2012;5(1):220-228.
13. Ho SY, Cabrera JA, Tran VH, Farre J, Anderson RH, Sanchez-Quintana D. Architecture of the pulmonary veins: relevance to radiofrequency ablation. *Heart*. 2001;86(3):265-270.
14. Chevalier P, Tabib A, Meyronnet D, et al. Quantitative study of nerves of the human left atrium. *Heart Rhythm*. 2005;2(5):518-522.
15. Katritsis DG. Autonomic ablation and neuromodulation: novel concepts in search of novel technology. *Pacing Clin Electrophysiol*. 2016;39(5):405-406.
16. Katritsis GD, Katritsis DG. Cardiac autonomic denervation for ablation of atrial fibrillation. *Arrhythm Electrophysiol Rev*. 2014;3(2):113-115.

17. Sanchez-Quintana D, Ho SY, Climent V, Murillo M, Cabrera JA. Anatomic evalua-
    tion of the left phrenic nerve relevant to epicardial and endocardial catheter
    ablation: implications for phrenic nerve injury. *Heart Rhythm.* 2009;6(6):764-768.
18. Delgado V, Di Biase L, Leung M, et al. Structure and function of the left atrium
    and left atrial appendage: AF and stroke implications. *J Am Coll Cardiol.*
    2017;70(25):3157-3172.
19. Gal P, Marrouche NF. Magnetic resonance imaging of atrial fibrosis: redefining
    atrial fibrillation to a syndrome. *Eur Heart J.* 2017;38(1):14-19.
20. Pighi M, Theriault-Lauzier P, Alosaimi H, et al. Fluoroscopic anatomy of right-sided
    heart structures for transcatheter interventions. *JACC Cardiovasc Interv.* 2018;11(16):
    1614-1625.
21. Mizusawa Y, Wilde AA. Brugada syndrome. *Circ Arrhythm Electrophysiol.*
    2012;5(3):606-616.
22. Zhang J, Sacher F, Hoffmayer K, et al. Cardiac electrophysiological substrate
    underlying the ECG phenotype and electrogram abnormalities in Brugada
    syndrome patients. *Circulation.* 2015;131(22):1950-1959.
23. Anderson RH, Smerup M, Sanchez-Quintana D, Loukas M, Lunkenheimer PP. The
    three-dimensional arrangement of the myocytes in the ventricular walls. *Clin
    Anat.* 2009;22(1):64-76.
24. Sánchez-Quintana D, Cabrera JA, Ho SY. Normal atrial and ventricular myocardial
    structures. In Camm AJ, Lüscher TF, Maurer G, Serruys SW, eds. ESC Textbook of
    Cardiovascular Medicine. 3rd ed. Oxford, UK: Oxford University Press; 2018.
25. Abrams DJ, Macrae CA. Long QT syndrome. *Circulation.* 2014;129(14):1524-1529.
26. Morita H, Wu J, Zipes DP. The QT syndromes: long and short. *Lancet.*
    2008;372(9640):750-763.
27. Sanchez-Quintana D, Cabrera JA, Farre J, Climent V, Anderson RH, Ho SY. Sinus
    node revisited in the era of electroanatomical mapping and catheter ablation.
    Heart. 2005;91(2):189-194.
28. Kurian T, Ambrosi C, Hucker W, Fedorov VV, Efimov IR. Anatomy and electro-
    physiology of the human AV node. *Pacing Clin Electrophysiol.* 2010;33(6):754-762.
29. Anderson RH, Mori S, Spicer DE, Sanchez-Quintana D, Jensen B. The Anatomy,
    Development, and Evolution of the Atrioventricular Conduction Axis. *J Cardiovasc
    Dev Dis.* 2018;5(3).
30. Katritsis DG, Josephson ME. Classification of electrophysiological types of atrioven-
    tricular nodal re-entrant tachycardia: a reappraisal. *Europace.* 2013;15(9):1231-1240.
31. Cabrera JA, Anderson RH, Macias Y, et al. Variable arrangement of the atrioven-
    tricular conduction axis within the triangle of Koch: Implications for permanent
    His bundle pacing. *JACC Clin Electrophysiol.* 2020;6(4):362-377.

4

Vascular Access and Catheter Placement

PATIENT PREPARATION

Patients should be studied in the postabsorptive state and after beta blockers or other antiarrhythmic agents have been discontinued for at least 5 days. Amiodarone should be withdrawn at least 2 months before the procedure if feasible. A transesophageal echocardiogram is recommended to exclude intracardiac thrombi in patients with atrial fibrillation (AF) or atrial flutter and is particularly important in such patients who have not been therapeutically anticoagulated for at least 3 to 4 weeks.

In most cases a diagnostic electrophysiology study (EPS) can be performed without sedation, but conscious sedation is appropriate when needed to attenuate anxiety.[1] Intravenous sedation now can be proceduralist (or operator) directed and nurse administered (i.e., the PDNA model).[2,3] An abundance of observational studies have indicated that sedation does not significantly affect basic electrophysiologic properties or inducibility of supraventricular tachycardia (SVT), with the possible exception of automatic atrial tachycardia.[4,5-7] For clinical purposes, this is true not only for the opiate-benzodiazepine combination but even for propofol, despite its dose-related depression of the sinus node and His-Purkinje conduction.[7] The opiate-benzodiazepine combination is safer than propofol but does not necessarily comprise only midazolam and fentanyl. Emulsified diazepam offers a less expensive alternative to midazolam and avoids the irritating effects of intravenously administered diazepam. Morphine or diamorphine

.ailable in the United Kingdom), which lacks the emetic effects morphine, are alternatives to fentanyl.[1] An initial dose of 5 mg .iazepam, followed by 5 mg diamorphine if needed, is usually adequate. However, individual drug and dosing choices depend on drug availability and legal environments in different countries and on the experience of the medical personnel. Dexmedetomidine, an α_2-adrenergic agonist, is an emerging, attractive sedative because of its short half-life and lack of respiratory depression, although it has been associated with cardiac conduction abnormalities and hypotension.[8]

FEMORAL VEIN PUNCTURE

The femoral veins can be used for insertion of all electrode catheters, including the coronary sinus (CS). Some operators prefer to use the internal jugular vein for the CS catheter. Local anesthesia is administered, and the femoral vein is cannulated. The vein lies just medial to the artery below the inguinal ligament. Many laboratories now require femoral vein cannulation under ultrasound guidance. If this is not feasible, access is accomplished by feeling the femoral artery pulse on the groin crease and puncturing at a point 2 cm medial to and 1 cm higher than the point of maximal impulse. A syringe half filled with heparinized flush solution is attached to the hub of a 18-gauge needle, which is advanced under negative pressure by withdrawing gently on the syringe, at a 45-degree angle from the skin surface. The needle is advanced while gentle aspiration is maintained on the syringe. If the need is inserted quickly, it may penetrate the front and back walls of the vein, reaching the pubic ramus. In this case the needle should be withdrawn slowly back into the vein lumen while maintaining suction. If the femoral artery is inadvertently punctured, the vein puncture is reattempted after 5 minutes of compression on the arterial puncture site.

JUGULAR VEIN PUNCTURE

If the femoral veins are inaccessible or not unsuitable, the internal jugular vein may be used. This is accomplished either by puncturing the vein 2 cm lateral to the carotid pulse in the neck, usually under ultrasound guidance, or by puncturing between the two heads of the sternocleidomastoid muscle that insert into the sternum and clavicle. The needle pierces the skin at the apex of the triangle formed by the two heads of the sternocleidomastoid muscle and is directed inferiorly and posteriorly at a 30-degree angle to the skin. It is important to keep the needle parallel to the midline to avoid the carotid artery. The former approach avoids the risk of pneumothorax at the expense of inadvertent puncture of the carotid artery. In this case 5 minutes of compression of the carotid artery puncture site artery is usually sufficient for hemostasis.

TRANSSEPTAL PUNCTURE

Transseptal access is obtained usually from the right femoral vein by using anatomic landmarks or transesophageal or intracardiac echocardiography. When echocardiographic assistance is not available, anatomic landmarks may be used. The transseptal sheath with the needle inside it, without protruding, is withdrawn from the superior vena cava on the atrial septum until it drops into the foramen ovale. Ideally, tenting of the fossa ovalis is confirmed by the ultrasound image or by contrast injection, after which the needle is advanced into the left atrium, ideally with continuous pressure monitoring. If the needle puncture is made through the fossa ovalis or its limbus (the "true" interatrial septum), the needle will always enter the left atrium (LA). However, if the needle is advanced through another part of the septum, entrance into the pericardial space or aorta is likely. A too anterior puncture risks entrance into the aorta, whereas a puncture that is too posterior risks entry into the pericardial space. If the needle inadvertently punctures the aorta, it usually can be simply withdrawn without adverse effects, unless the dilator and sheath have been advanced over the needle and into the aorta.

During redo ablation procedures, scarring at the previous transseptal site can make the puncture more difficult. This might be overcome by changing the needle curve from a small curve to a large curve design with an extra-sharp tip.[9] In the presence of a dilated left atrium, atrial angiography using a modification of the initial method described by Inoue for percutaneous mitral commissurotomy may be of help (Fig. 4.1).[10] When a difficult transseptal puncture is anticipated, intracardiac echocardiography has been shown to significantly reduce the rate of hemopericardium and tamponade (Fig. 4.2).[11]

After penetration of the septum, a pressure line is connected to the needle to ensure recording of left atrial pressure.

ernatively, a small-gauge wire with a J curve (e.g., SafeSept) advanced past the tip of the needle and positioned within a eft pulmonary vein to confirm that the needle is in the left atrium (Fig. 4.3). If this is confirmed, the sheath and the needle are gently pushed forward, the needle is withdrawn, and a long J-curve guidewire is inserted and positioned with a left pulmonary vein to allow safe passage of the sheath into the left atrium. The SafeSept is particularly useful in the case of a redundant membrane that results in a higher risk of perforation of the posterior wall or left atrial appendage when the needle in pushed and suddenly jumps into the LA. If the foramen ovale is thick or the procedure is truly necessary in patients with an atrial patch, the extra-sharp BRK-1 transseptal needle with intracardiac echocardiographic guidance and SafeSept wire, or radiofrequency-assisted puncture,[12] may be helpful.

The sheath should receive a continuous infusion of heparinized saline to prevent thrombi and air emboli. Diagnostic or ablation catheters can then safely be introduced into the left atrium after heparinization. The target activated clotting time (ACT) depends on the nature of the procedure. Ablation of a left-sided accessory pathway usually requires no more than a single heparin bolus of 3000 to 5000 units of heparin. For AF ablation procedures, most operators prefer a heparin bolus and continuous infusion to rapidly attain and maintain an ACT of 350 ms.

The most common complication of transseptal puncture is cardiac tamponade, with an average incidence of approximately 1%. It is usually treated by pericardiocentesis and drainage for 24 to 72 hours, even in anticoagulated patients. Surgical drainage and repair of the puncture site sometimes are necessary. Advanced age, female sex, and AF ablation are risk factors for pericardial tamponade.[13,14]

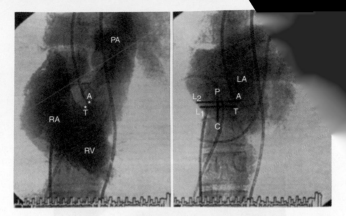

FIG. 4.1. Transseptal puncture. The end of the tricuspid valve at systole *(T)* is determined on a stop-frame frontal right atrial angiographic image *(left panel)* and translated to a stop-frame left atrial image *(right panel)*. On the latter image, an imaginary horizontal line is drawn from point T until it intersects the right lateral edge of the left atrium (L1). A vertical line is drawn at the midpoint between T and **L**1 (the midline), and its intersection with the caudal edge of the left atrium is regarded as point C. The puncture site *(P)* is determined on the midline at about a vertebral body height above point C. When the left atrial silhouette is clearly visible landmark for the upper end of the tricuspid valve *(T)* is substituted with the position of the aortic valve *(A)* marked by the tip of an arterial pigtail catheter touching the valve. An imaginary horizontal line is drawn from point A to point **L**2, the site where the line intersects the right lateral edge of the left atrium *(right panel)*. A vertical line (the midline) is drawn at the midpoint between A and **L**2, and its intersection with the caudal edge of the left atrium is regarded as point C. The puncture site is determined on the midline at a point about a vertebral body height above point C. This primary target puncture site is memorized in relation to the vertebral bodies.

LA, Left atrium; *PA,* Pulmonary artery; *RA,* right atrium; *RV,* right ventricle. (Hung JS. Atrial septal puncture technique in percutaneous transvenous mitral commissurotomy: mitral valvuloplasty using the Inoue balloon catheter technique. *Cathet Cardiovasc Diagn.* 1992;26: 275-284.)

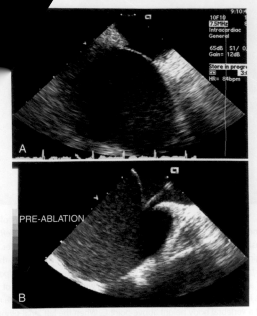

FIG. 4.2. ICE-assisted trans-septal puncture. *Upper panel,* Identification of the interatrial septum by intracardiac echocardiography (ICE). *Lower panel,* Puncture of the septum under ICE guidance.

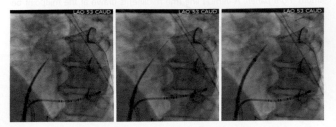

FIG. 4.3. The SafeSept technique. Atraumatic introduction of transseptal dilator and sheath into the left atrium over through-the-needle 0.014-inch J wire.

EPICARDIAL ACCESS

Percutaneous epicardial access is increasingly being performed to facilitate catheter ablation of ventricular tachycardias (VTs) with epicardial circuits, difficult cases of idiopathic VTs, and, rarely, focal atrial tachycardia and accessory pathways that cannot be successfully targeted endocardially.[15-17] It consists of two layers: the *visceral pericardium* or epicardium, a serous layer that is adjacent to the heart and proximal great vessels; and the *parietal pericardium,* which is formed by the outer fibrous sac and the continuation of the visceral pericardium as it reflects back near the origin of the great vessels to form the inner layer of the parietal pericardium. The visceral and parietal layers are separated by the pericardial cavity, which in healthy people contains 15 to 50 mL of serous physiologic fluid.[18] The thickness of the parietal pericardium varies from 0.8 to 2.5 mm.[17] Partial left (70%) or right (17%) pericardial absence may occur in 0.0001% of patients.[18,19] Thus cardiac magnetic resonance imaging or cardiac computed tomography (CT) is always recommended before undertaking the procedure. Furthermore, pericardial access is limited by pericardial sinuses and recesses around the veins and great arteries[20] and may not be feasible in patients with prior open heart surgery.

Anticoagulation should be discontinued or reversed before the procedure,[21] although in experienced centers epicardial ablation may be performed on anticoagulation to allow simultaneous endocardial ablation.[16]

The starting place for entrance into the skin is approximately 1 cm below the subxiphoid process for an anterior approach and right under the rib margin adjacent to the xyphoid for a posterior approach (Figs. 4.4, 4.5, and 4.6). For pericardial access, an anterior approach or a posterior approach can be used.[16] The anterior approach allows easier access to the anterior surface of the heart and ventricles and is safer than the posterior. It is associated with an increased risk for puncture of the superior epigastric artery or left internal mammary artery, and in certain situations (i.e., history of cardiac surgery and/or anterior sternotomy), a posterior puncture approach is preferred. The posterior approach allows easier access to the inferior ventricular walls and posterior LA walls but has the potential for causing intraabdominal bleeding through an inadvertent puncture of the diaphragm and the subdiaphragmatic structures.[17] If the patient has had previous epicardial ablation with potential pericardial adhesions, a surgical pericardial window is preferable. Prior coronary artery bypass surgery is a relative contraindication for picardial ablation unless coronary anatomy is well defined and access to the VT circuit on the opposite side of the heart is possible. Prior cardiac valvular surgery is also a relative contraindication given the potential for significant adhesions that limit access and, even if obtained, limit the ability to map freely.[16]

The anterior approach involves a shallow angle to the skin (<45 degrees) and the posterior approach involves a deeper angle (>45 degrees). A 17G Tuohy needle (150 mm) is placed under local anesthesia with the tip pointing toward the left shoulder and a brief fluoroscopic imaging in right anterior oblique (RAO) projection that will assess the angle of entry in the base to apical axis. The needle should always be advanced over the diaphragm because the latter is a highly vascular structure. Performing left anterior oblique (LAO) or left lateral fluoroscopy can assess the approximate angulation needed in anterior-to-posterior axis. Once the best considered direction needed is assessed, the needle can be advanced through the skin toward the outer silhouette of the heart, and targeting the space bordered by the sternum, the pericardium, and the dome of the diaphragm. When the needle reaches the heart border, ventricular pulsations will be transmitted from the needle tip. Premature ventricular contractions may also be seen. At this point the needle stylet is removed, a Luer-Lok syringe with undiluted contrast is connected, a small amount of contrast is injected to confirm the location of the needle tip within the pericardium, and a long guidewire is advanced through the needle. Most of the long guidewire should be advanced around the pericardium space. Fluoroscopy is used to identify the guidewire crossing multiple chambers that do share valves to rule out entrance into a cardiac chamber. This is usually easiest to appreciate in the LAO projection because the wire will outline the silhouette of the heart border. Intracardiac echocardiography can be used to identify the guidewire in the pericardial space and to confirm that it is not in the cardiac chambers. At this point, a long sheath can be advanced over the guidewire. Deflectable sheaths can be useful during mapping and ablation in the pericardial space.[16]

The mapping/ablation catheter is advanced into the pericardial space though the sheath. Epicardial voltage maps need to be interpreted with caution. Dense epicardial fat decreases the recorded voltage despite normal epicardium below the fat. These regions of dense fat are often found at the base of the heart and along major branches of the epicardial coronary arteries. Multiple angiographic views are recommended to assess the relative position of the coronary arteries. A distance of an ablation target site at least 5 mm away from a coronary

vessel is recommended.[21] Real-time integration of m
derived coronary anatomy and a CARTOUNIVU mc
used to better integrate the coronary anatomy with the ele
map. Left phrenic nerve injury is another concern, and h
pacing is performed before ablation along the anatomic cou.
nerve to assess proximity of the nerve.

The catheter needs to point toward the visceral pericardium
away from the parietal pericardium during mapping and ablati
Epicardial fat can impede lesion delivery to the myocardium of inter
est. The ablation catheter energy delivery electrode can heat up quickly,
reaching a temperature cutoff and limiting power delivery, because of
lack of blood flow in the pericardium. Therefore cooling the ablator tip
with irrigation is recommended to deliver adequate power. The irrigation rate may not need to be as high as required at the endocardial
surface (usually it is 5 to 7 mL/min), and care must be maintained to
adequately drain accumulating fluid to prevent cardiac compression.[16]

Complications of epicardial ablation are hemopericardium (incidence 5% to 10%) as a result of right ventricular perforation or coronary
artery injury, which may require surgical intervention; intraabdominal
bleeding; phrenic nerve injury; and postprocedural pericarditis.[17]

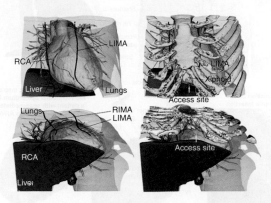

FIG. 4.4. Epicardial access. The layers traversed by the needle include the skin, superficial fascia, anterior rectus sheath/linea alba, rectus abdominis muscle, and posterior rectus sheath. The risk of damaging the artery is increased if the needle entry
or direction is too lateral. The left lobe of the liver is near the xiphisternum and may
be particularly at risk in patients with congestive heart failure and hepatomegaly.
RCA, right coronary artery; *LIMA*, left internal mammary artery; *RIMA*, right internal mammary
artery. (Lim HS, et al. Safety and prevention of complications during percutaneous epicardial access for the ablation of cardiac arrhythmias. *Heart Rhythm.* 2014;11:1658–1665.)

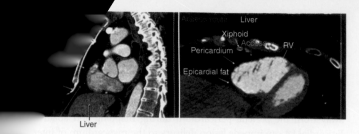

FIG. 4.5. Magnetic resonance imaging views for anterior pericardial access. (*Left panel:* Sagittal view; *right panel:* transverse view.) The needle traverses the superficial fascia, anterior rectus sheath, rectus abdominis muscle, and posterior rectus sheath and then over the dome of the diaphragm before reaching the fibrous and parietal serous layers of the pericardium.

RV, Right ventricle. (Lim HS, Sacher F, Cochet H, et al. Safety and prevention of complications during percutaneous epicardial access for the ablation of cardiac arrhythmias. *Heart Rhythm.* 2014;11:1658-1665.)

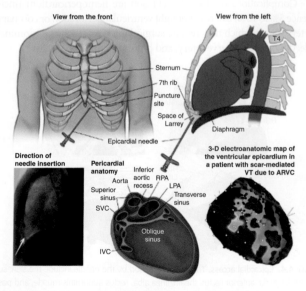

FIG. 4.6. Percutaneous access approach into the pericardial space.
ARVC, Arrhythmogenic right ventricular cardiomyopathy; *IVC,* inferior vena cava; *LPA,* left pulmonary artery; *RPA,* right pulmonary artery; *SVC,* superior vena cava; *VT,* ventricular tachycardia. (Modified from Aryana A, Tung R, d'Avila A. Percutaneous epicardial approach to catheter ablation of cardiac arrhythmias. *JACC Clin Electrophysiol.* 2020;6:1-20.)

CATHETER PLACEMENT

For a basic EPS, catheters are introduced under fluoroscopic visualization into the high right atrium (HRA-quadripolar), across the tricuspid valve to record a right-sided His-bundle electrogram (His-decapolar), the coronary sinus (CS-decapolar), and the right ventricular apex (RV-quadripolar). The His bundle may also be recorded from the left side of the septum, which is approached retrogradely through the aorta, or with a transseptal approach (Fig. 4.7). Many laboratories prefer to use three catheters for diagnosis of suspected SVT. This is achieved by using the CS catheter for atrial pacing instead of a fourth catheter in the right atrium. For the study of bradycardias, two catheters (HRA and His) are sufficient. For programmed electrical stimulation of the ventricle a single catheter may be enough, but an additional His may be needed for establishment of the ventricular origin of the arrhythmia. Anticoagulation is not usually necessary for diagnostic EPSs unless the left atrium or left ventricle is entered.

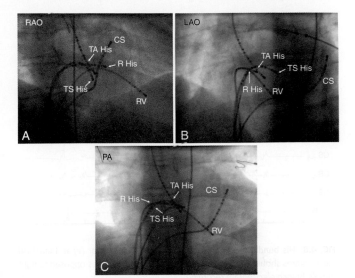

FIG. 4.7. Recording electrodes. Position of the electrodes at the high right atrium, His bundle, coronary sinus and RV apex, as seen in the (A) right anterior oblique (RAO) projections, (B) left anterior oblique *(LAO)*, and (C) posteroanterior *(PA)*,.

CS, Coronary sinus; *R His,* right septal His; *RV,* right ventricle; *TA His,* left septal His recorded through a transaortic catheter; *TS His,* left septal His recorded through a transseptal catheter.

HRA

The usual site for recording and stimulation is the high posterolateral wall of the right atrium at the junction of the SVC in the region of the sinus node (Fig. 4.8). If signals are inadequate or pacing thresholds are high because of atrial disease, the septal site at the area of Bachman's bundle can be used.

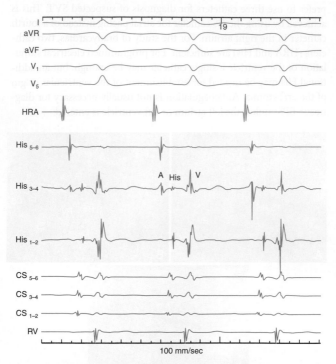

FIG. 4.8. His bundle electrogram recording. Both ventricular (V) and atrial (A) electrograms should be clearly visible to ensure His bundle as opposed to right bundle branch electrogram recording.

I, III, aVR, aVF, V1, V5, electrocardiography leads; *CS,* coronary sinus; *His,* His bundle potential recorded from the right septum; *HRA,* high right atrium; *RV,* right ventricle.

RV

The RV catheter is advanced across the tricuspid annulus with counterclockwise torque to the RV apex. Because the RV apex may appear inferior to the left ventricle (LV) apex, catheters in the RV apical position may be confused for an extracardiac position. For engaging the right ventricular outflow tract, clockwise torque is needed.

His Bundle

For recording of the His bundle electrogram the catheter is inserted into the RV as superior as possible across the tricuspid valve and is slowly withdrawn with clockwise torque to keep the electrodes in contact with the septum until an atrial and a His bundle depolarization are present (see Fig. 4.7). The His bundle deflection appears as a rapid biphasic or triphasic spike, 15 to 25 ms in duration, interposed between local atrial and ventricular electrograms.[22] When only atrial and ventricular electrograms are apparent, the catheter has to be moved to a more superior position across the tricuspid valve and rotated slightly clockwise. When no clear A is visible, a right bundle potential can be recorded 30 ms or less in front of the QRS and should not be mistaken for the His bundle depolarization (Fig. 4.9).

When a recording of the His bundle cannot be obtained from the right septum, mapping of the His bundle can be accomplished from the left side of the septum through the femoral artery or via transseptal access (Fig. 4.10).[23]

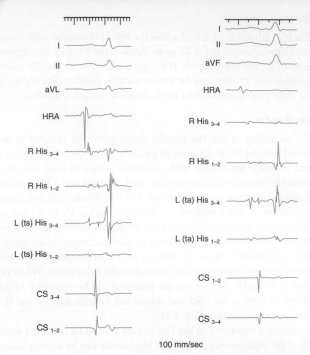

100 mm/sec

FIG. 4.9. Recording of the His bundle branch potential from the right or left septum. For the left septal approach either retrograde insertion of the catheter through the aortic valve or a transseptal approach may be tried. The transseptal access allows easier exploration of the posterior part of the septum.

I, II, aVL, aVF, electrocardiography leads; *L(ta) His,* His bundle potential recorded from the left septum via a transaortic approach; *L(ts) His,* His bundle potential recorded from the left septum via a transseptal approach; *R His,* His bundle potential recorded from the right septum.

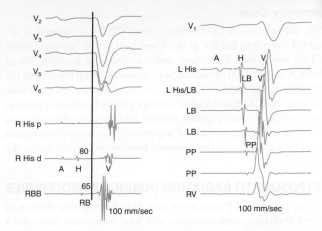

FIG. 4.10. Right and left bundle branch recording. *Left,* Recording of a His bundle depolarization from the right septum. The HV interval is 80 ms (normal range 35–55 ms). The more distal poles of the catheter record a right bundle branch potential as indicated by the absence of an atrial electrogram, consistent with a location distal to the His bundle depolarization (RB to V 65 ms). *Right,* Recording of a His bundle depolarization from the left septum. A decapolar catheter is inserted retrogradely across the aortic valve and records activity from the basal to apical septum. Note recording of the left bundle and Purkinje potentials by the electrodes that are deeper in the LV.

A, atrial electrogram; *L His,* His bundle potential recorded from the left septum; *L His/LB,* is bundle or left bundle branch potential recorded from the left septum; *LB,* left bundle branch; *PP,* Purkinje potential; *RBB,* right bundle branch; *R His d,* distal His bundle potential recorded from the right septum; *R His p,* proximal His bundle potential recorded from the right septum; *V,* ventricular potential. (Modified from Sarabanda AV, Gali WL, Gomes GG. Bundle branch reentry: a novel mechanism for sustained ventricular tachycardia in Chagas heart disease. *HeartRhythm Case Rep.* 2018;4:293-297; and Upadhyay GA, Cherian T, Shatz DY, et al. Intracardiac delineation of septal conduction in left bundle-branch block patterns. *Circulation.* 2019;139:1876-1888.)

Coronary Sinus

For cannulation of the coronary sinus (CS), the catheter is inserted deep into the RV at the lower part of the tricuspid valve (TV), and is then withdrawn under a clockwise traction. When both A and V electrograms appear, thus indicating the area of the CS ostium, the catheter has to be advanced and turned clockwise to enter the CS. A deflectable catheter greatly facilitates cannulation, which is usually always feasible. In extremely difficult cases or with suspected congenital anomalies, a coronary angiogram may be used to reveal the anatomic position of CS that drains the contrast.

EXPOSURE TO RADIATION DURING EP PROCEDURES

In the past, long EP procedures such as radiofrequency ablation of atrial fibrillation, were associated with long fluoroscopy times and a risk of radiation-related adverse effects.[24] The widespread use of electroanatomic mapping systems and intracardiac ultrasound have resulted in a drastic reduction in radiation exposure to patients. The risk to operators and patients is also reduced by the use of low-intensity fluoroscopy at a reduced frame rate of two to three frames per second. A growing number of operators now are performing EP procedures, including all types of radiofrequency ablation procedures and transseptal puncture, using a zero-fluoroscopy approach.

The implementation of ALARA (as low as reasonably achievable) protocols is strongly recommended for all EP procedures.[25]

References

1. Katritsis DG. Conscious sedation for diagnostic electrophysiology and catheter ablation of supraventricular tachycardia. *Europace.* 2019;21(1):3-4.
2. Gerstein NS, Young A, Schulman PM, Stecker EC, Jessel PM. Sedation in the electrophysiology laboratory: a multidisciplinary review. *J Am Heart Assoc.* 2016;5(6).
3. Gaitan BD, Trentman TL, Fassett SL, Mueller JT, Altemose GT. Sedation and analgesia in the cardiac electrophysiology laboratory: a national survey of electrophysiologists investigating the who, how, and why? *J Cardiothorac Vasc Anesth.* 2011;25(4):647-659.
4. Lai LP, Lin JL, Wu MH, et al. Usefulness of intravenous propofol anesthesia for radiofrequency catheter ablation in patients with tachyarrhythmias: infeasibility for pediatric patients with ectopic atrial tachycardia. *Pacing Clin Electrophysiol.* 1999;22(9):1358-1364.

5. Yip AS, McGuire MA, Davis L, et al. Lack of effect of midazolam on inducibility of arrhythmias at electrophysiologic study. *Am J Cardiol.* 1992;70(6):593-597.

6. Lau W, Kovoor P, Ross DL. Cardiac electrophysiologic effects of midazolam combined with fentanyl. *Am J Cardiol.* 1993;72(2):177-182.

7. Fazelifar A, Eskandari A, Hashemi M, et al. Deep sedation in patients undergoing atrioventricular nodal reentry tachycardia ablation. *Res Cardiovasc Med.* 2013;2(4):176-179.

8. Slupe AM, Minnier J, Raitt MH, Zarraga IGE, MacMurdy KS, Jessel PM. Dexmedetomidine sedation for paroxysmal supraventricular tachycardia ablation is not associated with alteration of arrhythmia inducibility. *Anesth Analg.* 2018.

9. Hu YF, Tai CT, Lin YJ, et al. The change in the fluoroscopy-guided transseptal puncture site and difficult punctures in catheter ablation of recurrent atrial fibrillation. *Europace.* 2008;10(3):276-279.

10. Hung JS. Atrial septal puncture technique in percutaneous transvenous mitral commissurotomy: mitral valvuloplasty using the Inoue balloon catheter technique. *Cathet Cardiovasc Diagn.* 1992;26(4):275-284.

11. Aldhoon B, Wichterle D, Peichl P, Cihak R, Kautzner J. Complications of catheter ablation for atrial fibrillation in a high-volume centre with the use of intracardiac echocardiography. *Europace.* 2013;15(1):24-32.

12. Hsu JC, Badhwar N, Gerstenfeld EP, et al. Randomized trial of conventional transseptal needle versus radiofrequency energy needle puncture for left atrial access (the TRAVERSE-LA study). *J Am Heart Assoc.* 2013;2(5):e000428.

13. Katritsis GD, Siontis GC, Giazitzoglou E, Fragakis N, Katritsis DG. Complications of transseptal catheterization for different cardiac procedures. *Int J Cardiol.* 2013;168(6):5352-5354.

14. Katritsis GD, Zografos T, Giazitzoglou E, Katritsis DG. Thrombotic cardiac tamponade after transseptal puncture. *HeartRhythm Case Rep.* 2015;1(2):39-40.

15. Lim HS, Sacher F, Cochet H, et al. Safety and prevention of complications during percutaneous epicardial access for the ablation of cardiac arrhythmias. *Heart Rhythm.* 2014;11(9):1658-1665.

16. Kumareswaran R, Marchlinski FE. Practical guide to ablation for epicardial ventricular tachycardia: when to get access, how to deal with anticoagulation and how to prevent complications. *Arrhythm Electrophysiol Rev.* 2018;7(3):159-164.

17. Aryana A, Tung R, d'Avila A. Percutaneous epicardial approach to catheter ablation of cardiac arrhythmias. *JACC Clin Electrophysiol.* 2020;6(1):1-20.

18. Shah AB, Kronzon I. Congenital defects of the pericardium: a review. *Eur Heart J Cardiovasc Imaging.* 2015;16(8):821-827.

19. Khandaker MH, Espinosa RE, Nishimura RA, et al. Pericardial disease: diagnosis and management. *Mayo Clin Proc.* 2010;85(6):572-593.

20. Chaffanjon P, Brichon P, Faure C, Favre J. Pericardial reflection around the venous aspect of the heart. *Surg Radiol Anat.* 1997;19(1):17-21.

21. Aliot EM, Stevenson WG, Almendral-Garrote JM, et al. EHRA/HRS Expert Consensus on Catheter Ablation of Ventricular Arrhythmias: developed in a partnership with the European Heart Rhythm Association (EHRA), a Registered Branch of the European Society of Cardiology (ESC), and the Heart Rhythm Society (HRS); in collaboration with the American College of Cardiology (ACC) and the American Heart Association (AHA). *Heart Rhythm.* 2009;6(6):886-933.

22. Josephson ME. Electrophysiologic evaluation of sinus node function. In: *Cardiac Clinical Electrophysiology*. Volter Kluwer Philadelphia, PA; 2015:72-85.

23. Katritsis DG, John RM, Latchamsetty R, et al. Left septal slow pathway ablation for atrioventricular nodal reentrant tachycardia. *Circ Arrhythm Electrophysiol*. 2018;11(3):e005907.

24. Pantos I, Patatoukas G, Katritsis DG, Efstathopoulos E. Patient radiation doses in interventional cardiology procedures. *Curr Cardiol Rev*. 2009;5(1):1-11.

25. Pass RH, Gates GG, Gellis LA, Nappo L, Ceresnak SR. Reducing patient radiation exposure during paediatric SVT ablations: use of CARTO(R) 3 in concert with "ALARA" principles profoundly lowers total dose. *Cardiol Young*. 2015;25(5):963-968.

5

Electrophysiology Hardware

ELECTRODE CATHETERS

Basic Mapping Catheters

Catheters used for electrophysiology studies (EPSs) and ablation are composed of multiple insulated wires encased in woven Dacron or polyurethane. Electrodes used in electrophysiology (EP) catheters are usually made of polished platinum-iridium alloy. Platinum is an inert and biologically safe metal with excellent electrical properties but is mechanically soft. The addition of iridium improves mechanical strength without affecting electrical performance.[1] Electrode catheters are typically available in 3 to 8 French (F) diameters and 110 to 120 cm long. Usually 6F quadripolar, hexapolar, or decapolar deflectable catheters composed of 2 mm long electrodes (with a distal tip of 1 or 2 mm) separated by 5-mm distances are used for conventional EPS in adults (Fig. 5.1). Deflectable catheters can be deflected in one or two directions (bidirectional) in the same plane. Smaller electrodes and narrow interelectrode distances (≤1 mm) may be needed for studying complex arrhythmias or multicomponent electrograms.

Advanced Mapping Catheters

The **Halo XP** is a 7F catheter that has been designed for electrophysiologic mapping of the tricuspid annulus during atrial flutter ablation procedures. The catheter has a high torque shaft with a halo-shaped tip section containing 10 pairs of platinum electrodes with a 2-18-2-8-2 mm arrangement (see Fig. 5.1). The **Lasso** 7F catheter is designed to record pulmonary vein potentials during

AF ablation procedures. A similar design is the Inquiry *AFocus II* catheter. It uses 20 small 1-mm electrodes for high-resolution mapping. The *PentaRay* is a 7F catheter with 5 soft, flexible 3F branches and 22 electrodes (1 mm long) in a 4-4-4 mm arrangement that allow higher mapping resolution.

Multipolar recording catheters have become the norm for electroanatomic mapping, and there have been multiple alternative mapping systems that have seen variable success. The *EnSite Array* catheter has 64 non-contact electrodes formed by breaks in the insulation of braided wires forming a woven basket around a saline-filled balloon. The *Advisor HD Grid* is a steerable mapping catheter with a grid-patterned configuration of 16 electrodes for faster data collection. It is used with the EnSite Precision mapping system. The *IntellaMap Orion* mapping catheter is a basketlike catheter designed for use with the Rhythmia mapping system. It offers higher resolution because of its 64-electrode structure. Other basket-like catheters, such as the *Constellation,* and the *TOPERA,* are also available. The *AcQMap,* a non-contact catheter using ultrasound-based technology to localise the catheter and produce the cardiac anatomy whilst recording charge instead of bipolar electrograms, is in an investigational stage at present. All these catheters are connected to the recording/ablation unit via cables specific to the configuration of the catheter.

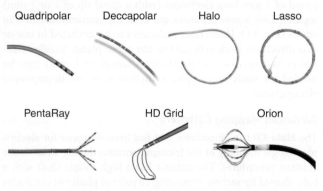

| Quadripolar | Deccapolar | Halo | Lasso |
| PentaRay | | HD Grid | Orion |

FIG. 5.1. Diagnostic electrophysiology catheters.

SHEATHS

Usually, ordinary sheaths are used for catheter insertion through the femoral veins. Long sheaths (63 cm) may be needed to gain access and attain stability in specific sites within the heart, such as for transseptal access to the left atrium or for positioning of the ablation catheters in the right free wall aspect of the tricuspid annulus. Some operators use two long sheaths in the left atrium for radiofrequency (RF) ablation of atrial fibrillation. A deflectable long sheath (Agilis Systems, Chesterfield, MO, USA) may be helpful for positioning and maintaining stability of ablation catheters.

ELECTROGRAM RECORDING AND PROCESSING

The hardware of the EP laboratory, apart from the catheters and connecting cables, consists of the recording and processing EP unit, a stimulator for programmed stimulation, the RF or other energy source generators, and low-resistance grounding patches connecting the RF generator to the patient.

Intracardiac electrograms need to be amplified and displayed in an environment of appropriate grounding and isolation to minimize interference offering a signal-to-noise factor of 20 decibels or more. Acquired signals are subjected to filtering that enhances parts of the frequency spectrum and rejects noise. With multiple devices connected, there is a leakage current flowing through the patient at a fundamental frequency of approximately 50 Hz that can produce artifacts on intracardiac signals. Wireless monitors near the laboratory and mobile phones exacerbate these artifacts. Thus the amplifiers used for recording intracardiac potentials apart from gain modification must have **high- and low-band pass filters** to permit appropriate attenuation of the incoming signals. Modern electronic systems allow a wide range of filtering, but most intracardiac recordings are clearly defined with filtering between 30 and 50 Hz for high pass and 400 and 500 Hz for low pass.

Recorded signals in the EP laboratory are usually **bipolar** because they are measured as a voltage difference between two electrodes. With the use of a 10-mm interelectrode distance, the normal left ventricular bipolar electrograms have an amplitude of 3 to 10 mV, with a duration of less than 70 ms.[2] However, these amplitudes depend on electrode size and spacing (Fig. 5.2).[3] Standard linear ablation catheters have a 3.5-mm distal electrode separated by 1 mm from a proximal 1-mm electrode, resulting in a center-to-center interelectrode spacing of 3.25 mm. As such, each bipolar electrogram represents an underlying tissue diameter ranging from 3.5 to 5.5 mm, depending on the angle of incidence (from perpendicular to parallel to the tissue, respectively).[4] This sampling resolution is often insufficient for identifying and selectively pacing channels of surviving myocardial bundles embedded in surrounding scar tissue. Thus, bipolar voltage amplitude depends on several factors such as the electrode size and the interelectrode distance, conduction velocity between the bipolar electrodes, and the wavefront of activation (Fig. 5.3). The use of multielectrode mapping catheters with smaller electrode and interelectrode spacing can increase the resolution of mapping, enhancing identification of surviving channels and macro–re-entrant circuits.[5]

When one of the electrodes is at distance from the cardiac structures, the voltage difference between the exploring and the distant (indifferent) electrode is referred to as a **unipolar** signal. Unipolar electrograms recorded from the endocardium have large field of view (antenna) that may potentially be helpful identifying abnormalities extending beyond the endocardium itself. Signals are obtained using a 10- to 30-Hz high-pass filter and are used for evaluation of epicardial disease, but there are no data that validate the source of the unipolar signal. Unipolar voltage and configuration are influenced by electrode size, noise, wave front of activation, wall thickness, and surrounding anatomical structures.[5]

Recorded electrograms are assessed at speeds of 100 or 200 mm/s (compared with 25 mm/s for the surface electrocardiogram). At the usual speed of 100 mm/s, 6000 mm are recorded within 1 minute or 60,000 ms. Thus a tachycardia cycle length (or pacing) of 600 ms indicates a heart rate of 100 beats per minute (bpm).

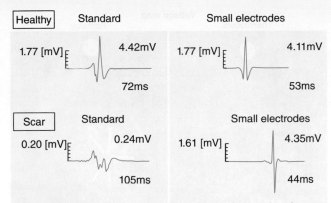

FIG. 5.2. Differences in bipolar electrogram (EGM) voltage and configuration depending on electrode size. Recordings from a standard 3.5-mm-tip electrode catheter (standard) and 0.8-mm electrode (small electrode). Recordings from healthy normal tissue and within scar are shown. In healthy tissue the amplitude and configuration of EGMs are similar. The only difference is a small increase in width using the standard catheter. In scar the standard catheter records a very low amplitude, broad multiphasic EGM, whereas the small electrode catheter records a normal EGM.

(Josephson ME. Electrophysiology at a crossroads: a revisit. *Heart Rhythm.* 2016;13:2317-2322.)

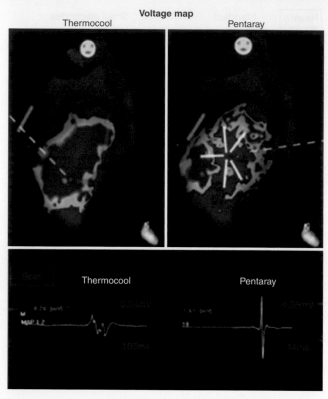

FIG. 5.3. The effect of electrode size and interelectrode spacing on electrograms. A voltage map with Thermocool *(top left panel;* 3.5 mm tip and 1 mm ring) and Pentaray *(top right panel;* each electrode 0.8 mm²) are shown. The red area is less than 0.5 mV. The bipolar signal recorded in the red area was 0.24 mV *(top left panel)* and was broad and fragmented. Recordings from the same site with a Pentaray show normal bipolar amplitude and width *(bottom panel).*
(Josephson ME, Anter E. Substrate mapping for ventricular tachycardia: assumptions and misconceptions. *JACC Clin Electrophysiol.* 2015;1(5):341-352.)

PACING

The typical power settings for conventional **programmed electrical stimulation,** at 60 to 300 bpm, are voltage twice the pacing threshold, current 1 to 2 mA, and 2-ms pulse width, at 100 ohm, usually delivered at 1 to 5 Hz.

References

1. Iravanian S, Langberg JJ. A review of bioelectrodes for clinical electrophysiologists. *Heart Rhythm*. 2019;16(3):460-469.
2. Cassidy DM, Vassallo JA, Marchlinski FE, Buxton AE, Untereker WJ, Josephson ME. Endocardial mapping in humans in sinus rhythm with normal left ventricles: activation patterns and characteristics of electrograms. *Circulation*. 1984;70(1):37-42.
3. Josephson ME. Electrophysiology at a crossroads: a revisit. *Heart Rhythm*. 2016;13(12):2317-2322.
4. Tschabrunn CM, Roujol S, Dorman NC, Nezafat R, Josephson ME, Anter E. High-Resolution Mapping of Ventricular Scar: Comparison Between Single and Multielectrode Catheters. *Circ Arrhythm Electrophysiol*. 2016;9(6).
5. Josephson ME, Anter E. Substrate mapping for ventricular tachycardia: assumptions and misconceptions. *JACC Clin Electrophysiol*. 2015;1(5):341-352.

6

Basic Intervals and Atrial and Ventricular Conduction Curves

BASIC INTERVALS

Basic intervals during sinus rhythm represent a quantitative assessment of the electrical activation of the heart. Normal atrial activation begins at the sinus node, spreads to the low atrium and atrioventricular (AV) junction, and then to the left atrium (Fig. 6.1). Occasionally, the low-right atrium is activated slightly later than the atrium recorded at the AV junction. Activation of the left atrium is mainly through the region of the central fibrous trigone at the apex of the triangle of Koch but also occurs through Bachmann's bundle, the midatrial septum at the fossa ovalis, and the coronary sinus. In the presence of a normal QRS duration, the normal activation times from the onset of ventricular depolarization to the electrogram recorded from the catheter placed near the right ventricular apex are 5 to 30 ms (Fig. 6.2).[1] The right ventricular (RV) free wall at the insertion of the moderator band into the anterior papillary muscle (apical third of the RV free wall) is typically the earliest site of RV activation and precedes the apical septum by 5 to 15 ms. This depends on if there is continuation of the right bundle branch (RBB) toward the apical septum (<25%) or if the apical septum is activated from Purkinje fibers coming off the RBB in the moderator band. Left ventricular endocardial activation begins at 0 to 15 ms after the onset of the QRS, and the duration of left ventricular endocardial activation ranges from 28 to 50 ms.[1] The midseptum and the inferior wall adjacent to the midseptum are the earliest areas of left ventricular endocardial activation, followed by the superior-basal aspect of the free wall. Activation then spreads radially from these breakthrough sites to activate the apex and then the base at the inferoposterior wall.

Basic intervals during sinus rhythm are measured on the His bundle recording electrograms in sinus rhythm at the usual recording speed of 100 mm/s, although a speed of 200 mm/s may also be used for better accuracy (Fig. 6.3). The most important criterion for reliable measurement is reproducibility. Care should be taken to ensure catheter stability during recordings by means of continuous verification against electrogram characteristics and, if needed, stored fluoroscopic or electroanatomic images

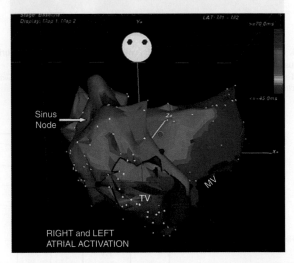

FIG. 6.1. Electroanatomic mapping of atrial normal conduction during sinus rhythm. (Josephson ME. *Cardiac Clinical Electrophysiology.* 5th ed. Riverwoods, IL: Wolters Kluwer; 2015.)

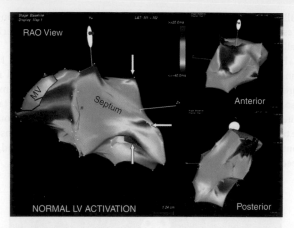

FIG. 6.2. Electroanatomic mapping of ventricular normal conduction during sinus rhythm.
LV, Left ventricle; *MV,* mitral valve; *RAO,* right anterior oblique. (Josephson ME. *Cardiac Clinical Electrophysiology.* 5th ed. Riverwoods, IL: Wolters Kluwer; 2015.)

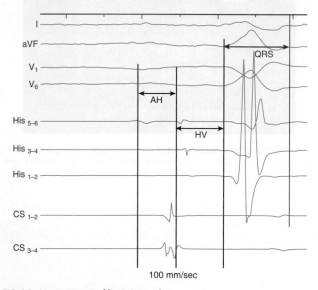

FIG. 6.3. Measurement of basic intervals.
I, aVF, V1, V6, Electrocardiogram leads; *CS,* coronary sinus; *His,* His bundle; *HRA,* high right atrium.

AH Interval

The AH interval represents conduction time from the low-right atrium at the interatrial septum through the AV node to the His bundle. It is measured from the earliest reproducible rapid deflection from baseline of the atrial activation to the earliest rapid deflection of the His bundle depolarization (see Fig. 6.3). Because the exact point within the atrial electrogram when the impulse encounters the AV node is not known, the AH interval is an approximation of AV nodal conduction time. The normal range is 55 to 150 ms.[2] The AH interval is sensitive to autonomic tone. A prolonged AH interval may indicate AV nodal disease or high vagal tone, whereas a shorter than normal AH can occur during sympathetic activation.

HV Interval

The HV interval represents conduction time from the proximal His bundle to the ventricular myocardium. It is measured from the earliest rapid deflection of the His bundle depolarization to the earliest onset of ventricular activation recorded from multiple surface electrocardiography (ECG) leads. If only one ECG channel is available, a V1 or V2 lead should be used because the earliest ventricular activity is usually recorded in one of these leads in the presence of a narrow QRS. Occasionally, however, and especially in the presence of a septal infarction, ventricular activation can occur before the onset of the QRS. Because anatomically the proximal portion of the His bundle begins on the atrial side of the tricuspid valve, the most proximal His bundle deflection is that associated with the largest atrial electrogram. Thus even if a large His bundle deflection is recorded in association with a small atrial electrogram, the catheter must be withdrawn to obtain a His bundle deflection associated with a larger atrial electrogram. This maneuver can on occasion markedly affect the measured HV interval and can elucidate otherwise inapparent intra-His block. In the absence of preexcitation, the normal HV interval is 35 to 55 ms.[2] Thus during sinus rhythm an apparent His deflection with an HV interval of less than 30 ms either reflects recording of a bundle branch potential or ventricular preexcitation. An apparent HV interval less than 35 ms in the absence of an atrial depolarization indicates that the presumed His bundle depolarization is actually an RBB potential, whereas a prolonged HV indicates infranodal AV conduction disease (see Chapter 9). Unlike the AH interval, the HV interval is not significantly affected by variations in autonomic tone.

QRS Interval

The QRS duration is measured on the surface ECG from the beginning of the q or R wave to the end of the QRS. Normal QRS duration is 120 ms or less.

PACING MANEUVERS

Incremental pacing and the introduction of programmed single or multiple extrastimuli during sinus or paced rhythms are essential for electrophysiology procedures. They are used to characterize the properties of the AV conduction system, detect arrhythmogenic substrates such as accessory pathways, assess inducibility of tachycardias, and provide clues to the facilitate the mechanism of tachycardia. Usually, ventricular pacing maneuvers are conducted before atrial pacing ones because the latter may induce atrial fibrillation. Autonomic manipulation with drugs such as isoprenaline or atropine may be needed to facilitate conduction and tachycardia induction.

Continuous pacing is delivered at a constant rate at a cycle length of 400 to 600 ms at atrial or ventricular sites.

Programmed electrical stimulation refers to pacing that is performed at a constant basic drive cycle length, most commonly 500 or 600 and 400 or 350 ms, for eight pulses (S1–S1), followed by the introduction of an extrastimulus (S2) and with stepwise reduction in the S1–S2 interval by 10-ms decrements until tissue (A or V or atrioventricular node [AVN]) refractoriness or S1–S2 of 200 to 220 ms is reached. Stimuli of 1 to 2 ms duration are delivered at twice the diastolic threshold. Double, triple, or more extrastimuli may be necessary for the induction of the clinical tachycardia.

Ramp pacing implies bursts of pacing with a gradual decrease of cycle length with each interval. It is used to induce or interrupt tachycardias.

REFRACTORY PERIODS

The refractoriness of a cardiac tissue can be defined by the response of that tissue to the introduction of premature stimuli.

The **effective refractory period (ERP)** of a cardiac tissue is the longest interval of the input into a part of the conduction system that fails to propagate through that tissue. For example, the atrial ERP is defined by the longest S_1S_2 interval that fails to capture the atrium.

The A_1A_2 interval of an atrial pacing beat that fails to display a His or V electrogram represents the AV nodal ERP.

The **relative refractory period (RRP)** is the longest coupling interval of a premature impulse that results in prolonged conduction of the premature impulse relative to that of the basic drive. Thus the RRP of the atrium is the longest S_1S_2 interval at which the S_2A_2 interval exceeds the S_1A_1 interval.

The **functional refractory period (FRP)** of a cardiac tissue is the minimum interval between two consecutively conducted impulses through that tissue. Because the FRP is a measure of output from a tissue, it is described by measuring points distal to that tissue. It follows that determination of the ERP of a tissue requires that the FRP of more proximal tissues be less than the ERP of the distal tissue; for example, the ERP of the His-Purkinje system can be determined only if it exceeds the FRP of the AVN. Thus the FRP of the AVN is the shortest H_1H_2 interval in response to any A_1A_2 interval.

ATRIOVENTRICULAR CONDUCTION CURVES

Atrial pacing maneuvers are used to study the properties of the AVN and to assess the inducibility of atrial arrhythmias.

Atrial pacing is most commonly performed from the high-right atrium in the region of the sinus node or from the coronary sinus. Programmed electrical stimulation is performed at a cycle length (S1–S1) of 500 to 600 and then 400 ms with an extra stimulus delivered after eight paced beats and at progressively shortened intervals (S1–S2), in 10- to 20-ms decrements, to a minimum of 200 ms or until atrial or AV nodal refractoriness is reached. Although there are several patterns of response to programmed atrial extrastimuli, characterized by differing sites of conduction delay and block and the coupling intervals at which they occur, the most common pattern is seen when the atrial impulse encounters progressively greater delay in the AVN without any change in infranodal conduction (Fig. 6.4). Block eventually occurs in the AVN or the atrium itself. Thus the normal response to atrial pacing is for the AH interval to gradually lengthen as the cycle length is decreased until AV nodal block occurs. This is the typical

decremental behavior of the AVN (Fig. 6.5). Decremental conduction may also be seen with slowly conducting posteroseptal accessory pathways (APs), atriofascicular bypass tracts, and nodofascicular/nodoventricular bypass tracts.

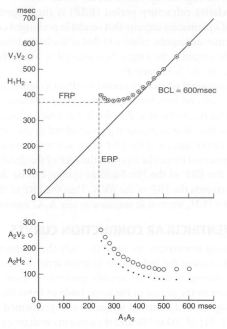

FIG. 6.4. **Usual pattern of normal AV conduction curves.** Normally the atrioventricular (AV) node displays a gradual conduction time prolongation with atrial extrastimulation, thus resulting in smooth conduction curves with progressive increment of the AH or HH intervals. Note the gradual increase of AH intervals with shortening of the coupling intervals A_1A_2.

ERP and FRP are the effective and functional refractory periods of the AV node. *ERP*, Effective refractory period; *FRP*, functional refractory period. (Katritsis D, Camm AJ. Clinical electrophysiological mechanisms of tachycardias arising from the atrioventricular junction. In: Macfarlane PW: Comprehensive Electrocardiography. 2nd Edition, Springer, 2011.)

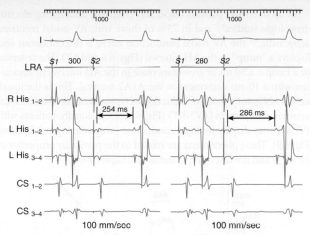

FIG. 6.5. Decremental conduction of the AV node. There is a continually increasing AH interval after progressively shorter extrasimulation intervals.
AV, Atrioventricular; *CS*, coronary sinus; *LRA*, low right atrium.

Depending on autonomic tone, abnormal AH prolongation or a prolonged AV nodal block cycle length (CL) can occur during atrial pacing in patients with normal conduction, and the administration of isoprenaline (boluses of 5–10 mcg intravenously [IV] or infusion of 2–5 mcg/min) may be necessary for the induction of a paroxysmal supraventricular tachycardia. Because of the marked effect of the autonomic nervous system on AV nodal function, AV nodal Wenckebach block occurs at a wide range of paced cycle lengths. In the absence of preexcitation, most patients in the basal state develop AV nodal Wenckebach block at paced atrial cycle lengths of 500 to 350 ms.[3] Occasionally, young, healthy patients develop Wenckebach block at relatively long-paced cycle lengths, presumably secondary to enhanced vagal tone, whereas others, with heightened sympathetic tone, conduct 1:1 at cycle lengths of 300 ms.

Infranodal conduction (HV interval) remains unaffected (or very slightly delayed) in the absence of conduction disease. Prolongation of the HV interval or infra-His block produced at gradually reduced paced cycle lengths of 400 ms or more are abnormal and probably signify impaired infranodal conduction (see Chapter 9). Infranodal block is not necessarily pathologic and can be due to functional block dependent on the Ashman ("long–short") phenomenon.

In up to 35% of patients (especially children) undergoing electro-physiologic studies[4-7] and in 75% of those with AV nodal reentrant tachycardia,[8,9] the AV nodal conduction curve is discontinuous and displays a "**jump**" in the AH interval (Figs. 6.6 and 6.7). The criterion for a jump is a 50 ms or greater increase in the AH interval in association with a 10-ms decrement in the A1A2 interval. This is the usual, but not obligatory, mode of induction of typical atrioventricular nodal reentrant tachycardia (AVNRT) (Fig. 6.8). Occasionally, patients with AVNRT may display multiple conduction jumps during atrial pacing (Fig. 6.9). These phenomena are related to the particular properties of the AVN and are discussed in detail in Chapter 14.

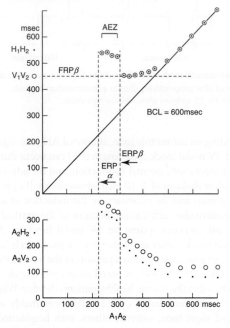

FIG. 6.6. **Discontinues AV conduction curve.** A sudden increment of AV nodal conduction time results in a discontinuous curve. The sudden increase of AH (jump) indicates refractoriness of one (β) pathway and conduction through another (α) pathway.

AV, Atrioventricular; *ERP*, Effective refractory period; *FRP*, functional refractory period. (Katritsis D, Camm AJ. Clinical electrophysiological mechanisms of tachycardias arising from the atrioventricular junction. In: Macfarlane PW: *Comprehensive Electrocardiography*. 2nd ed. New York, NY: Springer; 2011.)

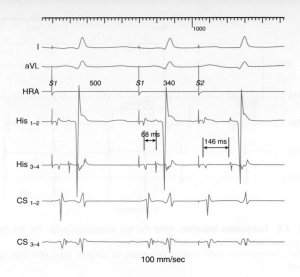

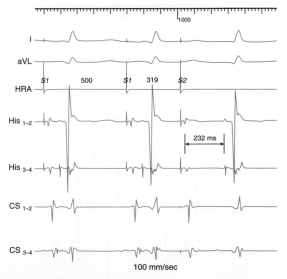

FIG. 6.7. Antegrade conduction jump. The extrastimulation-evoked AH interval of 232 ms exceeds the immediately previous AH extrastimulation-evoked AH interval (146 ms) by more than 50 seconds.

CS, Coronary sinus; *HRA*, high right atrium.

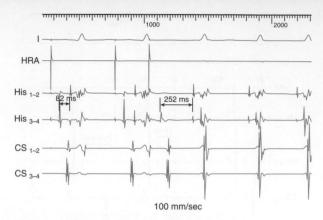

FIG. 6.8. Tachycardia induction. After the last extrastimulus (S), the AH gets prolonged and a tachycardia (AVNRT) is induced.
AVNRT, Atrioventricular nodal reentrant tachycardia; *CS,* coronary sinus; *HRA,* high right atrium.

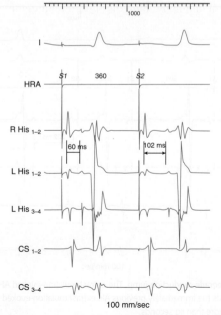

FIG. 6.9, cont'd

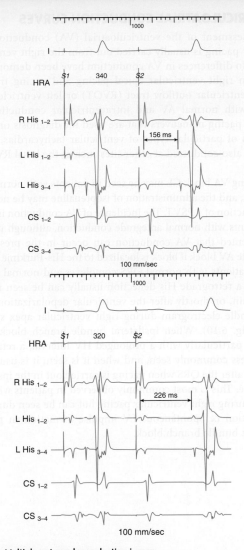

FIG. 6.9. Multiple antegrade conduction jumps.
CS, Coronary sinus; *HRA,* high right atrium.

VENTRICULOATRIAL CONDUCTION CURVES

For assessment of the ventriculoatrial (VA) conduction, ventricular pacing is usually carried out from the right ventricular apex. No differences in VA conduction have been demonstrated between right ventricular apical pacing and pacing from the right ventricular outflow tract (RVOT) or left ventricle in patients with normal AV and intraventricular conduction. For certain pacing maneuvers that are used for diagnosis or for induction of particular types of ventricular tachycardias, pacing may be also conducted at other sites such as the basal RV or the RVOT.

A long VA block CL may be seen in patients with normal conduction, and the administration of isoprenaline may be necessary for induction of a PSVT. The incidence of VA conduction is higher in patients with normal antegrade conduction, although it is well documented that VA conduction can occur in the presence of complete AV block if block is localized to the His-Purkinje system.

In patients with normal QRS complexes and normal HV intervals, a retrograde His deflection usually can be seen in front of, within, or shortly after the ventricular depolarization in the His bundle electrogram during right ventricular apex stimulation (Fig. 6.10). When ipsilateral bundle branch block is observed, particularly with a prolonged HV interval, a retrograde His is less commonly seen, and when it is seen, it is usually inscribed after the QRS when pacing is carried out in the ipsilateral ventricle. This is most commonly observed in patients with RBB block during right ventricular pacing but can be seen during LV stimulation or spontaneous LV impulse formation in patients with left bundle branch block.

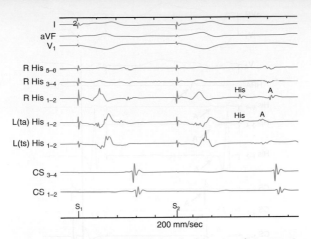

FIG. 6.10. Recording of a retrograde His bundle electrogram during V pacing.
I, aVF, V5, Electrocardiogram leads; *CS,* coronary sinus; *HRA,* high right atrium; *L(ta) His,* His bundle recorded from the left septum through a transaortic approach; *L(ts) His,* His bundle recorded from the left septum through a transseptal approach; *R His,* His bundle recorded from the right septum.

Pacing for the investigation of presumed SVT is as described with atrial pacing. Programmed ventricular stimulation with a single extrastimulus is performed until the retrograde AV nodal refractory period is reached. The retrograde atrial activation sequence should be examined. In the absence of a retrogradely conducting AP, the atrial electrogram recorded in the His bundle electrogram is usually earliest (Fig. 6.11). However, sometimes, particularly at short coupling intervals, earliest retrograde activation is recorded at the ostium or proximal portion of the coronary sinus (CS)[10] (Fig. 6.12). This retrograde activation sequence can also be observed in the presence of a concealed septal accessory pathway with decremental properties.

When a 10-ms decrement in the V1V2 interval is associated with a 50 ms or greater increase in the VA interval, this is evidence of dual AV nodal pathways (retrograde jump). Retrograde dual AV nodal pathways can be observed in patients with AVNRT but sometimes occur in individuals without AVNRT (Fig. 6.13).

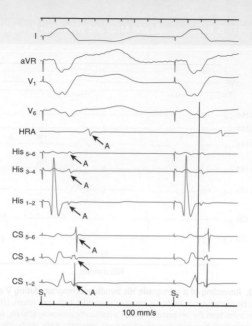

FIG. 6.11. Normal atrial retrograde activation sequence during V pacing. Earliest atrial retrograde activation is recorded by the His bundle electrode *(vertical line)*.
I, aVR, V1, V6, Electrocardiogram leads; *CS,* coronary sinus; *His,* His bundle; *HRA,* high right atrium.

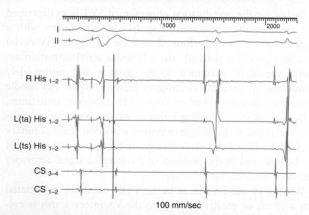

FIG. 6.12. Normal atrial retrograde activation sequence during V pacing. The earliest atrial retrograde activation is recorded almost simultaneously by the right His bundle electrode and the CS electrode. However, left septal His recordings reveal the left septum (at the His area) as the site of the earliest atrial retrograde activation *(vertical line)*.
I, II, Electrocardiogram leads; *CS,* coronary sinus; *HRA,* high right atrium; *L(ta) His,* His bundle recorded from the left septum through a transaortic approach; *L(ts) His,* His bundle recorded from the left septum through a transseptal approach; *R His,* His bundle recorded from the right septum.

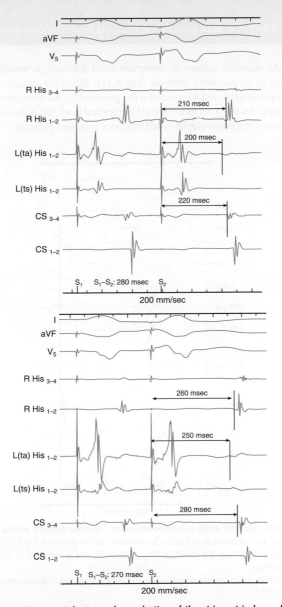

FIG. 6.13. Decremental retrograde conduction of the atrioventricular node. A retrograde conduction jump is demonstrated.

I, aVF, V5, Electrocardiogram leads; *CS,* coronary sinus; *HRA,* high right atrium; *L(ta)His,* His bundle recorded from the left septum through a transaortic approach; *L(ts) His,* His bundle recorded from the left septum through a transseptal approach; *R His,* His bundle recorded from the right septum.

An eccentric pattern of retrograde atrial activation is strong evidence of an accessory pathway (Fig. 6.14). When the earliest atrial retrograde activation is recorded at the proximal CS but even the distal CS precedes the A recorded at the His (vertical line), this indicates the presence of a posteroseptal or left posterior accessory pathway.

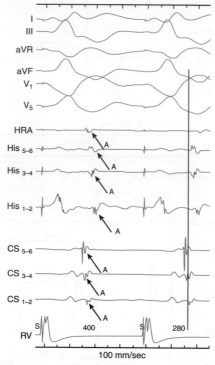

FIG. 6.14. Eccentric atrial retrograde activation sequence during V pacing. The earliest atrial retrograde activation is recorded by the proximal the CS (CS$_{5-6}$) electrode, but even the distal CS (CS$_{5-6}$) precedes the A recorded at the His *(vertical line)*.

I, II, aVF, aVR, V\i, V5, Electrocardiogram leads; *CS,* coronary sinus; *HRA,* high right atrium; *RV,* right ventricle.

For induction of VT, the Wellens protocol or other versions (simplified or accelerated protocols) are used.[11-14] A detailed discussion of their clinical significance is provided in Chapter 16.

References

1. Josephson ME. Description of electrograms. In: *Clinical Cardiac Electrophysiology.* 5th ed. Wolters Kluwer; Philadelphia, PA, 2015.
2. Josephson ME. Measurement of conduction Intervals. In: *Clinical Cardiac Electrophysiology.* 5th ed. Wolters Kluwer; Philadelphia, PA; 2015.
3. Josephson ME. Programmed stimulation. In: *Clinical Cardiac Electrophysiology.* 5th ed. Wolters Kluwer; Philadelphia, PA; 2015:35-69.
4. Casta A, Wolff GS, Mehta AV, et al. Dual atrioventricular nodal pathways: a benign finding in arrhythmia-free children with heart disease. *Am J Cardiol.* 1980;46(6): 1013-1018.
5. Denes P, Wu D, Dhingra R, Amat-y-Leon F, Wyndham C, Rosen KM. Dual atrioventricular nodal pathways. A common electrophysiological response. *Br Heart J.* 1975;37(10):1069-1076.
6. Thapar MK, Gillette PC. Dual atrioventricular nodal pathways: a common electrophysiologic response in children. *Circulation.* 1979;60(6):1369-1374.
7. Brugada P, Heddle B, Green M, Wellens HJ. Initiation of atrioventricular nodal reentrant tachycardia in patients with discontinuous anterograde atrioventricular nodal conduction curves with and without documented supraventricular tachycardia: observations on the role of a discontinuous retrograde conduction curve. *Am Heart J.* 1984;107(4):685-697.
8. Katritsis DG, Camm AJ. Atrioventricular nodal reentrant tachycardia. *Circulation.* 2010;122(8):831-840.
9. Katritsis DG, Josephson ME. Classification of electrophysiological types of atrioventricular nodal re-entrant tachycardia: a reappraisal. *Europace.* 2013;15(9):1231-1240.
10. Katritsis DG, Becker A. The atrioventricular nodal reentrant tachycardia circuit: a proposal. *Heart Rhythm.* 2007;4(10):1354-1360.
11. Brugada P, Wellens HJ. Comparison in the same patient of two programmed ventricular stimulation protocols to induce ventricular tachycardia. *Am J Cardiol.* 1985;55(4):380-383.
12. Morady F, DiCarlo L, Winston S, Davis JC, Scheinman MM. A prospective comparison of triple extrastimuli and left ventricular stimulation in studies of ventricular tachycardia induction. *Circulation.* 1984;70(1):52-57.
13. Hummel JD, Strickberger SA, Daoud E, et al. Results and efficiency of programmed ventricular stimulation with four extrastimuli compared with one, two, and three extrastimuli. *Circulation.* 1994;90(6):2827-2832.
14. Morady F, DiCarlo Jr LA, Baerman JM, de Buitleir M. Comparison of coupling intervals that induce clinical and nonclinical forms of ventricular tachycardia during programmed stimulation. *Am J Cardiol.* 1986;57(15):1269-1273.

7

Electroanatomic Mapping and Magnetic Guidance Systems

ELECTROANATOMIC MAPPING
THEORETICAL CONSIDERATIONS

During conventional electrophysiology (EP) procedures, catheters are manually navigated with the use of single or bi-plane fluoroscopy. An inherent limitation of fluoroscopic navigation is that orientation of the catheter relative to the cardiac anatomy can only be appreciated in two dimensions. Thus it may make complex procedures challenging and is associated with radiation exposure for both patient and physician. In 1996 Ben-Haim and Josephson published a report of a new technology referred to as nonfluoroscopic in vivo navigation and mapping (Fig. 7.1).[1] Navigation was achieved by a magnetic sensor inserted in an EP recording catheter and magnetic field radiators placed below the operating bed. This discovery led to an era of innovation with several three-dimensional (3D) **electroanatomic mapping (EAM)** systems being developed for clinical use in the EP laboratory.

A fundamental principle of 3D EAM is the ability to collect anatomic (location) and electrical (electrograms) data simultaneously. This means that as the catheter connected to the 3D EAM system is moved in a cardiac chamber, serial recording of location data allows replication of the catheter tip's location in real time on a computer monitor. When location data are acquired at specific anatomic locations, a meshlike geometry can be created that replicates the chamber's anatomy. As location data are being collected, the catheters also record electrograms. Acquired electrograms can be displayed on the 3D chamber anatomy at their collected location coordinates. Each electrogram can be annotated for **local activation time (LAT)** or **amplitude (voltage)** and the annotation displayed, following a color code, on the map. Therefore, during this mapping process, the operator creates a 3D electroanatomic map of the chamber of interest (Fig. 7.2A).

Impedance-based location measurements (or a combination with magnetic field–based technology) are also used by some 3D EAM systems. This is performed by emitting a small current from the catheter electrodes and sensor patches placed on the patient. The resulting current ratio recorded at each sensor, per electrode, allows calculation of location data and consequent catheter visualization and mapping.

EAM has rendered mapping and ablation of complex arrhythmias, such as postoperative right atrial flutters and ventricular tachycardia (VT), feasible when previously this was a challenge.[2,3] Randomized ablation trials using EAM in patients with supraventricular tachycardia have demonstrated similar acute procedural success rates and reduced fluoroscopy time.[4,5] EAM is also useful for activation and voltage mapping and for tagging locations of specific electrograms of interest that allow substrate-modification ablation approaches (see Chapter 16).

The three systems used in clinical practice for EAM are the **CARTO** mapping platform (currently in its CARTO 3 version 7), the **EnSite Precision** platform, and the **Rhythmia HDx** system, which has the capability to record and map from 64 electrodes simultaneously.

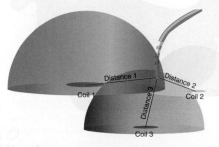

FIG. 7.1. The locatable catheter is composed of tip and ring electrodes and a location sensor totally embedded within the catheter. A location pad is composed of three coils that generate a magnetic field that decays as a function of distance from that coil. The sensor measures the strength of the field, and the distance from each coil (D1, D2, D3) can be measured. The location of the sensor is determined from the intersection of the theoretical spheres whose radii are the distances measured by the sensor.

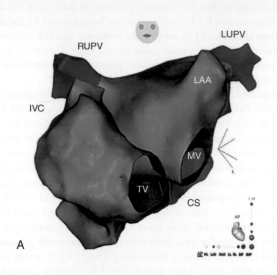

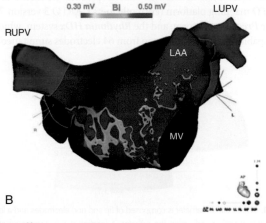

FIG. 7.2, Cont'd

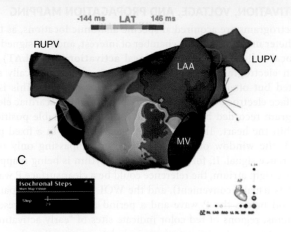

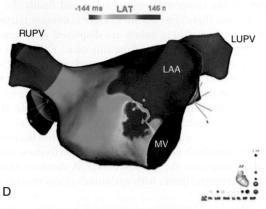

FIG. 7.2. (A) An anatomic map of the right atrium (RA) and left atrium (LA), as well as the coronary sinus (CS), pulmonary veins (PV), and left atrial appendage (LAA), is shown. This was collected using CARTO 3 v6 with the CONFIDENSE module during atrial tachycardia, with a cycle of 303 ms. (B) Bipolar voltage map of the LA during tachycardia, with limits from 0.30 mV to 0.50 mV. (C) Isochronal map of the left atrium during tachycardia. (D) LAT map of the same tachycardia. Note how in both (C) and (D) the early colors (red), meet the late colors (purple) to suggest a mitral isthmus dependent macroreentry.
LAT, Local activation time; *LUPV,* left upper pulmonary vein; *MV,* mitral valve; *RUPV,* right upper pulmonary vein.

ACTIVATION, VOLTAGE, AND PROPAGATION MAPPING

Electrograms are acquired at specific anatomic locations, as the catheter moves across the chamber of interest, and is assigned to a local activation timing. The **local activation time (LAT)** of each electrogram is then compared with an automatically selected but often user-modified stable fiducial point. This is a surface electrocardiography (ECG) lead, or an intracardiac electrogram recorded by a diagnostic catheter in a stable position within the heart. The comparison occurs within in a fixed period, the window of interest (WOI), encompassing only one reference signal. If, for example, sinus rhythm is being mapped in the right atrium, the reference could be a clear surface P wave (V1 is usually convenient), and the WOI would have to span a period before the P wave and a period after it. With present systems, regions of red color indicate sites of "early activation" and activation becomes progressively later proceeding through the colors of the rainbow to yellow-green and finally the blue and purple hues that define the sites of late activation relative to the reference point. These colors are displayed as a time bar adjacent to the 3D map. Thus, if the annotated LAT of an electrogram is "early" in the window compared with the reference signal (i.e., occurs before it), it will be assigned a red color to be displayed as on the 3D map. As signals get later compared with the reference, the color eventually will change to purple. If colors are missing, then, a portion of the window has not been mapped with EGMs, either because the window has been set up incorrectly, mapping has been insufficient, or activation encompasses more time than the window covers. A common example of this is a perimitral flutter with epicardial conduction over the coronary sinus (CS).[6]

Two other concepts pertain to activation mapping: isochrones and propagation. **Isochronal mapping** is a type of LAT mapping whereby color coding is done based on groups of EGMs with the same LAT (isochrones) as opposed to depicting and annotating each EGM distinctly. The maps appear similar, but crucially the area of a color (i.e., how much tissue is activated simultaneously) is purported to correlate to conduction speed (Fig. 7.2C and D).

Voltage maps of the recorded electrograms can be created with colors representing the maximal bipolar/unipolar voltage amplitude. These maps provide a method by which to quantify cardiac

scarring and have significant value in modern cardiac EP procedures (Fig. 7.2B).

Mapping during arrhythmia also allows the creation of an actual
propagation map of the tachycardia. This is a "moving" version of
LAT that displays spread of activation wave front throughout a
cardiac cycle as a live wave front traversing the cardiac chamber. It allows visual appreciation of the mapped arrhythmia mechanism and a
visual estimation of relative conduction velocity through various sites.

PRACTICAL POINTS OF 3D MAPPING

Several problems can influence accuracy and should be eliminated
as much as possible during the mapping process. They include the
inherent noise of the location system, the reproducibility of the
fiducial point on the ECG, the reproducibility of cardiac mechan-
ics on a beat-to-beat basis, and gating of image acquisition to the
cardiac cycle and respiratory phase.[7] Maps created using EAM
systems are also subject to additional variability depending on accurate annotation of electrogram qualities, consistent catheter
contact with tissue, distributed sampling of the entire structure of
interest, density of location "points" in the map, type of rhythm
being mapped, direction of activation wave front propagation, and
the size and spacing of the electrodes used to acquire the data.[8]

Patient Movement and Respiratory Stability

A basic requirement of accurate 3D EAM maps is that the patient
remains still throughout the entire procedure. CARTO has argu-
ably developed the most accurate navigation technology based on
magnetic localization, which, as discussed, depends on creating a
matrix of location data based on the reach of the intracardiac catheter in the magnetic field. However, this approach means it is also
most sensitive to patient movements relative to the magnetic field,
despite it also using impedance-based localization technology via
sensor patches on the patient. EnSite Precision and Rhythmia
HDx rely less on magnetic localization, using impedance primarily, and therefore are less sensitive to patient movements. However,
localization by impedance is heavily limited by even minor changes
in tissue characteristics (e.g., tidal volume or fluid status) that occur continuously during EP procedures, as well as background
current noise.[9,10] If a patient moves during mapping, the entire
collected map will "shift" with respect to where the heart and the

catheters truly lie. This is a challenge to correct, by moving either patches, equipment, or the patient, and further mapping of the same map impossible. Many operators employ general anesthesia to avoid problems related to patient movement

Movement of the catheter caused by inspiration and expiration can be problematic when precise ablation is needed. Although patient tidal volumes can be controlled during general anesthesia procedures, it is preferable to employ technology available within the 3D EAM systems. All major system use thoracic impedance measurements to calculate respiratory motion and allow location data or EGM only during a predefined phase of respiration (typically end expiration).

Another challenge to accurate localization of catheters and anatomy by 3D EAM is the nonuniformity of cardiac anatomy in patients. For example, an extremely dilated left ventricle (LV) in a patient with scar-related VT may mean that the LV apex is "out of range" of the mapping range of any system.

Reference Electrogram

During activation mapping, the electrical fiducial point needs to be stable and have a clearly reproducible annotation point. With atrial tachycardias, a stable intracardiac atrial electrogram such as a CS catheter electrogram is usually chosen because the P wave can be indistinct on the body surface ECG. With VTs, a large, reproducibly identifiable component of a QRS complex is typically chosen.[11] Advances in 3D EAM systems can also take advantage of specific algorithms to identify the best reference signal from the body surface or stable intracardiac signals. Once selected, 3D EAM systems will annotate the reference signal automatically for the duration of the case. It is critically important, before mapping starts, to assess the automatic annotation of this signal because it cannot be changed after acquisition of the first point, to avoid map distortion. For voltage mapping, the reference can be any reliable and stable signal; errors in timing annotation are less important because the variable mapped is amplitude. However, because voltage and activation are almost always collected simultaneously, a stable reference selection should mark the start of any 3D mapping procedure.

Once the fiducial point is selected, it will provide time 0 ms within the WOI of any activation map. Fig. 7.3 shows how changing the reference while mapping the same rhythm (in this case an atrial tachycardia), changes the appearance of the LAT map. These differences are critical because the LAT map appearance guides ablation.

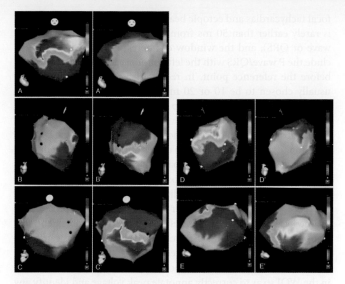

FIG. 7.3. Two electroanatomic activation maps of the same macroreentrant left atrial tachycardia (left atrial flutter) created with two different temporal references are shown. In each panel, orientation of the left atrium is indicated by the orientation of the face at the top of the panel and the small heart in the lower left corner. (A) to (E), "Earliest" activation (red) is seen in the roof of the left atrium and then proceeds down the septal and lateral walls, with latest activation at the interolateral left atrium. (A') to (E') show the same tachycardia, but the map is constructed based on a reference point that is 120 ms later than selected for (A) through (E). Notice that the activation sequence has significantly changed, with "earliest" activation (red region) at the inferior portion of the left atrium.
(Del Carpio Munoz F, Buescher TL, Asirvatham SJ. Three-dimensional mapping of cardiac arrhythmias: what do the colors really mean? *Circ Arrhythm Electrophysiol.* 2010;3:e6-11.)

Window of Interest

The WOI is defined by specifying an interval around the reference point, with symmetric or asymmetric boundaries, within which the mapping system records electrical signals for annotation. The WOI usually covers most of the cardiac cycle length in duration but strictly no more than one cardiac cycle in time—that is, not more than two reference signals.

Determination of the WOI is based on the rhythm being mapped when the diagnosis is known or clinically suspected. In focal tachycardias and ectopic beats, the true early site of activation is rarely earlier than 50 ms from the start of the surface ECG (P wave or QRS), and the window of interest is easily chosen to include the P wave/QRS with the left boundary beginning 40 to 50 ms before the reference point. In reentrant tachycardias the WOI is usually chosen to be 10 or 20 ms less than the tachycardia cycle length, and different methods to position it around the reference point have been proposed.

For atrial macroreentry, the most used calculation is the DePonti equation,[12] which is calculated to center the WOI around activation occurring in the mid-diastolic pathway supporting reentry. However, a practical approach is choosing a timing interval slightly less than the tachycardia cycle and distributing this evenly around the reference, which is 0 ms. Another common practical approach is to set the left boundary at 40 ms before P-wave onset and extend forward for the remainder of the cycle. For ventricular substrate mapping during sinus or atrially paced rhythms, the principle is to include the entire ventricular component of activation and restoration in the WOI so as to correctly annotate peak voltage and identify any abnormally late activation. Therefore the WOI should exclude atrial activation and can be symmetric or asymmetric, depending on the reference chosen. During ventricular pacing, care must be taken to exclude the stimulation artifact from the WOI (even if chosen as the reference) to avoid its annotation as true voltage.

It is important to consider certain common errors regarding the WOI as illustrated in Fig. 7.4. If the WOI is too short, for any rhythm, a certain section of activation will be "missed." This may not be a significant problem when mapping a focal tachycardia, where the most important information is the pattern of activation after breakout; however, in the case of reentry or even late potential mapping, this can change the map dramatically because the entire circuit or channel may not be visualized. Conversely, if the WOI is too large, areas of adjacent early activation and late activation may be labeled as the same. Another common pitfall of mapping of a reentrant tachycardia with a 3D mapping system is the perception that the site of slow conduction that facilitates tachycardia perpetuation is the zone where the "earliest" activation sites meet the "latest" ones (early meets late area). Although in some cases this might be correct, many times it is not. The activation timing of a site depends on the positioning of the WOI around the reference point; thus the "early meets late" zone is also dependent on this factor.

For reentrant tachycardias, the WOI is typically specified such that the sum of the intervals approximates the tachycardia cycle length, but the window settings specifying how much of the cycle length being mapped should be shown as being before or after a particular reference electrogram is arbitrary. Two different operators may correctly choose two different windows of reference, again giving rise to two different locations for "red areas" for the same tachycardia. It is evident that the red or "early" site is an entirely arbitrary location for macroreentrant arrhythmias.[11] Fig. 7.5 illustrates the effect of the choice of WOI in a case of focal (microreentrant) VT in a patient with operated tetralogy of Fallot.[13] Activation map is suggestive of reentry between the tricuspid annulus and this low-voltage region with an early-meets-late pattern. The scale bar shows that the earliest and latest activation times span the whole window. A closer look at Fig. 7.5B (left) shows that QRS is broad and the reference point is toward the second half of the QRS. Therefore the annotation window begins at approximately equal to 20 ms ahead of QRS onset. Activation occurring 30 ms ahead of QRS onset would then be marked in the end of the window and mimic macroreentry. Reannotating the points using a window of -170 to $+80$ ms clearly shows a focal onset with centrifugal activation.

LAT1: CORRECT (EMPIRICAL) WOI, CORRECT REFERENCE

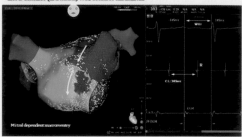

LAT3: LONG WOI, CORRECT REFERENCE

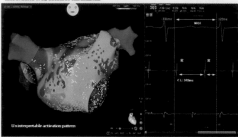

LAT2: CORRECT (DePonti) WOI, CORRECT REFERENCE

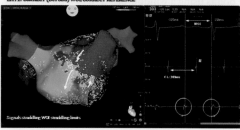

LAT4: SHORT WOI, CORRECT REFERENCE

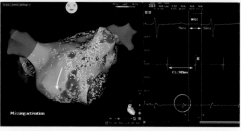

FIG. 7.4. Effects of changing the WOI in the same tachycardia. This is a perimitral macroreentry with a cycle length of 303ms mapped with a PentaRay catheter. (light blue, bottom line). Also shown are the V2 ECG lead (yellow), and CS (dark blue). LAT1: This is an "optimal" version of the LAT map. The early meets late area is present on the anterior LA wall and the color scheme suggests activation rotating around the mitral valve annulus, in a counter clockwise direction (large white arrows).The WOI has been calculated empirically, as 290ms (13ms less than the tachycardia) and split equally around the mapping reference signal, R (CS 5,6). The early area is suggestive of the "exit" site of this reentrant circuit. A signal from this area (EGM) is shown on the right panel, and a small yellow arrow demonstrates its LAT annotation point within the WOI as early. Note that this signal is abnormal/fractionated. Entrainment from this site was consistent with perimitral reentry, and, radiofrequency energy applications to these signals led to tachycardia termination. LAT2: The WOI has been calculated using the DePonti method. The map is very similar with LAT1, but the early area seen in LAT1 now also contains points annotated as slightly later in the cycle (green and blue colors in the map). These small errors, that suggest activation moving in an opposite direction (small white arrow close to the mitral annulus on the map) might be explained by the signals encircled on the right panel. These atrial signals "straddle" the time interval of the WOI. Therefore there are situations where a signal from the "next" beat may encroach within the mapped WOI, and lead to missanotation. Usually, this leads to minor changes of the map, but may produce significant changes depending on the tachycardia mapped. LAT3 and LAT4 are examples of incorrect WOI settings. A very short WOI in LAT3 leads to missed atrial activation occurring during a tachycardia cycle but not being mapped. This is visually appreciated as a lack of late (purple) colors in the LAA. In LAT4 the WOI is too long and therefore more than one cycle contribute to the map, which is uninterpretable.

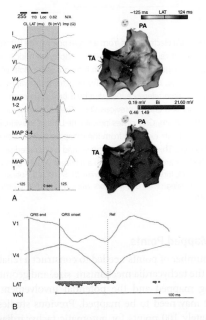

FIG. 7.5, Cont'd

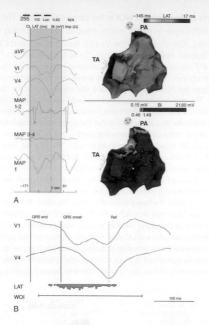

FIG. 7.5. *Upper panel:* (A) Electrograms from a single point at the left with activation late in the window and a local activation time (LAT) map in the middle with a pattern of early meets late. A voltage map is shown on the right with cutoffs of 1.5 and 0.46 mV for scar and dense scar, respectively. (B) Two electrocardiography leads from a single cycle along with time reference indicated by a *broken line* and other lines indicating the QRS onset and end of previous QRS. The chosen window of interest (WOI) is shown at the bottom. *Gray circles* indicate the LATs of individual points. This figure was plotted using data exported from the mapping system. *Lower panel:* (A) and (B) Reannotated map. The same map is shown and is organized similar to upper panel. However, the LATs are reannotated with a different WOI (−170 to +80 ms). *PA,* Pulmonary annulus; *TA,* tricuspid annulus. (Selvaraj RJ, Shankar B, Subramanian A, et al. Chasing red herrings: making sense of the colors while mapping. *Circ Arrhythm Electrophysiol.* 2014;7:553-556.)

Number of Mapped Points

The required number of points needed to construct a reliable map is dependent on the tachycardia mechanism, size, and geometry of the chamber being mapped and the potential involvement of other chambers that may need to be mapped. Previous studies suggests that approximately 100 points for automatic tachycardias and 200 points for reentrant arrhythmias are usually taken in a given chamber.[11] However, in current clinical practice with automated point collection systems, these numbers are far higher and routinely reach the thousands. When point collection is manual, it is important to ensure that every electrogram collected is from the same cardiac rhythm and with appropriate catheter contact. Point coverage is equally important. Large unmapped areas between points leads to the systems interpolating data in these areas. Interpolation is a particular problem in activation mapping, where the area occupied by an isochrone is related to conduction velocity and can lead to a false impression of rapid conduction or a large area of the heart all activating isochronally. Other examples of interpolation errors relate to backward wave fronts on reentrant propagation maps, particularly near areas where early activation meets late activation.

Most systems are able to collect a comparable amount of points (nearing 20,000) per map, with the exception of Rhythmia HDx, which can accommodate more than 100,000 and produce very high-resolution maps.

Mapped Rhythm and Automated Point Collection

Each 3D electroanatomic map can only display one distinct rhythm (which is why, to an extent, atrial fibrillation cannot be "mapped"). This is because the reference and WOI are set before acquisition of the first point. The reference cannot be changed prospectively in most systems; however, the WOI can. Because the reference and WOI are determined for a specific rhythm, this must be monitored closely during the procedure. Certain rhythm changes will have no impact because they occur outside the WOI and are not included in the map. A catheter-induced premature ventricular contraction (PVC) will fall into the set WOI, and if not noticed, collected points during the PVC will affect the appearance of the map, which can often skew the appearance of substrate maps. Therefore care must be taken when mapping to ensure points are collected only during the appropriate rhythm.

There are, however, automated algorithms, used by all three major mapping systems, to ensure point collection occurs in a prespecified rhythm only to aid the operators. These are typically a set of operator-specific collection filters. The **CONFIDENSE** module of CARTO allows the user to set point collection criteria such as matching reference morphology, beat-to-beat cycle length, and LAT of the reference and an impedance-based tissue proximity indication to ensure contact. These filters are selected before mapping but can be changed throughout and, while catheters are navigated in the heart, displayed as a traffic light system to the operator indicating when criteria are met or not to allow or block point collection.[14]

Finally, all major systems are moving to develop methods for simultaneously mapping more than one rhythm.

Annotation

Either bipolar or unipolar electrograms can be annotated for activation time and amplitude. Amplitude is typically easier to annotate because it is a maximal or minimal measurement. Activation time is typically automatically annotated to the maximal dv/dt. That is the component of the electrogram deflection where maximal amplitude and maximal change in activation time occur—or the maximal negative unipolar derivative—and is considered to reflect peak depolarization of tissue underlying the recording electrode. However, in cases where there is a pronounced far-field electrogram component, such as near atrioventricular valve annuli or where electrograms are fractionated, split, or very delayed, determination of the dv/dt can be erroneous. Annotation of activation to maximal or minimal deflections is equally challenging. Certain automatic systems exist to overcome this issue. *EnSite Precision* has developed an algorithm that annotates the latest deflection of an electrogram. *CARTO 3 (HD COLOURING)* automatically calculates the time between electrogram annotations and displays them as a white area, indicating a line of block. Conversely, signals separated by a wide range of LAT have red area between them to signify an early-meets-late area (Fig. 7.6).[15] Regardless, operators have to assess annotation of points during the case to ensure accurate, and interpretable, maps.

Rhythmia (Lumipoint algorithm) analyzes the complete electrogram tracing to determine activity at each location and therefore includes nearfield signals in its analysis. A window of interest may be used to highlight regions of the map that activate within a certain time within the cycle. This allows maps to be automatically reannotated within specific windows of interest to identify late and/or fractionated potentials, as well as the putative isthmuses of re-entrant circuits.

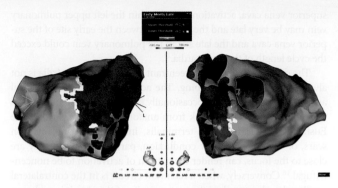

FIG. 7.6. The same tachycardia from Fig. 7.4 is displayed with the additional early and extended early meets late function on CARTO 3 v6. *White lines* indicate areas of conduction block and *red lines* areas of true early-meets-late site in the reentry circuit. The thresholds reflect the percent difference in local activation time (LAT) within the window of interest, between two points, to be marked accordingly.

FOCAL VERSUS MACROREENTRANT TACHYCARDIAS

In focal tachycardias the cycle length of the tachycardia is longer than the time required for activation of the chamber of origin. An activation sequence map of the chamber shows activation during only a portion of the tachycardia cycle length, typically less than 50%.[16,17] With macroreentrant tachycardias, some part of the chambers is electrically activated at any given time during the cardiac cycle. A complete and carefully performed activation map accounts for the entire tachycardia cycle length.[16] Thus, the 3D electroanatomic maps look very different with focal and macroreentrant atrial tachycardias and VTs. With a focal tachycardia, an early point of activation with centrifugal uniform spread from that site is expected, whereas with reentry the circuit should be visualized, and the mapped cycle length is very close or equal to the cycle length of the tachycardia. However, in very diseased hearts, there may be bystander regions of very late activation that actually activate simultaneously with the next beat of tachycardia at the site of the reentrant circuit. The difference between one electrogram within the circuit and another bystander site activating very late may exceed the cycle length of the tachycardia. This finding may occasionally occur in automatic tachycardias also. When both atria are being mapped and the origin of tachycardia is in the myocardial extensions within the superior vena cava, activation points within the left upper pulmonary vein may be very late and the interval between the early site of the superior vena cava and the late site in the pulmonary vein could exceed the cycle length of the tachycardia.[16]

The distinction between a reentrant and a focal tachycardia is not always clear from 3D mapping. The activation sequence of a focal automatic tachycardia can occasionally be confusing and interpreted as reentry. Conduction block from anatomic obstacles, such as the Eustachian ridge or crista terminalis, intrinsic scarring, incision scars, or regions with slow conduction, particularly when they are close to the focus, can render the pattern of activation to be noncentrifugal.[16] Conversely, when a reentrant circuit is in the contralateral cardiac chamber or when the vast majority of the circuit is midmyocardial or epicardial, a point source emanation appears, mistakenly leading to the diagnosis of automatic tachycardia.[16] When the mapping process reveals a focal pattern, one should appreciate the individual timing of the earliest mapped electrogram compared with the surface deflection (P wave/R wave, depending on the chamber of interest), and if no distinct early potentials are noticed and a wide area of similarly prematurity is present, an origin in a neighboring structure or on the epicardial surface should be considered.

3D ELECTROANATOMIC MAPPING AND IMAGE REGISTRATION

Electroanatomic mapping systems may be capable of merging computed tomographic (CT)/cardiac magnetic resonance (CMR) imaging volume data sets with acquired electroanatomic maps and simultaneously displaying them within the same coordinate system.[18,19] Registration of preacquired CT and CMR images can be imprecise.[20] The main limitation is that imaging typically is performed at least 1 day before the ablation procedure and the cardiac chambers, being in constant motion, may not align accurately with the intraprocedural 3D map created with the mapping system. Nevertheless, this technology can be particularly useful when performing PVC ablation with a LV origin, particularly if near the LV summit, because coronary anatomy often lies in close proximity of the PVC exit and potential ablation site. The 3D maps can also be merged with fluoroscopic images, a function that is used to facilitate AF and PVC ablation.

An intracardiac ultrasound catheter can be used with the mapping system to further define cardiac geometry within the mapping field, and image volumes from the ultrasound system appear more accurate than those of merged CT/CMR images.[21,22] Coregistration of electroanatomic mapping and ECG imaging that allows noninvasive reconstruction of epicardial unipolar electrograms using heart–torso geometry and body surface potentials is also under study, especially for unstable VTs.[23] Other imaging features of 3D electroanatomic mapping include an ability to visualize selected sheaths (as well as catheters) and to begin mapping from the groin. In certain patient populations, therefore, particularly pediatric, complete avoidance of fluoroscopy with the aid of 3D EAM systems may become clinically routine.

BEYOND ACTIVATION AND VOLTAGE MAPPING

In recent years, 3D EAM systems have included novel mapping methods separate from voltage and activation mapping. On the CARTO3 platform, **Ripple Mapping** is annotation-independent approach to mapping that eliminates the need for a window of interest. Collected electrograms are portrayed as bars on the cardiac anatomy, allowing for visualization of the entire electrogram (Fig. 7.7). When the map is played, the bars appear in EGM sequence, relative to a reference, and an unlimited time of activation, or number of beats, can be viewed in this way. Ripple mapping has been shown to improve outcomes for atrial tachycardia, compared with LAT mapping, in a randomized clinical trial.[24] A similar tool exists on the EnSite Precision system but is still dependent on annotation and the WOI.

Coherence is a new feature on the CARTO 3 v7 system that displays an activation map integrated with a conduction vector map.[25] Clinical evaluation is still pending on this new technology.

New mapping systems are also being developed. Notably, the **Acutus Mapping** system proposes mapping of electrical dipoles, or charge density (coulombs/cm), between areas, calculated from the amplitude of unipolar potentials, instead of typical bipolar electrograms, from the cardiac chambers. This is achieved by noncontact mapping (via a basket-type catheter) of the chamber of interest. The anatomy and localization are performed by use of ultrasound emitted from crystals on the basket catheter.[26] The Acutus system is being assessed in atrial tachycardia and atrial fibrillation patients.

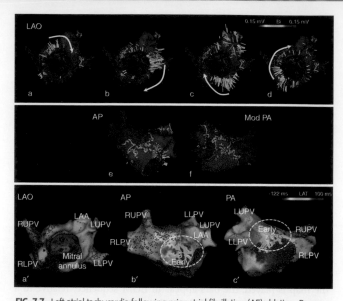

FIG. 7.7. Left atrial tachycardia following prior atrial fibrillation (AF) ablation. Because of the presence of two "early" sites on the local activation time map, the propagation pattern was difficult to interpret. No Ripple bars were seen at less than 0.15 mV; tissue less than this threshold was displayed in red and greater than this threshold in purple. The left atrium is seen in LAO with the mitral valve en face. (A) to (D) A Ripple wave front rotated clockwise around the mitral annulus. A line of ablation between the mitral annulus and left lower pulmonary vein terminated atrial tachycardia.

AP, Anteroposterior; *LAA,* Left atrial appendage; *LAO,* Left anterior oblique; *LLPV,* Left lower pulmonary vein; *LUPV,* Left upper pulmonary vein; *Mod PA,* Modified posteroanterior view; *PA,* Posteroanterior view; *RLPV,* Right lower pulmonary vein; *RUPV,* Right upper pulmonary vein. (Katritsis G, Luther V, Kanagaratnam P, et al. Arrhythmia mechanisms revealed by ripple mapping. *Arrhythm Electrophysiol Rev.* 2018;7(4):261-264.)

MAGNETIC GUIDANCE SYSTEMS

Mapping by manual catheter manipulation requires skill, and outcomes can be heavily dependent on operator experience. Remote or robotic catheter navigation are aimed at eliminating the need for manual catheter manipulation, achieving precise catheter movement and improved catheter stability independent from the operator's manual catheter manipulation skill. Several technologies have been developed to achieve these goals. The Niobe Stereotaxis magnetic navigation system remotely controls the tip of a proprietary ablation catheter using changes in magnetic field direction from large rotating earth magnets (see Fig. 7.6).[27] This system can be combined with robotic catheter manipulation components (Vdrive system) to control various diagnostic catheters remotely as well. Other systems also exist. Published studies suggest that magnetic navigation is a viable alternative to manual catheter navigation.[28-32] There is no evidence that outcomes of ablation are improved by use of a magnetic navigation system.

References

1. Ben-Haim SA, Osadchy D, Schuster I, Gepstein L, Hayam G, Josephson MA. Nonfluoroscopic, In vivo navigation and mapping technology. *Nat Med.* 1996;2(12):1393-1395.

2. Jais P, Shah DC, Haissaguerre M, et al. Mapping and ablation of left atrial flutters. *Circulation.* 2000;101(25):2928-2934.

3. Josephson Me, Anter E. Substrate mapping for ventricular tachycardia: assumptions and misconceptions. *Jacc Clin Electrophysiol.* 2015;1(5):341-352.

4. Sporton SC, Earley MJ, Nathan AW, Schilling RJ. Electroanatomic versus fluoroscopic mapping for catheter ablation procedures: a prospective randomized study. *J Cardiovasc Electrophysiol.* 2004;15(3):310-315.

5. De Ponti R, Salerno-Uriarte JA. Non-fluoroscopic mapping systems for electrophysiology: the 'tool or toy' dilemma after 10 years. *Eur Heart J.* 2006;27(10):1134-1136.

6. Schaeffer B, Hoffmann BA, Meyer C, et al. Characterization, mapping, and ablation of complex atrial tachycardia: initial experience with a novel method of ultra high-density 3D mapping. *J Cardiovasc Electrophysiol.* 2016;27(10):1139-1150.

7. Gepstein L, Hayam G, Ben-Haim SA. A novel method for nonfluoroscopic catheter-based electroanatomical mapping of the heart. in vitro and in vivo accuracy results. *Circulation.* 1997;95(6):1611-1622.

8. Cronin EM, Bogun FM, Maury P, et al. 2019 HRS/EHRA/APHRS/LAHRS Expert Consensus statement on catheter ablation of ventricular arrhythmias. *Heart Rhythm.* 2019.

9. Koutalas E, Rolf S, Dinov B, et al. Contemporary mapping techniques of complex cardiac arrhythmias—identifying and modifying the arrhythmogenic substrate. *Arrhythm Electrophysiol Rev.* 2015;4(1):19-27.

10. Bourier F, Fahrig R, Wang P, et al. Accuracy assessment of catheter guidance technology in electrophysiology procedures: a comparison of a new 3D-based fluoroscopy navigation system to current electroanatomic mapping systems. *J Cardiovasc Electrophysiol.* 2014;25(1):74-83.

11. Del Carpio Munoz F, Buescher TL, Asirvatham SJ. Three-dimensional mapping of cardiac arrhythmias: what do the colors really mean? *Circ Arrhythm Electrophysiol.* 2010;3(6):E6-11.

12. De Ponti R, Verlato R, Bertaglia E, et al. Treatment of macro-re-entrant atrial tachycardia based on electroanatomic mapping: identification and ablation of the mid-diastolic isthmus. *Europace.* 2007;9(7):449-457.

13. Selvaraj RJ, Shankar B, Subramanian A, Nair K. Chasing red herrings: making sense of the colors while mapping. *Circ Arrhythm Electrophysiol.* 2014;7(3):553-556.

14. Liang JJ, Elafros MA, Muser D, et al. Comparison of left atrial bipolar voltage and scar using multielectrode fast automated mapping versus point-by-point contact electroanatomic mapping in patients with atrial fibrillation undergoing repeat ablation. *J Cardiovasc Electrophysiol.* 2017;28(3):280-288.

15. Iden L, Weinert R, Groschke S, Kuhnhardt K, Richardt G, Borlich M. First experience and validation of the extended early meets late (EEML) tool as part of the novel carto software hd coloring. *J Interv Card Electrophysiol.* 2020.

16. Del Carpio Munoz F, Buescher TL, Asirvatham SJ. Teaching points with 3-dimensional mapping of cardiac arrhythmia: mechanism of arrhythmia and accounting for the cycle length. *Circ Arrhythm Electrophysiol.* 2011;4(1):E1-3.

17. Liuba I, Walfridsson H. Activation mapping of focal atrial tachycardia: the impact of the method for estimating activation time. *J Interv Card Electrophysiol.* 2009;26(3):169-180.

18. Dong J, Dickfeld T, Dalal D, et al. Initial experience in the use of integrated electroanatomic mapping with three-dimensional mr/ct images to guide catheter ablation of atrial fibrillation. *J Cardiovasc Electrophysiol.* 2006;17(5):459-466.

19. Dong J, Calkins H, Solomon SB, et al. Integrated electroanatomic mapping with three-dimensional computed tomographic images for real-time guided ablations. *Circulation.* 2006;113(2):186-194.

20. Zhong H, Lacomis Jm, Schwartzman D. On the accuracy of cartomerge for guiding posterior left atrial ablation in man. *Heart Rhythm.* 2007;4(5):595-602.

21. Okumura Y, Henz BD, Johnson Sb, et al. Three-dimensional ultrasound for image-guided mapping and intervention: methods, quantitative validation, and clinical feasibility of a novel multimodality image mapping system. *Circ Arrhythm Electrophysiol.* 2008;1(2):110-119.

22. Khaykin Y, Skanes A, Whaley B, et al. Real-time integration of 2d intracardiac echocardiography and 3d electroanatomical mapping to guide ventricular tachycardia ablation. *Heart Rhythm.* 2008;5(10):1396-1402.

23. Graham AJ, Orini M, Zacur E, et al. Evaluation of ecg imaging to map hemodynamically stable and unstable ventricular arrhythmias. *Circ Arrhythm Electrophysiol.* 2020;13(2):E007377.

24. Luther V, Agarwal S, Chow A, et al. Ripple-at study. *Circ Arrhythm Electrophysiol.* 2019;12(8):E007394.

25. Anter E, Duytschaever M, Shen C, et al. Activation mapping with integration of vector and velocity information improves the ability to identify the mechanism and location of complex scar-related atrial tachycardias. *Circ Arrhythm Electrophysiol.* 2018;11(8):E006536.

26. Grace A, Willems S, Meyer C, et al. High-Resolution noncontact charge-density mapping of endocardial activation. *Jci Insight.* 2019;4(6).

27. Faddis MN, Blume W, Finney J, et al. Novel, Magnetically guided catheter for endocardial mapping and radiofrequency catheter ablation. *Circulation.* 2002;106(23):2980-2985.

28. Akca F, Theuns DA, Abkenari LD, De Groot NM, Jordaens L, Szili-Torok T. Outcomes Of repeat catheter ablation using magnetic navigation or conventional ablation. *Europace.* 2013;15(10):1426-1431.

29. Shauer A, De Vries Lj, Akca F, et al. Clinical Research: remote magnetic navigation vs. manually controlled catheter ablation of right ventricular outflow tract arrhythmias: a retrospective study. *Europace.* 2018;20(Suppl_2):Ii28-Ii32.

30. Skoda J, Arya A, Garcia F, et al. Catheter ablation of ischemic ventricular tachy-cardia with remote magnetic navigation: stop-vt multicenter trial. *J Cardiovasc Electrophysiol.* 2016;27 Suppl 1:S29-37.

31. Kawamura M, Scheinman MM, Tseng ZH, Lee BK, Marcus GM, Badhwar N. Comparison of remote magnetic navigation ablation and manual ablation of idiopathic ventricular arrhythmia after failed manual ablation. *J Interv Card Electrophysiol.* 2017;48(1):35-42.

32. Qian P, De Silva K, Kumar S, et al. Early and long-term outcomes after manual and remote magnetic navigation-guided catheter ablation for ventricular tachy-cardia. *Europace.* 2018;20(Suppl_2):Ii11-Ii21.

8

Physics of Ablation

RADIOFREQUENCY ABLATION

Radiofrequency (RF) ablation induces tissue necrosis by heating the targeted tissue. Most cardiac ablation systems deliver RF energy between a unipolar platinum-iridium electrode at the tip of the ablation catheter and a large dispersive grounding patch on the patient's skin, typically on the abdomen or thigh (Fig. 8.1). Ablation catheters also have electrodes to record electrical activity from within the heart (Fig. 8.2). When the catheter is placed at the target site, alternating current (AC) in the RF range (500 to 1000 kHz) is applied to the tip electrode. As RF current passes from the tip of the ablation catheter to the grounding patch, resistive heating occurs in the intervening tissue at a rate proportional to the square of current density.[1] Current density is highest in the immediate vicinity of the ablation catheter tip, which has a small surface area. As a result, significant resistive heating occurs only at the catheter tip–tissue interface and in a small volume of surrounding tissue. Deeper lesions result from conductive heating of myocardium adjacent to the site of resistive heating.[1] Application of electric current of any frequency will result in tissue heating; however, higher frequencies (in the MHz range) are transmitted to tissues distant from the electrode, and heat dissipation can occur over a much larger tissue mass, whereas lower frequencies can lead to stimulation of cardiac muscle and nerves, resulting in arrhythmias and pain.[1]

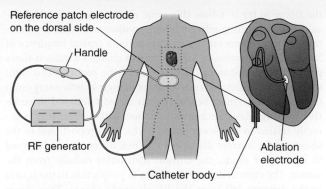

FIG. 8.1. Schematics of cardiac radiofrequency (RF) ablation system. A cardiac RF catheter is inserted and steered to the target site inside the heart and a ground pad is placed on the patient's back.
(Panescu D, Whayne JG, Fleischman SD, et al. Three-dimensional finite element analysis of current density and temperature distributions during radio-frequency ablation. *IEEE Trans Biomed Eng.* 1995;42:879-890.)

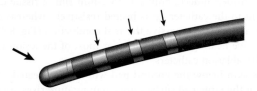

FIG. 8.2. Cardiac radiofrequency (RF) ablation catheter (7F = 2.3 mm diameter). The RF electrode at the tip (*large arrow*, 4 mm length) creates the ablation zone, and the mapping electrodes *(small arrows)* record electrical activity from within the heart.

Heat Generation in Tissue

The electrode at the tip of the catheter is not insulated, and electric energy can travel into the targeted tissue surrounding the probe. Because the electrical energy is delivered in the form of alternating current, the electric field created within the tissue periodically reverses direction (Fig. 8.3). This causes the ions in the tissue to try to follow this same alternating path, which results in ions drifting relative to one another and relative to neutral particles. These rapid movements (for a typical frequency of 500 kHz the direction of ion movement changes a million times per second) result in collisions between the particles that limit their drift velocities and convert some of their kinetic energy into thermal energy. This phenomenon is called **frictional** or **resistive heating.** Resistive heat production within the tissue is directly related to RF power density, which is proportional to the square of the current density (I^2). When RF energy is delivered in a unipolar mode, the current distributes radially from the source. The current density decreases in proportion to the square of the distance (r^2) from the RF electrode source. Thus direct resistive heating of the tissue decreases in relation with the distance from the electrode to the fourth power.[1,2] Hence, doubling the distance from the catheter tip reduces resistive heating by 94%. Because of the rapid reduction in heating with distance, lesions created by RF energy are typically small and well circumscribed.[1] Deeper tissue heating occurs solely as a result of heat conduction from the narrow radius of volume heating around the electrode.[2] Indeed, only a 1- to 2-mm rim of tissue directly adjacent to the catheter tip is heated resistively, whereas deeper tissues are heated by passive thermal conduction (Fig. 8.4). This conductive heating is responsible for most of the lesion volume from RF ablation catheters.

The skin below the ground pad will also be heated, but because of the large pad surface area, temperature rises are low. A single application lasts typically 45 to 120 seconds and produces an ablation lesion 5 to 10 mm in diameter. The operator can control the size of the lesion by varying the time period and intensity of application, contact force, and the size of the ablation electrode. Generally there are three methods to control applied intensity[1]: (1) **power control,** in which electrical voltage applied to the RF electrode is adjusted to keep applied RF power constant; (2) **temperature control,** in which one or more thermal sensors (either thermocouples or thermistors) are integrated in the RF electrode, typically near the tip, and the applied RF power is adjusted to keep the measured temperature at a defined target value; and (3) **impedance control,** in which RF power is adjusted depending on tissue impedance, which is measured between the RF electrode and the ground pad. Most ablation catheters employ temperature control, where temperature measured within the electrode tip is used to adjust applied RF power. The location of maximum tissue temperature is a few mm from the catheter tip and is affected by local intracardiac blood flow, which considerably affects tissue heating and resulting size of the ablation zone. In general, larger ablation zones are possible at locations with high flow rate because of increased convective cooling.[3-5] A major consideration for RF ablation is that catheter tip temperature can differ substantially from underlying tissue temperature because of the complex relationship between RF heating of adjacent tissue and convective cooling from intracavitary blood flow. This can result in a measured catheter tip temperature that is significantly lower than true tissue temperature, especially with larger-tipped catheters, which are exposed to more convective cooling because of their larger surface area. In fact, tissue temperatures can exceed 100°C, even while a much lower temperature is recorded from the catheter tip. This can boil fluid within the tissue, resulting in an explosive steam pop, damage to adjacent structures, crater formation, cardiac perforation, and tamponade. Catheters of different lengths and diameters are commercially available depending on desired size of the ablation zone. Newer catheter designs employ internal cooling to increase ablation zone size.

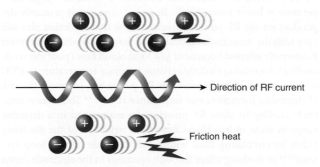

FIG. 8.3. Alternating radiofrequency current is supplied to the tissue through the tip of the catheter, and the resulting ion agitation causes ion friction, which in turn causes heat production (frictional heating).

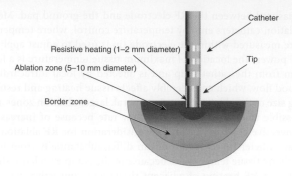

FIG. 8.4. Transfer of thermal energy during radiofrequency ablation.

Irrigation

When catheter ablation is performed under temperature control, RF power is regulated to maintain a constant electrode–tissue interface temperature (commonly 55°C or 60°C).[6] The ablation electrode–tissue interface temperature is dependent on the opposing effects of heating from the tissue and cooling by the blood flowing around the electrode.[7-9] At any given electrode–tissue interface temperature, the RF power delivered to the tissue is significantly reduced in areas of low blood flow.[8] The reduced cooling associated with low blood flow causes the electrode to reach the target temperature at lower power levels. Because lesion size is primarily dependent on the RF power delivered to the tissue,[10] lesion size will vary with the magnitude of local blood flow. Areas where lesion size is adversely affected because of low local blood flow (poor electrode cooling), increasing electrode–tissue interface temperature to 65°C or 70°C only minimally increases RF power and increases the risk of thrombus formation and impedance rise.[8,11,12] To increase electrode cooling to allow RF power to be maintained in a desirable range in areas of low blood flow, fluid irrigation of the electrode either by circulating fluid within the electrode (closed loop system)[13,14] or flushing saline through openings in the electrode (open irrigation system)[7,15] is used (Fig. 8.5). The "active electrode cooling" by irrigation allows sustained RF power, even at sites with low blood flow, to produce deeper lesions.[6]

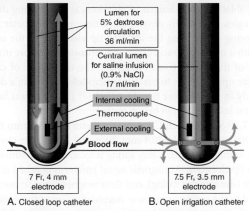

FIG. 8.5. Schematic representation of the irrigated electrode catheters. (A) Closed-loop irrigation 7F catheter, 4-mm tip electrode with an internal thermocouple. A dextrose solution at room temperature circulates continuously through the tip electrode, cooling the ablation electrode internally. (B) Open irrigation 7.5F catheter, 3.5-mm tip electrode with an internal thermocouple and six irrigation holes located around the electrode. Heparinized normal saline at room temperature irrigates through the electrode and six irrigation holes during each radiofrequency application, providing internal and external electrode cooling.
(Yokoyama K, Nakagawa H, Wittkampf FH, et al. Comparison of electrode cooling between internal and open irrigation in radiofrequency ablation lesion depth and incidence of thrombus and steam pop. *Circulation.* 2006;113:11-19.)

Electrode–Tissue Contact Force

Lesion generation in cardiac RF catheter ablation is dependent on the interaction between electrode and contacting tissue. The contact force (CF) between the catheter tip and the target tissue is a key factor to safe and effective lesion formation.[16,17] Insufficient CF may result in an ineffective lesion, whereas excessive CF may result in complications such as heart wall perforation, steam pop, thrombus formation, or esophageal injury.[18] Despite its importance, CF cannot be measured directly with available ablation catheters; thus other measures have been used as surrogates for CF, including the pattern of motion of the catheter tip under fluoroscopy, the amplitude of the unipolar and bipolar potentials, and impedance.[19] To measure catheter–tissue CF in real time during catheter mapping and RF ablation, two designs of ablation catheters using different technologies have been developed. One type of catheter uses a small spring connecting the ablation tip electrode to the catheter shaft with a magnetic transmitter and sensors to measure microdeflection of the spring (SmartTouch).[20] The other type of catheter uses three optical fibers to measure microdeformation of a deformable body in the catheter tip (TactiCath).[16] Both systems have CF resolution less than 1 g in bench testing.[16,21]

The 7.5F **SmartTouch CF** sensing catheter has a 3.5-mm tip electrode with six small holes (0.4 mm diameter) around the circumference for saline irrigation. A tiny spring is located just proximal to the ablation tip electrode. A magnetic signal emitter is attached to the tip electrode (distal to the spring), and three magnetic sensors are located proximal to the spring to measure microdeflection of the spring. The microdeflection is computed to the magnitude and angle of CF every 25.6 ms (Fig. 8.6).[20] CF is displayed both continuously and as the average value (over 1 second) on an electroanatomic mapping system. This catheter also has a magnetic location sensor for conventional electroanatomic mapping. CF catheters have resulted in improved long-term outcomes compared with traditional non-CF catheters.[22,23]

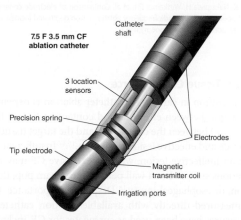

7.5 F 3.5 mm CF ablation catheter

Catheter shaft

3 location sensors

Precision spring

Tip electrode

Electrodes

Magnetic transmitter coil

Irrigation ports

FIG. 8.6. SmartTouch. A small spring coil connects the tip electrode to the catheter shaft. A magnetic signal emitter is located distal to the spring. Three magnetic location sensors, positioned just proximal to the spring, measure the microdeflection of the spring to compute the force (magnitude and angle) on the tip electrode.

The 7.5F **TactiCath** force sensor consists of a deformable body (elastic polymer) and three optical fibers (diameter of 0.125 mm) to measure microdeformations that correlate with force applied to the catheter tip (Fig. 8.7).[16] Infrared laser light (wave lengths 1520 to 1570 nm) is emitted through the proximal end of the three optical fibers. The light is reflected by fiber Bragg gratings on the deformable body at the distal end of the optical fibers, near the tip of the catheter. Applying CF to the tip of the catheter produces a microdeformation of the deformable body, causing the fiber Bragg gratings to either stretch or compress, which changes the wavelength of the reflected light. The change of wavelength is proportional to the CF applied to the tip. By monitoring the wavelength of the reflected light in the three fibers, the system is able to calculate and display the vector of the CF (magnitude and angle) at time intervals of 100 ms.

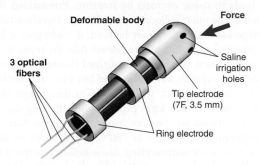

FIG. 8.7. TactiCath. The force sensor includes three optical fibers attached to a deformable body. Force on the deformable body changes the periodicity of the fiber Bragg gratings' refractive index pattern, which changes the reflected wavelength of light in the three optical fibers. The consequent change in the reflected wavelength is proportional to the contract force applied to the tip.

Microelectrodes

The **Qdot,** (THERMOCOOL SMARTTOUCH SF-5D) Catheter incorporates 3 microelectrodes, each with a surface area of 0.167 mm^2 embedded at the distal circumference of a standard 3.5-mm open-irrigated catheter.[24] In addition to recording from smaller tissue size, the microelectrodes record data at multiple angles relative to the vector of propagation (from parallel to perpendicular), which increases the ability to detect surviving myocardial bundles. Intial clinical experience has been promising.[25,26]

CRYOABLATION

Cryothermal ablation freezes tissue in a discrete and focused fashion to destroy cells in a precisely targeted area.[27] Cryoballoon ablation is widely used for pulmonary vein (PV) isolation in patients with persistent or paroxysmal AF.[28] Cryothermal ablation is based on the expansion of a cryorefrigerant (nitrous oxide, N_2O) into a double-lumen balloon in a single-step mode, which leads to tissue necrosis by freezing. Pressurized N_2O is delivered to the inner balloon via an ultrafine injection tube. As the refrigerant enters the inner balloon, it undergoes a liquid-to-gas phase change. Just before release into the inner balloon, the cryorefrigerant is further pressurized through a restriction tube and then expands into a region of low pressure. Because of the Joule-Thomson effect, which refers to the change in temperature observed when a gas expands while flowing through a restriction without any heat exchange, the temperature of the cryorefrigerant drops as low as –80°C. The cryorefrigerant absorbs heat from the surrounding tissue before returning to the console through a lumen maintained under vacuum. Cryoablation has been incorporated into a balloon-based catheter for efficient PV isolation.

The **Arctic Front** cryoballoon system has been commercially available since 2010. The cryoballoon catheter (Fig. 8.8) contains (1) an inner and outer balloon, (2) a central lumen for a guidewire for positioning and support, (3) a central tube for contrast injection to ensure adequate positioning and PV occlusion, (4) a thermocouple at the proximal end of the balloon to monitor inner balloon temperature, (5) a dual pull-wire mechanism that facilitates catheter deflection, and (6) a small-diameter circular diagnostic catheter for monitoring of pulmonary vein potentials. In addition, the catheter contains several redundant safety systems. For example, a constant vacuum is applied between the inner and outer balloon to ensure the absence of cryorcfrigerant leakage into the systemic circulation in the event of a breach in the integrity of the inner balloon. During ablation, circumferential lesions are created with two to three applications of coolant for 240 to 360 seconds each. The second-generation cryoballoon incorporated several technical improvements, including eight injection tubes, compared with four in the first-generation cryoballoon, and a more distal location of the injection ports on the catheter shaft (Fig. 8.9). These modifications enable a larger and more uniform freezing zone covering the entire northern hemisphere of the balloon.[29] From a practical perspective, this cooling feature facilitates the procedure by enabling contact of the ice cap with the PV antrum, even if the catheter balloon shaft is not parallel to the targeted vein. In addition, it enhances proper contact of the ice cap even if the PV antrum has an uncommon shape. A third-generation cryoballoon has been with a 40% shorter catheter tip. This feature provides improved maneuverability and allows a more proximal retraction of the circular catheter during ablation and thus a higher rate of real-time PV recordings.[30] The **POLARx** is another similar cryoballoon.

Cryoablation has been also used with ablation catheters such as the steerable 9F **Freezor** for the treatment of supraventricular tachycardia,[31] atrioventricular (AV) nodal reentrant tachycardia,[32] and ablation of the AV node.[33]

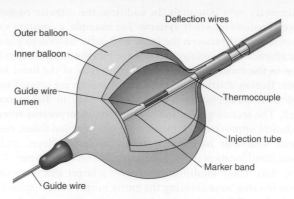

FIG. 8.8. Components of the cryoballoon catheter: A pressurized cryorefrigerant (N_2O) expands at a region of low pressure, which cools the inner balloon at temperatures as low as −80° C, which in turn cools the outer balloon at temperatures of −40°C to −50°C.
(Andrade JG, Dubuc M, Guerra PG, et al. The biophysics and biomechanics of cryoballoon ablation. *Pacing Clin Electrophysiol.* 2012;35:1162-1168.)

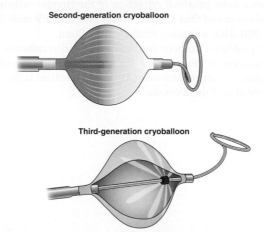

Second-generation cryoballoon

Third-generation cryoballoon

FIG. 8.9. The second generation has eight injection ports, more distal location of injection tubes and broader and homogeneous freezing zone (northern balloon hemisphere). The third generation has similar features to the second generation and 40% shorter catheter tip, which provides improved maneuverability and a higher rate of real-time electrogram recordings by the diagnostic catheter.

LASER ABLATION

Light amplification by stimulated emission of radiation (laser) is a device that generates a beam of light of a single wavelength that is highly collimated and coherent, which means that all waves are in phase with one another in both time and space. When laser light interacts with matter, it is absorbed and converted into heat, which can be used to ablate and create scar tissue. When using laser energy for lesion formation, the laser ablation catheter does not need to exert pressure on the tissue and contact force is not a factor in whether a laser lesion is transmural.[34] In addition, laser energy can be adjusted when ablating tissues of varying thickness, with higher energy applied to thicker tissue and lower energy applied to thinner structures in the heart.[35] Clinically, laser light is applied via an open-irrigated electrode laser mapping and ablation (**ELMA**) catheter.[36] The laser used is the Nd:YAG with a continuous wavelength of 1064 nm, which can produce deep lesions; however, for safe laser application without collateral damages to adjacent structures of the heart, energy settings adapted to the thickness of the myocardial wall are applied.[35]

A novel ablation technology being evaluated for PV isolation is endoscopic laser ablation (**EAS**).[37] The EAS system features a 980-nm diode laser and a multilumen catheter with a compliant, inflatable balloon at the tip (Fig. 8.10). Before ablation the deflated balloon is advanced into the left atrium, inflated with radiopaque deuterium oxide, and wedged against the ostium of a PV. An endoscope is introduced into the left atrium and live images are used to guide ablation. The infrared laser can be aimed radially or at variable angles toward the catheter tip to create point-by-point circumferential lesions with a green "aiming beam." The energy does not react with the deuterium in the balloon but causes heating of water molecules and coagulation necrosis of atrial tissue.[19] A second-generation laser balloon has been introduced to optimize tissue contact and visibility.[38]

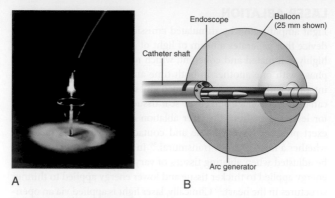

FIG. 8.10. Visually guided ablation catheter. Shown are the ablation catheter with the projected green arc of the aiming beam (A) and a schematic showing the location of the endoscope at the proximal end of the balloon (B).

(Reddy VY, Neuzil P, Themistoclakis S, et al. Visually-guided balloon catheter ablation of atrial fibrillation: experimental feasibility and first-in-human multicenter clinical outcome. *Circulation.* 2009;120:12-20.)

PULSED FIELD ABLATION

Electroporation is another modality for catheter ablation. It uses pulsed field ablation, a nonthermal ablative modality in which ultrarapid (<1 second) electrical fields are applied to target tissue.[39] This destabilizes cell membranes by forming irreversible nanoscale pores and leakage of cell contents, culminating in cell death. It can be performed without general anesthesia, reduces the risk of damaging adjacent structures, and in clinical practice on patients with AF has been shown to result in durable PV isolation (Fig. 8.11).[40] The advantages of this approach for AF ablation are that, theoretically at least, it avoids damage of the esophagus and phrenic nerve that are at danger during RF and cryoablation of the PVs.

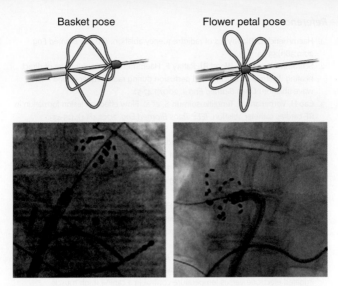

FIG. 8.11. The Pulsed Field Ablation catheter is shown over a guidewire with its splines in either the basket deployment pose *(left)* or the flower petal deployment pose *(right)*. *(Bottom)* The fluoroscopic images show the catheter in either of these poses, situated at the ostium of the left superior pulmonary vein (PV, *left*) and the right inferior PV *(right)*.

(Reddy VY, Neuzil P, Koruth JS, et al. Pulsed field ablation for pulmonary vein isolation in atrial fibrillation. *J Am Coll Cardiol.* 2019;74(3):315-326.)

ETHANOL ABLATION

Transarterial coronary ethanol ablation has also been a treatment option for drug- and RF-refractory arrhythmias. Retrograde coronary venous ethanol ablation has been used as an alternative to transarterial ablation to avoid pitfalls of arterial cannulation and perfusion. The technique is promising, especially from arrhythmias arising in the LV summit.[41,42]

STEREOTACTIC CARDIAC RADIOABLATION

Stereotactic cardiac radiotherapy is a new option for ablation of arrhythmias such as ventricular tachycardia where traditional ablation offers limited success. Noninvasive electrophysiology-guided cardiac radioablation has been reported, and the preliminary results are promising (ENCORE-VT trial).[43]

References

1. Haemmerich D. Biophysics of radiofrequency ablation. *Crit Rev Biomed Eng.* 2010;38(1):53-63.

2. Schramm W, Yang D, Wood BJ, Rattay F, Haemmerich D. Contribution of direct heating, thermal conduction and perfusion during radiofrequency and microwave ablation. *Open Biomed Eng J.* 2007;1:47-52.

3. Cao H, Vorperian VR, Tungjitkusolmun S, et al. Flow effect on lesion formation in RF cardiac catheter ablation. *IEEE Trans Biomed Eng.* 2001;48(4):425-433.

4. Hogh Petersen H, Chen X, Pietersen A, Svendsen JH, Haunso S. Lesion dimensions during temperature-controlled radiofrequency catheter ablation of left ventricular porcine myocardium: impact of ablation site, electrode size, and convective cooling. *Circulation.* 1999;99(2):319-325.

5. Burkhardt JD, Natale A. New technologies in atrial fibrillation ablation. *Circulation.* 2009;120(15):1533-1541.

6. Yokoyama K, Nakagawa H, Wittkampf FH, Pitha JV, Lazzara R, Jackman WM. Comparison of electrode cooling between internal and open irrigation in radiofrequency ablation lesion depth and incidence of thrombus and steam pop. *Circulation.* 2006;113(1):11-19.

7. Nakagawa H, Yamanashi WS, Pitha JV, et al. Comparison of in vivo tissue temperature profile and lesion geometry for radiofrequency ablation with a saline-irrigated electrode versus temperature control in a canine thigh muscle preparation. *Circulation.* 1995;91(8):2264-2273.

8. Matsudaira K, Nakagawa H, Wittkampf FH, et al. High incidence of thrombus formation without impedance rise during radiofrequency ablation using electrode temperature control. *Pacing Clin Electrophysiol.* 2003;26(5):1227-1237.

9. Kongsgaard E, Steen T, Jensen O, Aass H, Amlie JP. Temperature guided radiofrequency catheter ablation of myocardium: comparison of catheter tip and tissue temperatures in vitro. *Pacing Clin Electrophysiol.* 1997;20(5 Pt 1):1252-1260.

10. Wittkampf FH, Hauer RN, Robles de Medina EO. Control of radiofrequency lesion size by power regulation. *Circulation.* 1989;80(4):962-968.

11. Jais P, Shah DC, Haissaguerre M, et al. Efficacy and safety of septal and left-atrial linear ablation for atrial fibrillation. *Am J Cardiol.* 1999;84(9A):139R-146R.

12. Zhou L, Keane D, Reed G, Ruskin J. Thromboembolic complications of cardiac radiofrequency catheter ablation: a review of the reported incidence, pathogenesis and current research directions. *J Cardiovasc Electrophysiol.* 1999;10(4):611-620.

13. Calkins H, Epstein A, Packer D, et al. Catheter ablation of ventricular tachycardia in patients with structural heart disease using cooled radiofrequency energy: results of a prospective multicenter study. Cooled RF Multi Center Investigators Group. *J Am Coll Cardiol.* 2000;35(7):1905-1914.

14. Cooper JM, Sapp JL, Tedrow U, et al. Ablation with an internally irrigated radiofrequency catheter: learning how to avoid steam pops. *Heart Rhythm.* 2004;1(3): 329-333.

15. Yamane T, Jais P, Shah DC, et al. Efficacy and safety of an irrigated-tip catheter for the ablation of accessory pathways resistant to conventional radiofrequency ablation. *Circulation.* 2000;102(21):2565-2568.

16. Yokoyama K, Nakagawa H, Shah DC, et al. Novel contact force sensor incorporated in irrigated radiofrequency ablation catheter predicts lesion size and incidence of steam pop and thrombus. *Circ Arrhythm Electrophysiol.* 2008;1(5): 354-362.

17. Thiagalingam A, D'Avila A, Foley L, et al. Importance of catheter contact force during irrigated radiofrequency ablation: evaluation in a porcine ex vivo model using a force-sensing catheter. *J Cardiovasc Electrophysiol.* 2010;21(7):806-811.

18. Wittkampf FH, Nakagawa H. RF catheter ablation: Lessons on lesions. *Pacing Clin Electrophysiol.* 2006;29(11):1285-1297.

19. Barnett AS, Bahnson TD, Piccini JP. Recent advances in lesion formation for catheter ablation of atrial fibrillation. *Circ Arrhythm Electrophysiol.* 2016;9(5):e003299.

20. Nakagawa H, Kautzner J, Natale A, et al. Locations of high contact force during left atrial mapping in atrial fibrillation patients: electrogram amplitude and impedance are poor predictors of electrode-tissue contact force for ablation of atrial fibrillation. *Circ Arrhythm Electrophysiol.* 2013;6(4):746-753.

21. Perna F, Heist EK, Danik SB, Barrett CD, Ruskin JN, Mansour M. Assessment of catheter tip contact force resulting in cardiac perforation in swine atria using force sensing technology. *Circ Arrhythm Electrophysiol.* 2011;4(2):218-224.

22. Reddy VY, Dukkipati SR, Neuzil P, et al. Randomized, Controlled Trial of the Safety and Effectiveness of a Contact Force-Sensing Irrigated Catheter for Ablation of Paroxysmal Atrial Fibrillation: Results of the TactiCath Contact Force Ablation Catheter Study for Atrial Fibrillation (TOCCASTAR) Study. *Circulation.* 2015;132(10):907-915.

23. Natale A, Reddy VY, Monir G, et al. Paroxysmal AF catheter ablation with a contact force sensing catheter: results of the prospective, multicenter SMART-AF trial. *J Am Coll Cardiol.* 2014;64(7):647-656.

24. Glashan CA, Tofig BJ, Tao Q, et al. Multisize Electrodes for Substrate Identification in Ischemic Cardiomyopathy: Validation by Integration of Whole Heart Histology. *JACC Clin Electrophysiol.* 2019;5(10):1130-1140.

25. Leshem E, Tschabrunn CM, Jang J, et al. High-Resolution Mapping of Ventricular Scar: Evaluation of a Novel Integrated Multielectrode Mapping and Ablation Catheter. *JACC Clin Electrophysiol.* 2017;3(3):220-231.

26. Reddy VY, Grimaldi M, De Potter T, et al. Pulmonary Vein Isolation With Very High Power, Short Duration, Temperature-Controlled Lesions: The QDOT-FAST Trial. *JACC Clin Electrophysiol.* 2019;5(7):778-786.

27. Khairy P, Dubuc M. Transcatheter cryoablation part I: preclinical experience. *Pacing Clin Electrophysiol.* 2008;31(1):112-120.

28. Kuck KH, Brugada J, Furnkranz A, et al. Cryoballoon or radiofrequency ablation for paroxysmal atrial fibrillation. *New Engl J Med.* 2016;374(23):2235-2245.

29. Andrade JG, Dubuc M, Guerra PG, et al. The biophysics and biomechanics of cryoballoon ablation. *Pacing Clin Electrophysiol.* 2012;35(9):1162-1168.

30. Heeger CH, Wissner E, Mathew S, et al. Short tip-big difference? First-in-man experience and procedural efficacy of pulmonary vein isolation using the third-generation cryoballoon. *Clin Res Cardiol.* 2016;105(6):482-488.

31. Friedman PL, Dubuc M, Green MS, et al. Catheter cryoablation of supraventricular tachycardia: results of the multicenter prospective "frosty" trial. *Heart Rhythm.* 2004;1(2):129-138.

32. Skanes AC, Dubuc M, Klein GJ, et al. Cryothermal ablation of the slow pathway for the elimination of atrioventricular nodal reentrant tachycardia. *Circulation.* 2000;102(23):2856-2860.

33. Dubuc M, Khairy P, Rodriguez-Santiago A, et al. Catheter cryoablation of the atrio-ventricular node in patients with atrial fibrillation: a novel technology for ablation of cardiac arrhythmias. *J Cardiovasc Electrophysiol.* 2001;12(4):439-444.

34. Weber HP, Sagerer-Gerhardt M. Open-irrigated laser catheter ablation: influence of catheter irrigation and of contact and noncontact mode of laser application on lesion formation in bovine myocardium. *Lasers Med Sci.* 2014;29(3):1183-1187.

35. Weber H, Sagerer-Gerhardt M. Open-irrigated laser catheter ablation: relationship between the level of energy, myocardial thickness, and collateral damages in a dog model. *Europace.* 2014;16(1):142-148.

36. Weber H, Sagerer-Gerhardt M, Heinze A. Laser catheter ablation of long- lasting persistent atrial fibrillation: Longterm results. *J Atrial Fibrillation.* 2017;10(2):1588.

37. Dukkipati SR, Cuoco F, Kutinsky I, et al. Pulmonary vein isolation using the visu-ally guided laser balloon: a prospective, multicenter, and randomized compari-son to standard radiofrequency ablation. *J Am Coll Cardiol.* 2015;66(12):1350-1360.

38. Heeger CH, Phan HL, Meyer-Saraei R, et al. Second-generation visually guided laser balloon ablation system for pulmonary vein isolation: learning curve, safety and efficacy- The MERLIN Registry. *Circ J.* 2019;83(12):2443-2451.

39. Edd JF, Horowitz L, Davalos RV, Mir LM, Rubinsky B. In vivo results of a new focal tissue ablation technique: irreversible electroporation. *IEEE Trans Biomed Eng.* 2006;53(7):1409-1415.

40. Reddy VY, Neuzil P, Koruth JS, et al. Pulsed field ablation for pulmonary vein isolation in atrial fibrillation. *J Am Coll Cardiol.* 2019;74(3):315-326.

41. Da-Wariboko A, Lador A, Tavares L, et al. Double-balloon technique for retro-grade venous ethanol ablation of ventricular arrhythmias in the absence of suitable intramural veins. *Heart Rhythm.* 2020.

42. Tavares L, Lador A, Fuentes S, al. e. Intramural Venous Ethanol Infusion for Refractory Ventricular Arrhythmias. Outcomes of a Multicenter Experience. *JACC EP.* 2020.

43. Robinson CG, Samson PP, Moore KMS, et al. Phase I/II Trial of electrophysiology-guided noninvasive cardiac radioablation for ventricular tachycardia. *Circulation.* 2019;139(3):313-321.

9

Investigation of Bradycardias

SINUS BRADYCARDIA

Sinus rates less than 60 beats per minute (bpm) are defined as bradycardia in adults.[1,2] Lower rates are common in well-trained athletes and occasionally in the young. During sleep the sinus rate may fall to 35 bpm with pauses up to 3 seconds and this is not considered abnormal.

Sinus arrhythmia usually refers to sinus cycle phasic variation that is related to the respiratory cycle and is normal.

Sinus arrest (sinus pauses) manifests itself as pauses with the PP interval containing the pause not being equal or multiple of the basic PP interval.

In *sinoatrial exit block* (first, second, or third degree) the atrium is not depolarized despite the sinus stimulus and the duration of the pause is a multiple of the basic PP interval, unless there is Mobitz I block out of the sinus node.

Wandering atrial pacemaker refers to shift of the dominant pacemaker from the sinus node to other atrial focus, usually lower at the crista terminalis.

Sinus node disease or *sick sinus syndrome* refers to any of the following conditions that may coexist:

1. Persistent spontaneous bradycardia less than 50 bpm not caused by drugs and with chronotropic incompetence— that is, inability to achieve 85% of the age-predicted maximum heart rate on the treadmill.[2,3]

2. Sinus pauses greater than 3 seconds while awake or greater than 5 seconds during sleep, either because of sinus arrest or exit block.
3. Alternating episodes of bradycardia usually after tachycardia (mostly atrial fibrillation).

ATRIOVENTRICULAR BLOCK

First-degree atrioventricular (AV) block is characterized by a PR interval greater than 200 ms. A narrow QRS complex indicates that the block is most probably at the AV node, whereas wide QRS can be seen with a block either at the node or His-Purkinje system.

Second-degree AV block is characterized by P waves not conducted to the ventricles.

Type I second-degree AV block (Mobitz I or Wenckebach) is progressively increasing PR intervals until a P wave fails to be conducted to the ventricles.

Type II second-degree AV block (Mobitz II) is *consecutive*, nonconducted P waves without visible changes in the PR interval (i.e., AV conduction time) before and after the blocked impulse, provided there is normal sinus rhythm. The diagnosis of type II block cannot be established if the first postblock P wave is followed by a shortened PR interval or is not discernible.

Third-degree (complete) AV block is when no P wave is conducted to the ventricles and ventricular contraction is maintained by a nodal or infranodal escape rhythm. Unless the escape rhythm is lower than the sinus rate, complete AV block cannot be differentiated from AV dissociation.

ATRIOVENTRICULAR DISSOCIATION

AV dissociation is independent beating of the atria and ventricles as a result of the following:

1. Slowing of the sinus rate that allows escape of a subsidiary or latent pacemaker.
2. Acceleration of a latent pacemaker, as happens in nonparoxysmal AV junctional tachycardia or ventricular tachycardia.
3. Complete heart block with junctional or ventricular escape rhythm.

INTRAVENTRICULAR BLOCK

Left bundle branch block (LBBB) and **right bundle block (RBBB)** lead to interventricular dyssynchrony.

RBBB may display normal axis or 180 degrees (common type or Wilson block). Left or extreme right axis deviation suggests coexistent hemiblock. Pure RBBB and bifascicular blocks are associated with S waves in leads I and aVL. An electrocardiography (ECG) pattern of RBBB in lead V1 with absent S wave in leads I and aVL indicates concomitant LBB delay and bilateral block.[4]

In mirror-image dextrocardia or dextroversion, relocating the V_1 through V_6 leads (with the V_1–V_6 leads placed in the V_{6R}–V_{3R}, V_1, and V_2 positions) is necessary for ECG interpretation (Fig. 9.1). Thus an apparent RBBB may actually be a LBBB in this setting.[5]

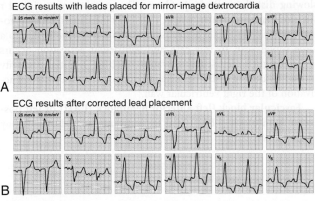

ECG results with leads placed for mirror-image dextrocardia

A

ECG results after corrected lead placement

B

FIG. 9.1. Electrocardiogram after correction in dextrocardia. (A) A 12-lead electrocardiogram (ECG) was obtained with the lead electrodes placed according to the anatomic condition of mirror-image dextrocardia. (B) The ECG leads were relocated, with the V_1 through V_6 leads placed in the V_{6R} through V_{3R}, V_1, and V_2 positions. The corrected 12-lead ECG shows an rS pattern in lead V_1 and slurred R waves in leads V_5 and V_6.

(Chang Q, Liu R, Feng Z. Bundle branch block site in a patient with a right-lying heart and wide QRS complex. *JAMA Intern Med.* 2019;179(2):254-256.)

LBBB may display normal or more often left axis deviation, which implies a worse prognosis. Right axis deviation may be seen in dilated cardiomyopathy. Current criteria for LBBB include a QRS duration 120 ms or longer, and this threshold is also used for CRT recommendations. However, certain patients may not have true complete LBBB but likely have a combination of left ventricular hypertrophy and left anterior fascicular block, and stricter criteria such as a QRS duration 140 ms or longer for men and 130 ms or longer for women, along with mid-QRS notching or slurring in two or more contiguous leads, have been proposed.[6] Septal conduction during LBBB is heterogenous. There may be complete block, usually high at the left-sided His fibers (left intra-Hisian block, and most amenable to corrective His bundle pacing) and, less commonly, more distally at the left bundle level, or conduction slowing distally to Purkinje fibers.[7] The presence of an initial r wave of 1 mm or greater in lead V_1 usually indicates intact left-to-right ventricular septal activation,[8] unless the r wave is due to a large septal scar. In this case and ventricular activation occurs without right-to-left septal activation resulting in initial positivity in lead V_1 during LBBB because of unopposed endoepicardial activation of the right ventricular wall.[9]

Fascicular block (left anterior hemiblock [LAH] or left posterior hemiblock [LPH]) lead to intraventricular dyssynchrony (Figs. 9.2 and 9.3).

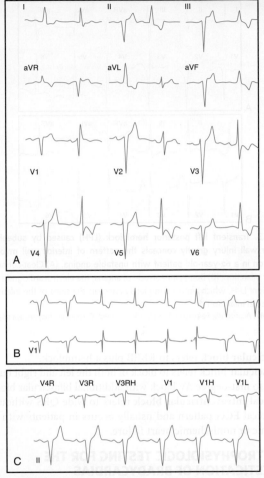

FIG. 9.2. Permanent right bundle branch block (RBBB) with intermittent left anterior hemiblock (LAH). The LAH conceals the signs of RBBB. (A) In every lead, the first beat shows LAH (plus RBBB), and the second beat shows RBBB alone. (B) Simultaneous recording of leads II and V$_1$. LAH is seen only in the first two beats and the last two beats. When LAH is absent, a typical RBBB pattern is uncovered. (C) The precordial chest leads recorded at the time when LAH was present (as seen in lead II) show the pattern of RBBB when V$_{3R}$ and V$_1$ were recorded one intercostal space above the normal level (V$_{3RH}$ and V$_{1H}$).

(Elizari MV, Acunzo RS, Ferreiro M. Hemiblocks revisited. *Circulation.* 2007;115:1154-1163.)

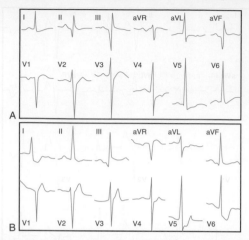

FIG. 9.3. Transient left posterior hemiblock (LPH) caused by subepicardial inferior wall injury greatly conceals the pattern of inferior wall myocardial infarction in a 62-year-old patient with unstable angina. (A) Clear-cut signs of inferior infarction. (B) During an episode of angina, the electrocardiogram shows a transient LPH, which almost completely conceals the signs of the inferior wall myocardial infarction.

(Elizari MV, Acunzo RS, Ferreiro M. Hemiblocks revisited. *Circulation.* 2007;115:1154-1163.)

Bifascicular block refers to RBBB plus a hemiblock.

Trifascicular block refers to block of both the left and right bundles or to first-degree AV block with additional bifascicular block.

Atypical intraventricular block refers to wide QRS without any typical ECG pattern and usually occurs in patients with ischemic or nonischemic heart failure.

ELECTROPHYSIOLOGIC TESTING FOR THE INVESTIGATION OF BRADYCARDIAS

In patients investigated for bradycardias either because of sinus node disease or AV conduction disturbances, the role of the electrophysiology study (EPS) is not well defined. Most of the time the clinical findings are sufficient to determine whether or not pacemaker implantation is indicated. However, there are certain occasions in which an EPS is helpful either for the establishment of diagnosis or for appropriate implementation of prophylactic pacing.

SINUS BRADYCARDIA

Early studies on limited patient cohorts suggested that the corrected sinus node recovery time (C-SNRT) may be useful in predicting the development of syncope and the need of permanent pacing in patients with bradycardia. A marked prolongation of the CSRT and an absent or blunted response to atropine and exercise suggest impaired sinus node function. However, a wide range of "normal" C-SNRT has been published, and it seems that only a very prolonged c-SNRT (>800 ms) has reasonable predictive ability.[10] When considering conventional upper limits, such as 500 to 550 ms, the sensitivity of the test in asymptomatic patients with dizziness or no symptoms who will need a pacemaker in the future is only 50% to 65%.[11] The sinoatrial conduction time (SACT) is an insensitive indicator, being prolonged in only 40% of patients with clinical findings of sinus node dysfunction.[12]

ATRIOVENTRICULAR CONDUCTION DISTURBANCES

Atrial premature beats may produce prolonged PR intervals caused by refractory fast pathway of the AV node, and nonconducted atrial premature beats can mimic AV block. The ECG appearance of first- or second-degree block may be due to junctional (His bundle) extrasystoles that are concealed (not conducted to the atria or ventricles) but render a portion of the conduction system refractory to propagation of a sinus beat. The presence of junctional premature depolarizations on the surface ECG suggests that concealed His bundle extrasystoles are responsible for the apparent AV block, but a His-bundle recording is the only method for positive identification (Fig. 9.4).

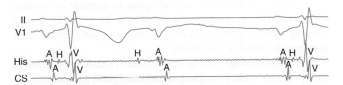

FIG. 9.4. Pseudo-type II infra-His block secondary to a concealed His bundle depolarization in a patient with RBBB and LAD.

II, V1, 12-lead electrocardiogram leads; *CS,* coronary sinus; *His,* His bundle. (Katritsis DG, Josephson ME. Electrophysiological testing for the investigation of bradycardias. *Arrhythm Electrophysiol Rev.* 2017;6:24-28.)

Anatomic Site of Block

High-grade block can occur anywhere in the AV conduction system, and usually if the **PR interval** is greater than 300 ms, the block is in the AV node. If the PR is less than 160 ms, the block is in the bundle of His or bundle branches.[13]

The **width of the QRS complex** and the configuration of conducted beats and/or escape beats are of only limited value in localizing the site of block. A narrow QRS complex is most compatible with an AV nodal or intra-His problem, and a wide QRS complex is most compatible with an infra-His problem, but a wide QRS complex can occur with AV nodal or intra-His disease in the presence of coexistent bundle branch block. However, approximately 70% of the time, Mobitz type II AV block (i.e., consecutive, nonconducted P waves without changes in the PR interval) is associated with bundle branch block. In 30% of cases of Mobitz II AV block (AVB), the QRS complex is narrow, consistent with block within the His bundle.[14] A pattern resembling a narrow QRS Mobitz type II AVB in association with an obvious Mobitz type I AVB pattern in the same recording makes block within the His less likely because a Wenckebach pattern in the His is fairly unusual.[14]

All Mobitz **type II AVBs** are infranodal, but not all infranodal blocks are associated with a Mobitz type II AVB pattern.[15] Although 2:1 or higher degrees of block (e.g., 3:1 and 4:1) have traditionally been classified as type II block, the site of those blocks cannot be reliably determined by the surface ECG. A 2:1 block in the context of bundle branch block does not necessarily indicate infranodal block because in 15% to 20% of patients the block is in the AV node.

If conduction improves with **atropine or exercise** or worsens with **carotid sinus massage**, the block is in the AV node. If AVB worsens with atropine or exercise or improves with carotid sinus massage, the block is infranodal.[13]

Simultaneous sinus slowing and AV block is indicative of vagotonic AVB in the AV node, even if a classic Mobitz I pattern is not present.

Symptomatic patients with Mobitz type I 2-degree AVB and a bundle branch block should also be considered for an EPS to determine the site of block. **Multiple levels of AV block** spontaneously or during pacing may also coexist in the same patient, and they can produce a confusing ECG picture that is difficult to interpret without an electrophysiology study.

Tachycardia-dependent AV block involves conduction block of early premature impulses, is a physiologic phenomenon often caused by high atrial rate. It has been attributed to refractoriness due to phase 3 repolarization *(phase 3 AV block)*, but this is disputable.[16]

Significant PR prolongation before and after block and prolonged PP intervals during ventricular asystole are indicative of vagal block in the AV node, which is benign condition responsible for vasodepressor syncope. On the other hand, **paroxysmal AV block** (pause- or bradycardia-dependent) is a pathologic phenomenon that occurs in the His-Purkinje system.[17,18] It is also called *phase 4 AV block,* but it may not depend on phase 4 depolarization.[16] The presence of paroxysmal AV block can be suspected by observing prolonged 3° AV block without sinus slowing that starts after a premature depolarization, but a definitive diagnosis requires His bundle recordings.[14]

Specific loss of function *SCN5A* **mutations** demonstrate varied competing gating effects that reduce sodium current density and enhance slow inactivation with selective slowing of conduction velocity in a way that may result in isolated progressive conduction system disease without provoking tachyarrhythmias.[19] Initial EPSs in mutations carriers with AV block revealed prolonged HV but normal AH intervals, thus suggesting infranodal block, but progressive AV block as a result of *SCN5A* mutations can be either nodal or infranodal and an EPS can be useful to make this distinction.

Several different types of muscular dystrophies, such as Emery-Dreifuss muscular dystrophy, limb girdle muscular dystrophy (Erb muscular dystrophy), myotonic dystrophy type 1 (Steinert disease), and desmin-related myopathy, are associated with progressive conduction defects. An EPS may identify patients in need of permanent pacing and improve survival of these patients.[20]

Prediction of High-Grade AV Block

HV interval. Bifascicular block, specifically RBBB with left-axis deviation, is the most common ECG pattern preceding complete heart block in adults.[12] Early studies on patients with bifascicular or trifascicular block reported an overall incidence of progression to complete heart block of approximately 1% to 2% per year.[21-24] Patients with syncope in particular may have a 17% cumulative incidence of complete AV block within the next 5 years.[23] The evaluation of the patient with bundle branch block or fascicular block necessarily involves testing the integrity of the remaining fascicle, and the simplest method of assessing this His-Purkinje reserve is the measurement of the HV intervals (normal ≤ 55 ms). In the presence of right bundle branch block, with or without additional fascicular block, the HV interval should be normal as long as conduction is unimpaired in the remaining fascicle. An LBBB usually prolongs the HV interval by approximately 10 ms. Most patients who go on to complete infranodal block have prolonged HV intervals (>70 ms).[22-24] Prolongation of the HV interval by 13 ms or more is strongly associated with second or third-degree AV block after transcatheter aortic valve replacement.[25] However, an HV greater than 70 ms may not independently predict development of complete heart block,[23] and approximately 50% of patients with RBBB and left anterior hemiblock and 75% of patients with LBBB have prolonged HV intervals.[26] Therefore an HV greater than 70 ms is nonspecific as a predictor of high-grade heart block. In our experience, approximately 70% of patients with HV intervals 100 ms or greater develop high-grade infranodal AVB within the next 2 years, and therefore this often is considered an indication for pacemaker implantation.

Of note, the surface ECG may not allow accurate assessment of the HV interval. Although a short PR interval (i.e., ≤160 ms) makes a markedly prolonged HV interval (i.e., ≥100 ms) unlikely, and a PR interval of more than 300 ms almost always means at least some AV nodal conduction abnormality,[13] intermediate values do not correlate with the HV interval (Fig. 9.5). In the presence of RBBB and left anterior hemiblock or LBBB with or without a superior axis, a normal PR interval can easily "conceal" a significantly prolonged HV interval, and a prolonged PR interval can be the result of a prolonged AH interval only (Figs. 9.6 and 9.7).

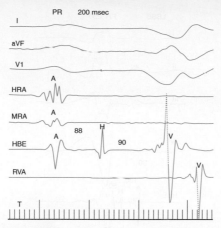

FIG. 9.5. Markedly prolonged HV interval in the presence of a normal overall PR interval. The PR interval is at the upper limits of normal (200 ms), and the QRS complex is prolonged with a pattern of interventricular conduction defect of the LBBB type. The HV interval is 90 ms.

HBE, His bundle electrogram; *HRA,* high right atrium; *MRA,* mid right atrium; *RVA,* right ventricular apex. (Katritsis DG, Josephson ME. Electrophysiological Testing for the Investigation of Bradycardias. *Arrhythm Electrophysiol Rev.* 2017;6:24-28.)

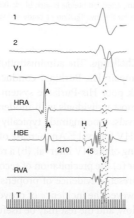

FIG. 9.6. Prolonged PR interval with a normal HV interval. The PR interval is 290 ms, and the QRS complex is prolonged with a pattern of right bundle branch block and left anterior fascicular block. The HV interval is normal at 45 ms, but the AH interval is prolonged at 210 ms.

HBE, His bundle electrogram; *HRA,* high right atrium; *RVA,* right ventricular apex. (Katritsis DG, Josephson ME. Electrophysiological testing for the investigation of bradycardias. *Arrhythm Electrophysiol Rev.* 2017;6:24-28.)

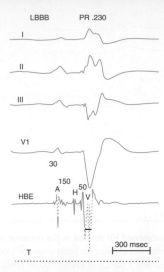

FIG. 9.7. Normal HV interval in left bundle branch despite PR prolongation and marked QRS complex widening. The PR interval is 230 ms and QRS complex 210 ms, yet the HV interval is normal (50 ms). The PR prolongation is due to AV nodal delay (AH interval = 150 ms).

HBE, His bundle electrogram; LBBB, left bundle branch block. (Katritsis DG, Josephson ME. Electrophysiological testing for the investigation of bradycardias. *Arrhythm Electrophysiol Rev.* 2017;6:24-28.)

Pharmacologic Challenge. The administration of pharmacologic agents known to impair His-Purkinje conduction (e.g., procainamide) may unmask poor His-Purkinje system reserve. In healthy individuals and in most individuals with moderately prolonged (55 to 80 ms) HV intervals, procainamide typically produces a 10% to 20% increase in the HV interval.[27] An increase of greater magnitude, including (a) doubling of the HV interval, (b) a resultant HV interval exceeding 100 ms, or (c) the precipitation of second- or third-degree infra-His block, represents evidence of propensity for spontaneous infra-His block. However, the incidence of provocation of AV block by procainamide is low, and the test may be useful in cases with borderline prolongation of the HV interval, but its diagnostic yield is rather limited.[28-30]

Other drugs may also be used to provide additional information about the His-Purkinje reserve. The value of adenosine or adenosine triphosphate (ATP) testing for induction of asystole because of latent sinus nodal disease AV block in patients investigated for unexplained syncope is not established, and these drugs have little or no effect on the His-Purkinje system.[31,32] However, there has been evidence that induction of cardiac pauses (because of AV block or sinoatrial block >10 seconds by an intravenous bolus of 20 mg ATP) indicates the need for DDD pacing in patients with unexplained syncope.[33,34] Adenosine might also be used, although its effects are not identical to those of ATP.[32,35]

Atrial Pacing. The use of atrial pacing to stress the His-Purkinje system provides further information beyond that of the baseline HV interval. Most normal patients will not exhibit second- or third-degree infranodal block at any time during incremental pacing, particularly at rates less than 150 bpm. Functional infranodal block because of a long-short sequence can be observed in patients without infranodal disease. However, second- or third-degree infranodal AVB *in the absence of a changing AH interval* at paced cycle lengths of 400 ms or greater and without a preceding long-short sequence is pathologic and is associated with a 33% rate of progression to high-grade AV block within the next 3 years.[22]

Box 9.1 presents the indications of EPS for diagnostic purposes in patients with apparent or suspected AV conduction abnormalities.

Box 9.1 Indications for Electrophysiology Study of Atrioventricular Block

1. Suspicion of concealed atrioventricular (AV) junctional extrasystoles
2. Asymptomatic type I second-degree AV block with bundle branch block
3. Asymptomatic second-degree AV block with bundle branch block
4. Questionable diagnosis of type II block with a narrow QRS complex
5. Suspicion of bradycardia-dependent (phase 4) infranodal block
6. Transient second-degree AV block with bundle branch block in patients with inferior myocardial infarction where the site of block is suspected to be in the His-Purkinje system rather than the AV node
7. Third-degree AV block with a fast ventricular rate
8. Progressive conduction disease as a result of neuromuscular disorders or suspected *SCN5A* mutations

---

Modified from Katritsis DG, Joephson ME. AV conduction abnormalities and AV blocks: role of EP testing. In: Camm AJ, Luscher T, Maurer G, Serruys P. *The ESC Textbook of Cardiovascular Medicine*. 3rd ed. Oxford, UK: Oxford University Press; 2019.

References

1. Olgin J, Zipes D. Specific arrhythmias. Mann DL, Zipes DP, Libby P, Bonow RO. *Braunwald's Heart Disease.* Philadelphia, PA: Elsevier; 2015:748-797.

2. Kusumoto FM, Schoenfeld MH, Barrett C, et al. 2018 ACC/AHA/HRS guideline on the evaluation and management of patients with bradycardia and cardiac conduction delay. *J Am Coll Cardiol.* 2019;74(7):932-987.

3. Katritsis D, Camm AJ. Chronotropic incompetence: a proposal for definition and diagnosis. *Br Heart J.* 1993;70(5):400-402.

4. Tzogias L, Steinberg LA, Williams AJ, et al. Electrocardiographic features and prevalence of bilateral bundle-branch delay. *Circ Arrhythm Electrophysiol.* 2014;7(4):640-644.

5. Chang Q, Liu R, Feng Z. Bundle branch block site in a patient with a right-lying heart and wide QRS complex. *JAMA Intern Med.* 2019;179(2):254-256.

6. Strauss DG, Selvester RH, Wagner GS. Defining left bundle branch block in the era of cardiac resynchronization therapy. *Am J Cardiol.* 2011;107(6):927-934.

7. Upadhyay GA, Cherian T, Shatz DY, et al. Intracardiac delineation of septal conduction in left bundle branch block patterns: mechanistic evidence of left intra-hisian block circumvented by his pacing. *Circulation.* 2019;139(16):1876-1888.

8. Padanilam BJ, Morris KE, Olson JA, et al. The surface electrocardiogram predicts risk of heart block during right heart catheterization in patients with preexisting left bundle branch block: implications for the definition of complete left bundle branch block. *J Cardiovasc Electrophysiol.* 2010;21(7):781-785.

9. Wellens HJ. Is the left bundle branch really blocked when suggested by the electrocardiogram? *Europace.* 2012;14(5):619-620.

10. Menozzi C, Brignole M, Alboni P, et al. The natural course of untreated sick sinus syndrome and identification of the variables predictive of unfavorable outcome. *Am J Cardiol.* 1998;82(10):1205-1209.

11. Gann D, Tolentino A, Samet P. Electrophysiologic evaluation of elderly patients with sinus bradycardia: a long-term follow-up study. *Ann Intern Med.* 1979;90(1):24-29.

12. Josephson ME. Electrophysiologic evaluation of sinus node function. In: *Clinical Cardiac Electrophysiology.* 5th ed. Wolters Kluwer; Philadelphia, PA, 2015.

13. Josephson ME, Wellens HJ. Episodic dizziness in a 74-year-old woman. *Heart Rhythm.* 2014;11(12):2329-2330.

14. Barold SS, Hayes DL. Second-degree atrioventricular block: a reappraisal. *Mayo Clin Proc.* 2001;76(1):44-57.

15. Antoniadis AP, Fragakis NK, Maligkos GC, Katsaris GA. Infra-Hisian block as cause of Wenckebach's phenomenon in an asymptomatic middle-aged man. *Europace.* 2010;12(6):898-902.

16. El-Sherif N, Jalife J. Paroxysmal atrioventricular block: are phase 3 and phase 4 block mechanisms or misnomers? *Heart Rhythm.* 2009;6(10):1514-1521.

17. Lee S, Wellens HJ, Josephson ME. Paroxysmal atrioventricular block. *Heart Rhythm.* 2009;6(8):1229-1234.

18. Shenasa M, Josephson ME, Wit AL. Paroxysmal atrioventricular block: Electro-physiological mechanism of phase 4 conduction block in the His-Purkinje sys-tem: a comparison with phase 3 block. *Pacing Clin Electrophysiol.* 2017;40(11):1234-1241.

19. Katritsis D. Progressive cardiac conduction disease. In: Zipes DP, Jalife J, eds. *Cardiac Electrophysiology: From Cell to Bedside.* 7th ed. Elsevier, Philadelphia, PA, 2017.

20. Wahbi K, Meune C, Porcher R, et al. Electrophysiological study with prophylactic pacing and survival in adults with myotonic dystrophy and conduction system disease. *JAMA.* 2012;307(12):1292-1301.

21. Dhingra RC, Palileo E, Strasberg B, et al. Significance of the HV interval in 517 patients with chronic bifascicular block. *Circulation.* 1981;64(6):1265-1271.

22. Dhingra RC, Wyndham C, Amat-y-Leon F, et al. Incidence and site of atrioven-tricular block in patients with chronic bifascicular block. *Circulation.* 1979;59(2):238-246.

23. McAnulty JH, Rahimtoola SH, Murphy E, et al. Natural history of "high-risk" bundle-branch block: final report of a prospective study. *N Engl J Med.* 1982;307(3):137-143.

24. Scheinman MM, Peters RW, Suave MJ, et al. Value of the H-Q interval in patients with bundle branch block and the role of prophylactic permanent pacing. *Am J Cardiol.* 1982;50(6):1316-1322.

25. Rivard L, Schram G, Asgar A, et al. Electrocardiographic and electrophysiological predictors of atrioventricular block after transcatheter aortic valve replacement. *Heart Rhythm.* 2015;12(2):321-329.

26. Josephson ME. Clinical Cardiac Electrophysiology. Clinical relevance of intraven-tricular conduction disturbances. *Clinical Cardiac Electrophysiology.* 5th ed. Wolters Kluwer; Philadelphia, PA, 2015.

27. Josephson ME, Caracta AR, Ricciutti MA, Lau SH, Damato AN. Electrophysiologic properties of procainamide in man. *Am J Cardiol.* 1974;33(5):596-603.

28. Gang ES, Denton TA, Oseran DS, Mandel WJ, Peter T. Rate-dependent effects of procainamide on His-Purkinje conduction in man. *Am J Cardiol.* 1985;55(13 Pt 1):1525-1529.

29. Tonkin AM, Heddle WF, Tornos P. Intermittent atrioventricular block: procain-amide administration as a provocative test. *Aust N Z J Med.* 1978;8(6):594-602.

30. Twidale N, Heddle WF, Tonkin AM. Procainamide administration during electro-physiology study—utility as a provocative test for intermittent atrioventricular block. *Pacing Clin Electrophysiol.* 1988;11(10):1388-1397.

31. Brignole M, Sutton R, Menozzi C, et al. Lack of correlation between the re-sponses to tilt testing and adenosine triphosphate test and the mechanism of spontaneous neurally mediated syncope. *Eur Heart J.* 2006;27(18):2232-2239.

32. Lerman BB, Belardinelli L. Cardiac electrophysiology of adenosine. Basic and clinical concepts. *Circulation.* 1991;83(5):1499-1509.

33. Brignole M, Gaggioli G, Menozzi C, et al. Adenosine-induced atrioventricular block in patients with unexplained syncope: the diagnostic value of ATP testing. *Circulation.* 1997;96(11):3921-3927.

34. Flammang D, Church TR, De Roy L, et al. Treatment of unexplained syncope: a multicenter, randomized trial of cardiac pacing guided by adenosine 5'-triphosphate testing. *Circulation*. 2012;125(1):31-36.

35. Fragakis N, Antoniadis AP, Saviano M, Vassilikos V, Pappone C. The use of adenosine and adenosine triphosphate testing in the diagnosis, risk stratification and management of patients with syncope: current evidence and future perspectives. *Int J Cardiol*. 2015;183:267-273.

10

Differential Diagnosis of Narrow-QRS (≤120 ms) Tachycardias

Narrow-QRS complexes (≤120 ms) are due to activation of the ventricles via the His-Purkinje system, consistent with origin of the arrhythmia above or within the His bundle. However, early activation of the His bundle can also occur in high septal ventricular tachycardias (VTs), thus resulting in relatively narrow-QRS complexes (110–140 ms).[1] In these cases the HV interval is less than 35 ms. Atrial fibrillation (AF) with rapid ventricular response may superficially resemble a regular narrow-QRS tachycardia, whereas focal or multifocal atrial tachycardia and atrial flutter may present as an irregular tachycardia as a result of varying atrioventricular (AV) conduction. Arrhythmias to be considered are presented in Box 10.1 and Fig. 10.1.

Box 10.1 Differential Diagnosis of Narrow-Qrs Tachycardias

NARROW-QRS (≤120 ms) TACHYCARDIAS

Regular

- Physiologic sinus tachycardia
- Inappropriate sinus tachycardia
- Sinus nodal reentrant tachycardia
- Focal AT
- Atrial flutter with fixed AV conduction
- AV nodal reentrant tachycardia
- Junctional ectopic tachycardia (or other nonreentrant variants)
- Orthodromic AV reentrant tachycardia
- Idiopathic VT (especially high septal VT)

Irregular

- AF
- Focal atrial tachycardia or atrial flutter with varying AV block
- Multifocal AT
- Junctional ectopic tachycardia (rare)

AF, Atrial fibrillation; *AV*, atrioventricular; *VT*, ventricular tachycardia.

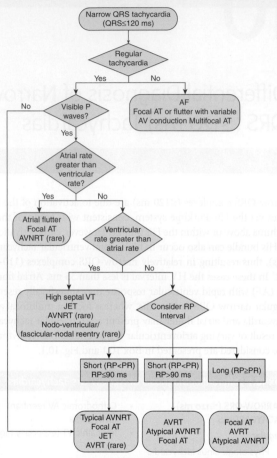

FIG. 10.1. Differential diagnosis of narrow-QRS tachycardia. Recording of a retrograde P wave should be sought by obtaining a 12-lead ECG and, if necessary, using the Lewis leads or even an esophageal lead connected to a precordial lead (V1) with use of alligator clamps. The 90-ms cutoff is a rather arbitrary number used for surface ECG measurements if P waves are visible and is based on limited data. In the electrophysiology laboratory the cutoff of the VA interval is 70 ms. JET may also present with AV dissociation.

AF, Atrial fibrillation; *AT,* atrial tachycardia; *AV,* atrioventricular; *AVNRT,* atrioventricular nodal reentrant tachycardia; *AVRT,* atrioventricular reentrant tachycardia; *ECG,* electrocardiogram; *JET,* junctional ectopic tachycardia; *RP,* RP interval; *VA,* ventriculoatrial; *VT,* ventricular tachycardia. (Brugada J, Katritsis DG, Arbelo E, et al. 2019 ESC Guidelines for the management of patients with supraventricular tachycardia: *Eur Heart J.* 2020;41(5):655-720.)

REGULAR NARROW-QRS (≤120 ms) TACHYCARDIAS

CLINICAL CHARACTERISTICS

Several clinical characteristics are useful for the appropriate diagnosis of a narrow-QRS tachycardia.[2] Atrial fibrillation (AF) is the most commonly treated substrate, followed by atrioventricular nodal reentrant tachycardia (AVNRT), atrial flutter, and atrioventricular reentrant tachycardia (AVRT), in patients referred for catheter ablation.[3-5] Thus AVNRT is the most common diagnosis in the presence of a regular narrow-QRS tachycardia. Women are more likely to be affected by AVNRT than men,[6-8] whereas the converse is true for AVRT.[6] A relationship to the menstrual cycle has been suggested,[9] and episodes are more frequent during pregnancy in women with preexisting supraventricular tachycardia (SVT).[10]

A sudden onset more likely points to AVNRT or AVRT, although an atrial tachycardia (AT) may also present in this way.[11] Reentrant tachycardias tend to last longer than AT episodes, which may occur in a series of repetitive runs.[11] Clear descriptions of pounding in the neck (the so-called frog sign) or "shirt flapping" would point to the possible competing influences of atrial and ventricular contraction on the tricuspid valve and to AVNRT as a likely cause.[7,12,13]

ELECTROCARDIOGRAPHIC DIFFERENTIAL DIAGNOSIS

In the absence of an electrocardiogram (ECG) recorded during the tachycardia, a 12-lead ECG in sinus rhythm may provide clues for the diagnosis of SVT.[14] The presence of preexcitation in a patient with a history of regular paroxysmal palpitations is suggestive of AVRT. The absence of apparent preexcitation does not rule out the diagnosis of AVRT because it may be due to a concealed accessory pathway (AP) that conducts only retrogradely or to an atriofascicular or nodofascicular/nodoventricular bypass tract that is not apparent during sinus rhythm. An ECG taken during tachycardia is very useful in the efficient diagnosis of SVT, although it may fail to lead to a specific diagnosis.[15]

Initiation and Termination of the Tachycardia

Sudden prolongation of the PR interval occurs in typical AVNRT after an atrial ectopic beat. An AT may also be initiated by an atrial ectopic beat but is not dependent on marked PR prolongation. Automatic, focal ATs are characterized by gradual acceleration (warm-up phenomenon) followed by deceleration (cool-down phenomenon)[16] and may also be incessant with short interruption by sinus beats. Premature atrial or ventricular beats may trigger AVRT. Premature ventricular complexes are a common trigger of atypical AVNRT but rarely induce typical AVNRT and or AT.

RP Interval

According to their P/QRS relationships, SVTs are classified as having short or long RP intervals. Short-RP SVTs are those with RP intervals shorter than half the tachycardia RR interval, whereas long-RP SVTs display RP greater than or equal to PR (Fig. 10.2). Rarely, recording of U waves during typical AVNRT may simulate a long-RP tachycardia.[17]

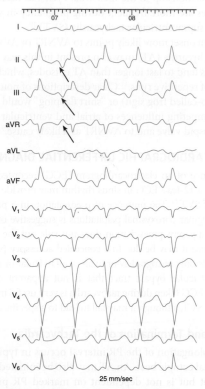

25 mm/sec

FIG. 10.2. A long-RP tachycardia. P waves are indicated by *arrows*. Inverse polarity of P waves indicates that this could represent atypical atrioventricular nodal reentrant tachycardia, atrioventricular reentrant tachycardia caused by a septal accessory pathway, or atrial tachycardia with a focus near the coronary sinus ostium.

On electrophysiologic study, a very short VA interval (≤70 ms) from the onset of the QRS to the atrial depolarization in the His bundle electrogram usually indicates typical AVNRT, or less commonly focal AT, but has also been reported in AVRT.[18] For surface ECG measurements, a cutoff interval of 90 ms has been shown to be useful and can be used if P waves are visible,[19] but data on actual RP measurement during various types of SVT are scarce.

P Wave Morphology

P waves similar to those in normal sinus rhythm suggest appropriate or inappropriate sinus nodal tachycardia, sinus nodal reentrant tachycardia, or focal AT arising close to the sinus node. P waves different from those in sinus rhythm and conducted with a PR interval equal to or longer than the PR in sinus rhythm are typically seen in focal AT but can also be seen in atypical AVNRT (Fig. 10.2). In AT the conduction to the ventricles may be fast (1:1) or slow (2:1 or more). The possibility of atrial flutter with 2:1 conduction should also be considered if the ventricular rate during SVT is approximately 150 beats per minute (bpm) because the atrial activity is usually 250 to 330 bpm. In the presence of antiarrhythmic medication in this setting, lowering the atrial rate may result in a higher ventricular rate in the absence of AV nodal blockade.

In the case of relatively delayed retrograde conduction that allows the identification of retrograde P waves, a pseudo r deflection in lead V1 and a pseudo S wave in the inferior leads are more common in typical AVNRT than in AVRT or AT.[20,21] These criteria are specific (91% to 100%) but modestly sensitive (58% and 14%, respectively).[20] A difference in RP intervals in leads V1 and III greater than 20 ms is also indicative of AVNRT rather than AVRT caused by a posteroseptal pathway.[21] The presence of a QRS notch in lead aVL has also been found as a reliable criterion suggesting AVNRT,[22] whereas a pseudo r in aVR was shown to have higher sensitivity and specificity than a pseudo r in V1 for the diagnosis of typical AVNRT.[23] However, in all referenced studies, cases of AT or atypical AVNRT were limited or entirely absent.

AV Block

AV block during a narrow-QRS-complex tachycardia is most common with atrial tachycardias, sometimes occurs with AVNRT, and rules out AVRT because the atria and ventricles are requisite parts of the reentry circuit (Fig. 10.3).

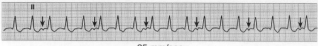

25 mm/sec

FIG. 10.3. Atrioventricular dissociation. P waves are indicated by *arrows*.

Bundle Branch Block

The development of bundle branch block (BBB) during SVT may also be helpful in the diagnosis of AVRT. BBB ipsilateral to the AP results ventriculoatrial (VA) prolongation of the VA interval as a result of lengthening of the reentry circuit attributable to transseptal conduction after conduction down the contralateral bundle.[24] Lengthening of the VA interval may or may not result in cycle length (CL) prolongation, depending on the behavior of the AH interval. An increase in the VA interval often is accompanied by a reciprocal shortening of the AH interval that minimizes an increase in CL.

Regularity of Tachycardia Cycle Length

The regularity of the RR interval should be assessed (Fig. 10.4).[14] Irregular tachycardias may represent focal or multifocal AT, focal AF, and atrial flutter with varying AV conduction. Patterns of irregularity can sometimes be found, such as in atrial flutter conducted with Wenckebach periodicity. Irregular arrhythmias, such as multifocal AT, typically display variable P-wave morphologies and varying PP, RR, and PR intervals. Atrial flutter can have fixed AV conduction and present as a regular tachycardia, and even AF may appear almost regular when very fast. Reentrant tachycardias, whether micro- or macroreentry, are usually regular. Incessant tachycardias may be the so-called permanent junctional reciprocating tachycardia (PJRT), focal AT, and, rarely, atypical AVNRT. CL alternans (also called RR alternans) may be seen in AVNRT, but these changes are less than 15% of the tachycardia CL.[25] If the irregularity exceeds 15% of the CL, a focal arrhythmia is much more likely.[26] QRS alternans initially was described to be an indicator of AVRT.[27,28] Subsequent studies have shown QRS alternans to be a rate-related phenomenon that is not specific to AVRT.[29]

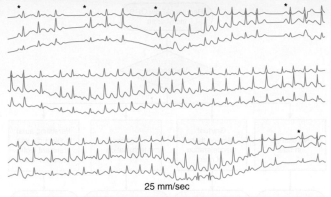

25 mm/sec

FIG. 10.4. Paroxysmal focal atrial tachycardia/atrial fibrillation. *Asterisks* indicate sporadic sinus P waves.

When there is CL variability in short-RP tachycardias, if the change in atrial CL precedes that change in the ventricular CL, this strongly favors atrial tachycardia. On the other hand, when the change in ventricular CL precedes the change in atrial CL, this strongly favors AVNRT or AVRT. During long-RP tachycardias, analysis of the sequence of change in CL in the atrium and ventricle is less helpful.[25,30] A fixed VA interval in the presence of variable RR intervals excludes AT.[15]

VAGAL MANEUVERS AND ADENOSINE

Vagal maneuvers (such as carotid sinus massage) and adenosine injection may help in clinical diagnosis, particularly in situations in which the ECG during tachycardia is unclear. Possible responses to vagal maneuvers and adenosine are shown in Fig. 10.5.

Termination of the arrhythmia with a P wave after the last QRS complex is very unlikely in AT, and most common in AVRT and typical AVNRT. Termination with a QRS complex is often seen in AT, and possibly in atypical AVNRT. Adenosine does not interrupt macroreentrant ATs (MRATs).[31] Fascicular VTs are verapamil sensitive but not adenosine sensitive. Most VTs, as opposed to SVTs, do not respond to carotid sinus massage, but a narrow-QRS VT originating at the left bundle branch and terminated with carotid sinus massage has been reported.[32]

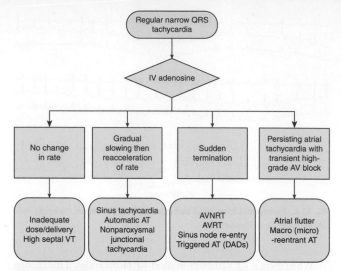

FIG. 10.5. Responses of narrow complex tachycardias to adenosine.
AT, Atrial tachycardia; *AV,* atrioventricular; *AVNRT,* atrioventricular nodal reentrant tachycardia; *AVRT,* atrioventricular reentrant tachycardia; *DADs,* delayed afterdepolarizations; *VT,* ventricular tachycardia. (Katritsis DG, Boriani G, Cosio FG, et al. EHRA/HRS/APHRS/SOLAECE consensus document on the management of supraventricular arrhythmias. *Europace.* 2017;19:465-511.)

ELECTROPHYSIOLOGY STUDY

At electrophysiology study, the differential diagnosis typically is between AVNRT, AVRT caused by a concealed or manifest accessory pathway, and atrial tachycardia. Automatic junctional tachycardia is rare in adults.[33] Nevertheless, differentiating AVNRT from junctional tachycardia is of clinical importance because ablation of the latter is associated with an increased risk of AV block. The distinction between AVNRT and a septal atrial tachycardia can be challenging, but various maneuvers should always lead to the correct diagnosis. We present the most useful and easily applicable maneuvers. A detailed discussion can be found elsewhere.[2]

Retrograde Atrial Activation Sequence During Tachycardia

AVNRT may display eccentric atrial activation and septal pathways may have decremental conduction properties and concentric retrograde atrial activation, thus making the differential diagnosis challenging. Although the retrograde atrial activation sequence is usually concentric in AVNRT, heterogeneity of both fast and slow conduction patterns has been well described, and all forms of AVNRT may display variable retrograde activation patterns.[34-36] Posterior or left septal fast pathways have been described in up to 7.6% in patients with typical AVNRT, and studies with left septal mapping indicate that left-sided retrograde fast pathways are used in a considerable proportion of patients with AVNRT (Fig. 10.6).[34] In atypical AVNRT, retrograde atrial activation can be quite eccentric and even suggestive of a left lateral accessory pathway.[37] Spontaneous changes of the VA interval without changes in the retrograde atrial activation sequence suggest different pathways for retrograde conduction in AVNRT.[38] Moreover, if this occurs with a stable ventricular rate, it suggests the atrium is not a necessary component of the reentry circuit and confirms the diagnosis of AVNRT.

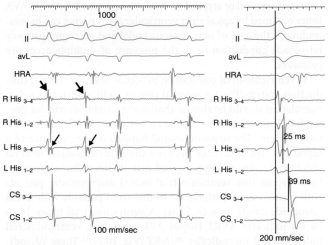

FIG. 10.6. Example of earliest retrograde atrial activation on the right septum preceding atrial activation on the left septum and coronary sinus ostium by 25 and 39 ms, respectively. Recording were obtained during an episode of typical atrioventricular nodal reentrant tachycardia that terminates spontaneously. The last tachycardia beat is not conducted to the atrium, thus revealing the actual components of the atrial electrogram on the right (thick arrows) and the left His recording electrode (thin arrows). The following sinus beat verifies identification of electrograms. Recordings are at 100 mm/sec on the left and 200 mm/sec on the right panel.

I, Lead I of the surface ECG, R His, right His bundle recording electrode; L His, left His bundle recording electrode; CS, coronary sinus. (Katritsis DG, Ellenbogen KA, Becker AE, et al. Atrial activation during atrioventricular nodal reentrant tachycardia: studies on retrograde fast pathway conduction. Heart Rhythm. 2006;3:993-1000, with kind permission.)

Ventricular Pacing During Sinus Rhythm

Ventriculoatrial conduction block, especially when it is not resolved with isoprenaline, rules out orthodromic AVRT.

VA Intervals. Atrial and ventricular conduction starts almost simultaneously in AVNRT, and VA times during tachycardia are therefore shorter than during ventricular pacing. Consideration of the ratio between the minimum ventriculoatrial interval during tachycardia and during ventricular pacing in sinus rhythm is useful. Ratios of 0.32 to 0.27 indicate typical AVNRT, 0.91 to 1.08 indicate AVRT using a posteroseptal pathway, and 0.94 to 1.29 indicate AVRT using an anteroseptal pathway.[39] Cases of atypical AVNRT, however, were not included in this study. A difference in the VA interval during tachycardia and right apical ventricular pacing greater than 90 ms has been reported to differentiate patients with typical or atypical AVNRT from those with AVRT.[40] VA times obtained by apical right ventricular (RV) pacing can be misleading in the case of simultaneous nodal and accessory pathway retrograde conduction or in the presence of multiple accessory pathways.

If ventriculoatrial conduction proceeds over the normal conduction system, the VA interval during right ventricular apical stimulation should be shorter than during right ventricular posterobasal stimulation because of earlier invasion of the His-Purkinje system. The opposite should happen in the presence of a septal AP. The difference between the ventriculoatrial interval obtained during apical pacing and that obtained during posterobasal pacing (the ventriculoatrial index) discriminates patients with posteroseptal pathway (>10 ms) from patients with nodal retrograde conduction (<5 ms). A ventriculoatrial index 10 to 70 ms indicates AVRT (septal AP), whereas a ventriculoatrial index −50 to 5 ms indicates AVNRT (Fig. 10.7).[41] These VA indices may not a reliable when there is coexistence of fast retrograde nodal conduction and a slow septal accessory pathway, conduction over a left lateral accessory pathway, and retrograde right BBB (RBBB) that delays atrial activation. A different activation sequence during RV pacing and SVT makes an atrial tachycardia highly likely.

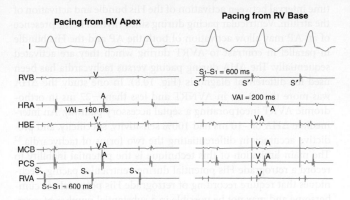

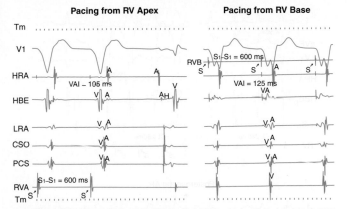

FIG. 10.7. Calculation of the ventriculoatrial index. *Upper panel:* Normal AVN conduction. The ventriculoatrial index is 160–200 = −40 ms. *Lower panel:* Posteroseptal AP. The ventriculoatrial index is 195 −125 = +70 ms.

AP, Accessory pathway; *AVN,* atrioventricular node; *HRA,* high right atrium; *HBE,* His bundle electrogram; *LRA,* low right atrium; *PCS,* proximal coronary sinus; *RVA,* right ventricular apex; *RVB,* right ventricular base; *Tm,* timelines. (Martinez-Alday JD, Almendral J, Arenal A, et al. Identification of concealed posteroseptal Kent pathways by comparison of ventriculoatrial intervals from apical and posterobasal right ventricular sites. *Circulation.* 1994;89:1060-1067.)

HA Intervals. During AVNRT, the HA interval represents the time interval between activation of the His bundle and activation of the atrium. Ventricular pacing during sinus rhythm in the presence of an AP may allow activation of both the AP and the His bundle in parallel in contrast to AVRT during which they are activated sequentially. The ΔHA during pacing versus tachycardia has been used for differential diagnosis (Fig. 10.8). In one study the ΔHA was more than 0 ms in AVNRT and less than −27 ms in orthodromic AVRT incorporating a septal accessory pathway. An intermediate ΔHA of –10 ms had 100% sensitivity, specificity, and predictive accuracy in differentiating the two forms of tachycardia.[42] The main limitation of this technique is the potential inability to record a retrograde His potential during ventricular pacing. Techniques that require recording of retrograde His potential are cumbersome and may not be possible in a substantial number of cases.

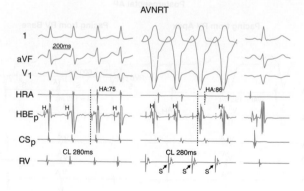

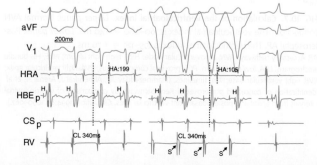

FIG. 10.8. ΔHA interval (Hapace-Hasvt). A ΔHA > 10 ms indicates atrioventricular nodal reentrant tachycardia rather than a posteroseptal accessory pathway. (Miller JM, Rosenthal ME, Gottlieb CD, Vassallo JA, Josephson ME. Usefulness of the delta HA interval to accurately distinguish atrioventricular nodal reentry from orthodromic septal bypass tract tachycardias. *Am J Cardiol.* 1991;68:1037-1044.)

Para-Hisian Pacing. Para-Hisian pacing during sinus rhythm is very useful for distinguishing between AV nodal and septal AP retrograde conduction.[43] An extranodal response through a septal accessory pathway is present when the retrograde atrial activation sequence and the stimulus to A interval during His bundle plus ventricular capture and during ventricular capture alone are the same (Figs. 10.9 and 10.10). Para-Hisian pacing is a sensitive and specific maneuver to establish the presence of a septal AP. However, it requires closely spaced bipolar electrodes (2-mm interelectrode spacing) for recording of retrograde His bundle activation and this may not be possible, especially in patients with very proximal RBBB.[43]

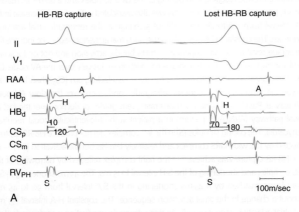

FIG. 10.9, cont'd

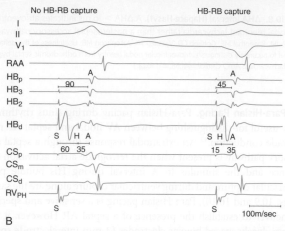

FIG. 10.9 Parahisan pacing demonstrating retrograde conduction over the AV node (AVN/AVN pattern). *A:* Para-Hisian pacing demonstrating retrograde conduction over the slow AV nodal pathway (AVN/AVN pattern). The pacing stimulus *(S)* in the left complex resulted in ventricular capture and HB-RB capture, producing a relatively narrow QRS complex and early activation of the His bundle *(H)*. HB-RB capture was lost in the right complex, resulting in widening of the QRS complex and a 60-ms increase in the S-H interval from 10 to 70 ms. This was also associated with a 60-ms increase in the S-A interval from 120 to 180 ms, without a change in the retrograde atrial activation sequence. The constant H-A interval (110 ms) and atrial activation sequence indicate that retrograde conduction was dependent on His bundle activation and not on local ventricular activation, indicating retrograde conduction exclusively over the AV node. Earlier atrial activation in the proximal coronary sinus electrogram (CS$_p$) than in the His bundle electrogram (HB$_p$) suggests retrograde conduction over the slow AV nodal pathway. *B:* Para-Hisian pacing demonstrating retrograde conduction over the fast AV nodal pathway (AVN/AVN pattern) in a patient with atrioventricular nodal reentrant tachycardia. The pacing stimulus *(S)* in the left complex did not produce HB-RB capture, reflected by the wide QRS complex and relatively late His bundle activation (S-H = 60 ms). HB-RB capture was achieved in the right complex reflected by narrowing of the QRS complex and shortening of the S-H interval to 15 ms. The 45-ms shortening in S-H interval was matched by a 45-ms shortening in the S-A interval from 90 to 45 ms, without a change in the atrial activation sequence. The constant H-A interval (35 ms) and atrial activation sequence indicate that retrograde conduction was dependent on activation of the His bundle and not on the local ventricular myocardium.

(Hirao K, Otomo K, Wang X, et al. Para-Hisian pacing. A new method for differentiating retrograde conduction over an accessory AV pathway from conduction over the AV node. *Circulation.* 1996;94:1027-1035.)

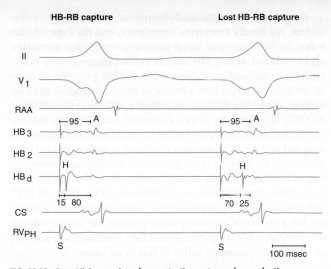

FIG. 10.10. Para-Hisian pacing demonstrating retrograde conduction over an anteroseptal accessory AV pathway (AP/AP pattern). HB-RB capture in the left complex resulted in an S-H interval of 15 ms. Loss of HB-RB capture in the right complex resulted in a 55-ms increase in S-H interval to 70 ms. The S-A interval remained fixed at 95 ms and the atrial activation sequence remained identical, indicating that retrograde conduction was dependent on the timing of ventricular activation and not on the timing of retrograde His-bundle activation.
(Hirao K, Otomo K, Wang X, et al. Para-Hisian pacing. A new method for differentiating retrograde conduction over an accessory AV pathway from conduction over the AV node. *Circulation.* 1996;94:1027-1035.)

Ventricular Pacing During Tachycardia

AVNRT and AVRT can always be terminated by overdrive ventricular pacing, whereas atrial tachycardia is rarely terminated.[44] Tachycardia termination by a ventricular extrastimulus that did not conduct to the atrium rules out an atrial tachycardia. The demonstration of AV dissociation by either atrial or ventricular pacing rules out AVRT, whereas the induction of the arrhythmia by ventricular extrastimulation makes atrial tachycardia extremely unlikely.

The development of BBB either spontaneously or after introduction of ventricular extrastimuli during AVNRT does not change the AA or HH intervals. A significant change in the VA interval with the development of BBB is diagnostic of orthodromic AVRT and localizes the pathway to the same side as the block.[33]

Tachycardia Resetting: His-Synchronous Ventricular Extrastimulation, His Bundle Premature Complexes, and the Preexcitation Index. In the presence of septal pathways, **ventricular extrastimuli introduced during His bundle refractoriness** during tachycardia (i.e., delivered coincident with the His potential or up to 50 ms before the His) may advance or delay subsequent atrial activation, depending on their decrement conduction properties. In AVNRT, atrial activity is not perturbed with His-synchronous ventricular depolarizations. Failure to reset the atria suggests, but does not prove, that an accessory pathway is not present or that it is relatively far from the site of premature stimulation. Demonstration of resetting excludes AVNRT unless the extrastimulus is delivered very close to inferior nodal extensions (Figs. 10.11–10.13).[45] This is a useful and easily performed maneuver. However, it identifies the presence of a pathway when positive but cannot rule out this possibility when negative. In addition, spontaneous variability in VA interval lessens the utility of this observation.

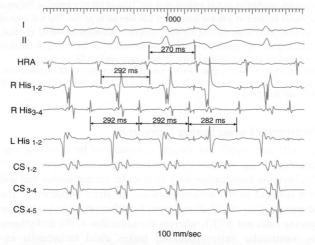

FIG. 10.11. Resetting of atrioventricular reentrant tachycardia because of a left posteroseptal accessory pathway. The tachycardia cycle length is 292 ms. At 270 ms a ventricular extrastimulus is delivered at a time when the His bundle is expected to be refractory and resets the next atrial electrogram (from 292 ms to 282 ms).

I, II, Electrocardiogram leads; *CS,* coronary sinus; *HRA,* high right atrium; *LHis:* His bundle recorded from the left septum; *RHis,* His bundle recorded from the right septum.

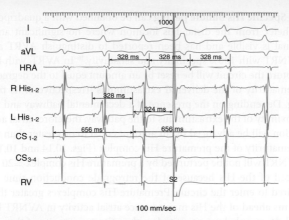

FIG. 10.12. His-synchronous ventricular extrastimulus. No resetting of typical atrioventricular nodal reentrant tachycardia with extrastimulation pacing from the right septum.

I, II, aVL, Electrocardiogram leads; *CS,* coronary sinus; *HRA,* high right atrium; *LHis,* His bundle recorded from the left septum; *RHis,* His bundle recorded from the right septum; *RV,* right ventricle.

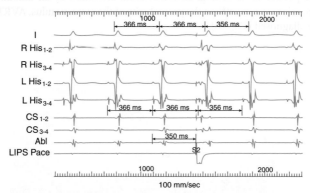

FIG. 10.13. For differential diagnosis purposes, His-synchronous ventricular extrastimuli must be delivered away from the AV nodal extensions. This is an example of resetting of atrioventricular nodal reentrant tachycardia by left inferoparaseptal extrastimuli that were delivered very close to the left inferior nodal extension. The His bundle electrogram is advanced by 10 ms.

I, Electrocardiogram lead; *Abl,* ablation catheter positioned at the area of the slow pathway; *AV,* atrioventricular; *CS,* coronary sinus; *HRA,* high right atrium; *LHis,* His bundle recorded from the left septum; *LIPS,* left inferoparaseptal; *RHis:* His bundle recorded from the right septum. (Katritsis DG, Becker AE, Ellenbogen KA, Giazitzoglou E, Korovesis S, Camm AJ. Effect of slow pathway ablation in atrioventricular nodal reentrant tachycardia on the electrophysiologic characteristics of the inferior atrial inputs to the human atrioventricular node. *Am J Cardiol.* 2006;97:860-865.)

Specific His bundle pacing can be obtained with a quadripolar catheter from the distal His location where no significant atrial signal is visible and has been reported to distinguish AVRT and AVNRT with 100% specificity and sensitivity.[46] In AVRT, with His capture the circuit will be reset by an amount equal to the degree of prematurity of the delivered extrastimulus irrespective of its timing. Depending on the presence of a decremental pathway and the proximity of the extrastimulus to the pathway, therefore, atrial activation will be advanced by an amount equal to or greater than the prematurity of the premature His complex (Figs. 10.14 and 10.15). AVNRT will not be perturbed by a premature His complex ≤20 ms ahead of the His because of the retrograde conduction time required to enter the circuit. Premature His complexes greater than 20 ms ahead of the His may advance atrial activity in AVNRT but will do so only by a quantity less than the prematurity of the premature His complex, also because of the retrograde conduction time necessary for the extrastimulus to enter the AVNRT circuit (Fig. 10.15). Thus if a premature His complex 20 ms or less ahead of the His perturbs tachycardia or if a premature His complex, irrespective of its timing, advances atrial activation by an amount equal to or greater than the prematurity of the extrastimulus, AVRT is diagnosed (Fig. 16).[46]

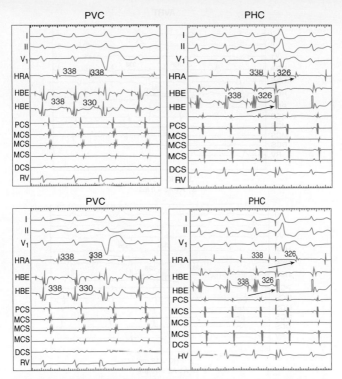

FIG. 10.14. Specific His bundle pacing. *Upper panel:* Supraventricular tachycardia (SVT) with concentric atrial activation, but the premature ventricular complex (PVC) timed to His refractoriness did not change the tachycardia and was nondiagnostic. A late premature His complex (PHC) (12 ms ahead of His) advances the tachycardia, establishing atrioventricular reentrant tachycardia (AVRT) diagnosis. *Lower panel:* SVT with eccentric atrial activation suggesting a left-sided accessory pathway, but atrioventricular nodal reentrant tachycardia is not definitively ruled out. An early PVC is able to advance the tachycardia but was not diagnostic of AVRT. An early PHC (52 ms ahead of His) advances the tachycardia by an equal amount, establishing AVRT diagnosis. The difference between His capture and non-His capture is apparent from narrowing of the QRS complex.

(Padanilam BJ, Ahmed AS, Clark BA, et al. Differentiating atrioventricular reentry tachycardia and atrioventricular node reentry tachycardia using premature His bundle complexes. *Circ Arrhythm Electrophysiol.* 2020;13:e007796.)

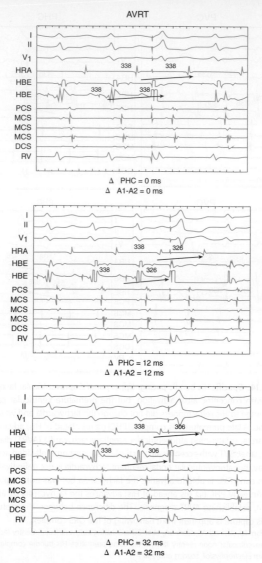

FIG. 10.15. Sequential premature His complexes (PHCs) in atrioventricular reentrant tachycardia (AVRT). Panels demonstrate the effects on AVRT based on the prematurity of the PHC. The A_1A_2 interval is advanced to the same degree of the prematurity of the PHC. *Red arrows* point to His to stimulus interval and A_1A_2 interval.

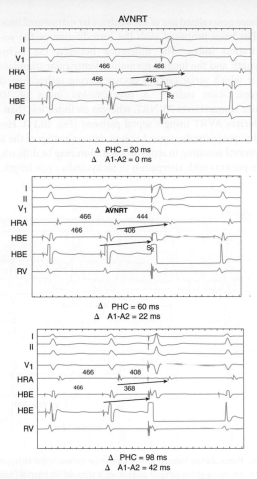

FIG. 10.15, cont'd Sequential PHCs in atrioventricular nodal reentrant tachycardia (AVNRT). Panels demonstrate the effects on AVNRT based on the prematurity of the PHC. The A_1A_2 interval is unaffected by a PHC 20 ms ahead of the His. Earlier PHCs advanced A_1A_2 interval but to a lesser degree than the prematurity of the PHC. *Red arrows* point to His-to-stimulus interval and A_1A_2 interval.

(Padanilam BJ, Ahmed AS, Clark BA, et al. Differentiating atrioventricular reentry tachycardia and atrioventricular node reentry tachycardia using premature His bundle complexes. *Circ Arrhythm Electrophysiol.* 2020;13:e007796.)

A more generalized use of the ventricular extrastimulation technique has been proposed with the introduction of the so-called **preexcitation index.** The difference between the tachycardia cycle length and the longest premature ventricular stimulation interval at which atrial capture occurs during tachycardia defines the preexcitation index.[47] A preexcitation index of 100 ms or greater characterizes AVNRT, whereas an index less than 45 ms characterizes AVRT using a septal pathway (Fig. 10.16). However, the technique is cumbersome because determination of the longest V_1V_2 interval resulting in atrial preexcitation may be difficult, especially in patients with alternation in tachycardia cycle length.

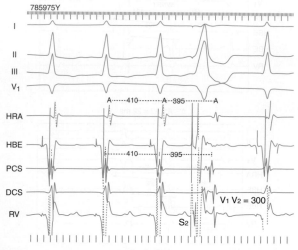

FIG. 10.16. Preexcitation index (PI). The difference between the tachycardia cycle length (410 ms) and the longest premature V stimulation interval (300 ms) at which atrial capture occurs during tachycardia. PI ≥ 100 ms: atrioventricular nodal reentrant tachycardia; PI < 45 ms: atrioventricular reentrant tachycardia using a septal pathway.

(Miles WM, Yee R, Klein GJ, Zipes DP, Prystowsky EN. The preexcitation index: an aid in determining the mechanism of supraventricular tachycardia and localizing accessory pathways. *Circulation.* 1986;74:493-500.)

Overdrive Ventricular Pacing. A useful criterion for the exclusion of atrial tachycardia is the atrial response on cessation of ventricular pacing associated with 1:1 ventriculoatrial conduction during tachycardia. Atrial tachycardia is associated with an A-A-V response, whereas AVNRT and AVRT produce an A-V response (Fig. 10.17).[48] This rule, however, has many exemptions. The His deflection should be considered in this respect because a late V electrogram might give an apparent AAV response that is actually A-H-A-V response in the presence AVNRT or AVRT, as opposed to A-A-H-V in the presence of atrial tachycardia (Fig. 10.18).[49] Apart from a long HV interval during slow–fast AVNRT that may cause atrial activation to precede ventricular activation, a very long AH interval exceeding the tachycardia cycle length may also produce a pseudo-A-A-V response (Fig. 10.19).[50] A pseudo-A-V response can also be seen with isoprenaline-increased automaticity of the AV junction such that junctional activity precludes conduction of the second A of A-A-V response to the ventricle (Fig. 10.20).[51] An A-A-V response also can be seen in AVNRT if there is a double fire after the last ventricular paced beat, with retrograde conduction through fast and slow AV nodal pathways (Fig. 10.21).[52]

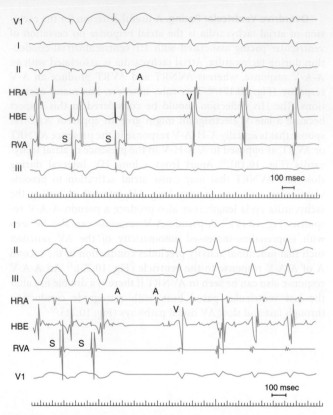

FIG. 10.17. Ventricular pacing during tachycardia. *Upper panel:* A-V response in typical AVNRT. *Lower panel:* A-A-V response upon cessation of ventricular pacing associated with 1:1 ventriculoatrial conduction that indicates atrial tachycardia.

(Knight BP, Zivin A, Souza J, et al. A technique for the rapid diagnosis of atrial tachycardia in the electrophysiology laboratory. *J Am Coll Cardiol.* 1999;33:775-781.)

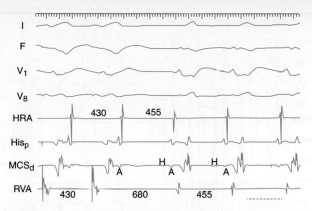

FIG. 10.18. Pseudo A-A-V response because of long HV (late V). Actually the response is A-H-A-V, and thus the tachycardia is atrioventricular nodal reentrant tachycardia or atrioventricular reentrant tachycardia.
(Vijayaraman P, Kok LC, Rhee B, Ellenbogen KA. Wide complex tachycardia: what is the mechanism? *Heart Rhythm.* 2005;2:107-109.)

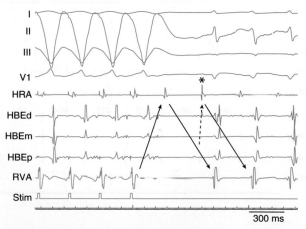

FIG. 10.19. Pseudo A-A-V response caused by long AH.
(Crawford TC, Morady F, Pelosi F. A long R-P paroxysmal supraventricular tachycardia: what is the mechanism? *Heart Rhythm.* 2007;4:1364-1365.)

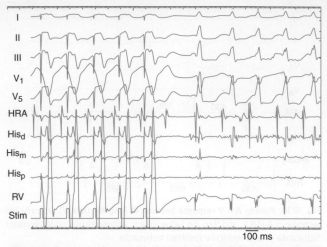

FIG. 10.20. Pseudo A-V response caused by isoprenaline-induced automaticity of the AV node.

(Kalra D, Morady F. Supraventricular tachycardia: what is the mechanism? *Heart Rhythm.* 2008;5:1219-1220.)

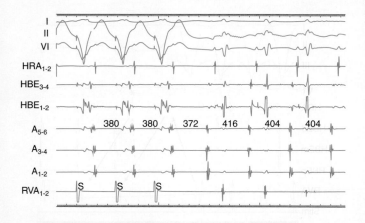

FIG. 10.21. Simultaneous fast and slow AV nodal pathway conduction. The first "A" is produced by retrograde conduction over a fast pathway, and the second "A" by retrograde conduction over a slow pathway.

(Kaneko Y, Nakajima T, Irie T, et al. V-A-A-V activation sequence at the onset of a long RP tachycardia: what is the mechanism? *J Cardiovasc Electrophysiol.* 2015;26:101-103.)

Tachycardia Entrainment. An RV apical pacing site is relatively close to the insertion of a septal accessory pathway as opposed to the AV junction and resetting and entrainment is much more common in AVRT than in AVNRT. When it is achieved, ventricular fusion during resetting or entrainment of tachycardia, indicated by QRS morphology different than that during ventricular pacing at sinus rhythm, occurs in AVRT because of septal pathways but not with AVNRT (Fig. 10.22).[53] This represents one of the initial attempts to establish the value of entrainment with and without fusion in the study of SVT. In AVRT with constant QRS fusion, the His bundle is depolarized by the anterograde wave front through the AV node, whereas in atypical AVNRT constant fusion is absent and the His bundle is depolarized by the retrograde paced wave front. Thus anterograde His bundle or septal ventricular resetting (capture at pacing cycle length) during RV entrainment has been found to be a criterion for AVRT, but it is indeterminate in up to 25% of patients.[54] Entrainment with stable QRS fusion requires stability of the tachycardia CL, and entrainment techniques are not always feasible.[48]

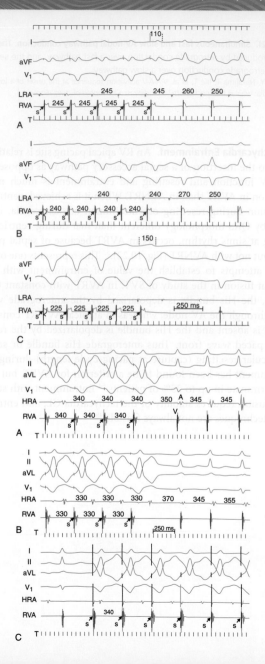

FIG. 10.22. Entrainment of supraventricular tachycardia. *Upper panels:* Entrainment during atrioventricular nodal reentrant tachycardia. (A) and (B) Last beats of a train of rapid ventricular pacing delivered during tachycardia and resulting in transient entrainment of tachycardia. (C) Pacing during sinus rhythm. Note that the QRS morphology is identical in all three panels (i.e., there is no ventricular fusion). *HRA,* High right atrium; *RVA,* right ventricular apex. *Lower panels:* Example of entrainment during orthodromic atrioventricular reentrant tachycardia. (A) and (B), Last beats of a train producing transient entrainment with resumption of tachycardia after cessation of pacing. Note a dramatic change in QRS morphology as a result of a slight change in pacing cycle length (from 245 ms in [A] to 240 ms in [B]), demonstrating ventricular fusion during entrainment. The change is even more notorious compared with the pacing train resulting in tachycardia termination (C). Again, as during resetting, an important increase in QRS duration can be observed as expression of ventricular fusion when (C) is compared with (A) (150 vs 110 ms).
LRA, Lateral right atrium; *RVA,* Right ventricular atrium. (Ormaetxe JM, Almendral J, Arenal A, et al. Ventricular fusion during resetting and entrainment of orthodromic supraventricular tachycardia involving septal accessory pathways. Implications for the differential diagnosis with atrioventricular nodal reentry. *Circulation.* 1993;88:2623-2631.)

Right ventricular pacing during SVT at a CL 10 to 40 ms shorter than the tachycardia CL produces progressive QRS fusion before the QRS morphology becomes stable and the tachycardia accelerates to the pacing CL when dealing with a septal bypass tract. This transition zone may be useful for differential diagnosis because tachycardia resetting most often occurs during this transition zone of QRS fusion in AVRT and only after this transition zone (i.e., fully paced QRS) in AVNRT (Fig. 10.23).[55] QRS fusion indicates that the His bundle is refractory. Therefore if a ventricular depolarization that has fused with the intrinsic QRS advances the next A, it is definitive evidence of the presence of an extranodal AP. In another similar study, acceleration of the tachycardia with more than one fully RV paced beats has been shown to indicate AVNRT with high accuracy (Fig. 10.24).[56] This maneuver can be used independent of entrainment success, or even when pacing terminates tachycardia. However, the end of the transition zone is marked by the first beat with a stable QRS morphology, and this is a subjective assessment. Pacing trains more than 40 ms shorter than tachycardia cycle length (TCL) or prematurity of the pacing train less than 80% TCL can result in an incorrect diagnosis of AVRT because the first fully paced beat is more likely to reset AVNRT, and the p wave occasionally can distort the QRS morphology, making it difficult to correctly recognize the end of the transition zone.[57] In addition, these techniques may be less useful with pathways remote from the pacing site.

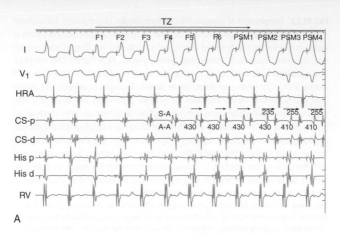

A

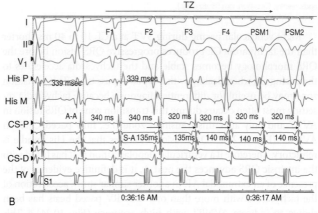

B

FIG. 10.23. Transition zone. (A) Atypical atrioventricular nodal reentrant tachycardia: Entrainment after the transition zone (TZ). Six QRS complexes demonstrate fusion (F1..F6) until QRS morphology becomes stable (PSM1...PSM4). After PSM3, S-A intervals *(arrows)* become fixed and atrial activation is advanced. (B) Atrioventricular reentrant tachycardia (septal accessory pathway): Entrainment during TZ. Fusion: (F1..F4), stable: (PSM1 and PSM2). After F2, the S-A interval *(arrows)* becomes fixed and atrial activation is advanced.

PSM indicates paced QRS with stable morphology; *HRA*, high right atrium; *His P*, His proximal; *His M*, His Mid; *CS-P*, CS proximal; and *CS-D*, CS distal. (AlMahameed ST, Buxton AE, Michaud GF. New criteria during right ventricular pacing to determine the mechanism of supraventricular tachycardia. *Circ Arrhythm Electrophysiol.* 2010;3:578-584.)

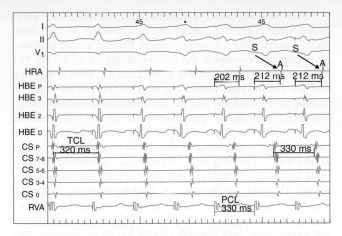

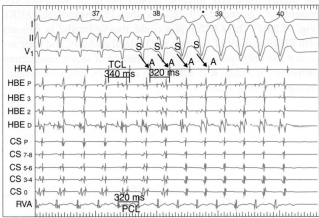

FIG. 10.24. Tachycardia acceleration (once fully captured RV pacing is achieved during tachycardia). *Upper panel:* Atrioventricular nodal reentrant tachycardia: Two beats to accelerate tachycardia cycle length (TCL) to the pacing cycle length (PCL). *Lower panel:* Atrioventricular reentrant tachycardia (right posteroseptal accessory pathway): One beat required to accelerate TCL to PCL.

(Dandamudi G, Mokabberi R, Assal C, et al. A novel approach to differentiating orthodromic reciprocating tachycardia from atrioventricular nodal reentrant tachycardia. *Heart Rhythm.* 2010;7:1326-1329.)

When the tachycardia is sustained and entrainable, the post-pacing interval (PPI) is helpful in distinguishing AVNRT from AVRT using a septal accessory pathway. Because a right ventricular pacing site is nearer to the reentry circuit for AVRT, the PPI more closely approximates the tachycardia CL than it does for AVNRT. For the same reason, the interval between the last ventricular pacing stimulus and the last entrained atrial depolarization (S-A) more closely approximates the VA interval measured during tachycardia. Patients with AVNRT have been reported to have (S-A)-VA intervals greater than 85 ms and PPI-TCL intervals greater than 114 ms (Fig. 10.25).[58] However, conventional entrainment techniques do not take into account pacing-induced incremental AV nodal conduction (i.e., in the postpacing A-H) that may alter the PPI. Thus a "corrected" PPI-TCL difference calculated by subtracting from it the difference of postpacing AH interval minus basic AH interval should be more accurate. The presence of a corrected PPI-TCL less than 110 ms indicates AVRT (Fig. 10.26).[59] These techniques could also be invalid in patients with RBBB and AVRT through a left lateral pathway, and their accuracy has been questioned in the presence of slowly conducting pathways (i.e., VA/R-R ≥ 40%), with up to 50% mistaken diagnoses reported (Fig. 10.27).[60]

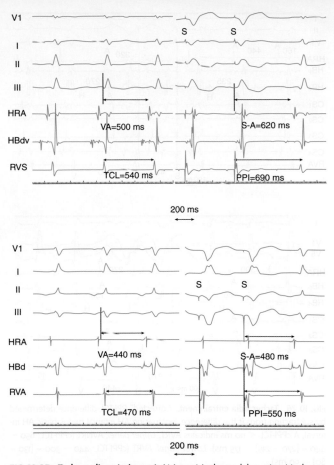

FIG. 10.25. Tachycardia entrainment. Atrioventricular nodal reentrant tachycardia is indicated by SA-VA intervals > 85 ms and PPI-TCL intervals > 114 ms. *Upper panel:* AVNRT (SA-VA = 120 ms, PPI-TCL = 150 ms). *Lower panel:* AVRT (SA-VA = 40 ms, PPI-TCL = 80 ms).

PPI, postpacing interval; *TCL,* tachycardia cycle length. (Michaud GF, Tada H, Chough S, et al. Differentiation of atypical atrioventricular node re-entrant tachycardia from orthodromic reciprocating tachycardia using a septal accessory pathway by the response to ventricular pacing. *J Am Coll Cardiol.* 2001;38:1163-1167.)

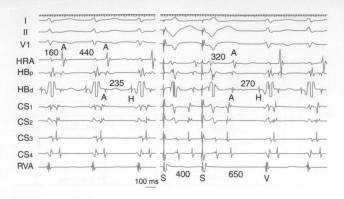

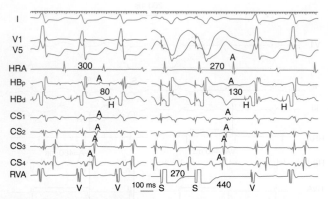

FIG. 10.26. Tachycardia entrainment. "Corrected" PPI-TCL difference determined by subtracting from it the difference: postpacing AH interval minus basic AH interval. A cPPI-TCL < 110 ms indicates AVRT. *Upper panel:* AVNRT (cPPI-TCL: 650 − 440 − [270 − 235] = 175 ms). *Lower panel:* AVRT (cPPI-TCL: 440 − 300 − [130 − 80] = 90 ms).

AVNRT, Atrioventricular nodal reentrant tachycardia; *AVRT,* atrioventricular reentrant tachycardia; *cPPI,* corrected PPI; *PPI,* postpacing interval; *TCL,* tachycardia cycle length. (Gonzalez-Torrecilla E, Arenal A, Atienza F, et al. First postpacing interval after tachycardia entrainment with correction for atrioventricular node delay: a simple maneuver for differential diagnosis of atrioventricular nodal reentrant tachycardias versus orthodromic reciprocating tachycardias. *Heart Rhythm.* 2006;3:674-679.)

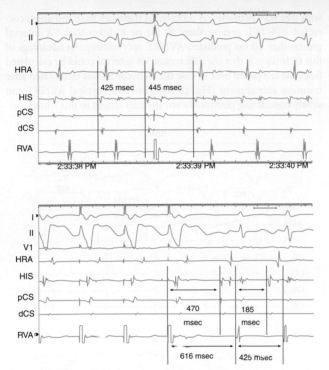

FIG. 10.27. Slowly conducting accessory pathway (VA/R-R> 0.4). The entrainment criteria are not valid. *Upper panel* AVRT. Right posteroseptal AP (His-synchronous V extrastimulus delays A. *Lower panel* AVRT. Right posteroseptal AP (SA-VA = 185 ms, PPI-TCL = 191 ms).

AP, Accessory pathway; *AVRT,* atrioventricular reentrant tachycardia; *PPI,* postpacing interval; *TCL,* tachycardia cycle length. (Bennett MT, Leong-Sit P, Gula LJ et al. Entrainment for distinguishing atypical atrioventricular node reentrant tachycardia from atrioventricular reentrant tachycardia over septal accessory pathways with long-RP [corrected] tachycardia. *Circ Arrhythm Electrophysiol.* 2011;4:506-509.)

Differential entrainment from the apex or the basal area of the right ventricle is also useful.[61] Since the RV apex is closer to the circuit in AVNRT than the base, the PPI after entrainment would also be shorter from the apex than the base of the right ventricle. Similarly, the stimulus-to-atrial interval after entrainment will be shorter. This would not be the case with accessory pathways, where the basal pacing site relative to the RV apex is variably related to the circuit, being closer than the RV apex with septal pathways and equidistant with free wall pathways. A differential (between base and apex) corrected PPI-TCL greater than 30 ms or a differential VA interval greater than 20 ms predicted AVNRT very reliably. An advantage of this technique is that the differential VA interval could be calculated from the last paced beat in case the tachycardia was terminated after transient entrainment (Fig. 10.28). However, atypical AVNRT and slowly conducting pathways were virtually absent in this study.

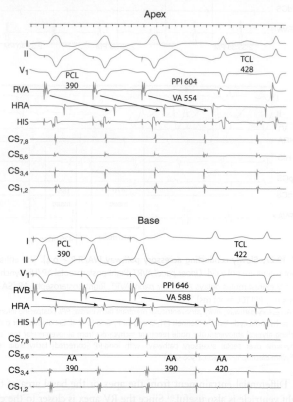

FIG. 10.28. Examples of differential entrainment responses in atypical fast–slow AVNRT. *(Upper panel)* Entrainment of atypical AVNRT from RVA at 390 ms and *(lower panel)* from RVB at 390 ms. Differential PPI-TCL and VA intervals are 42 ms and 34 ms, respectively. Panels are arranged from top to bottom as electrocardiographic leads I, II, and V1, and bipolar electrograms from the RVA, high right atrium *(HRA)*, His bundle *(His)*, or RVB and coronary sinus *(CS)* proximal (9,10) to distal (1,2). PCL, PPI, TCL, and VA are shown. The PPI is measured from the last pacing stimulus to the return cycle electrogram (RVA or RVB) and the TCL deducted to produce the PPI-TCL.

FIG. 10.28, cont'd The VA is measured from the last pacing stimulus to the last entrained HRA electrogram.

AVNRT, Atrioventricular nodal reentrant tachycardia; *HRA,* high right atrium; *PCL,* pacing cycle length; *PPI,* pacing cycle length; *TCL,* tachycardia cycle length; *RVA,* right ventricular apex; *RVB,* right ventricular base; *VA,* ventriculoatrial interval (Segal OR, Gula LJ, Skanes AC, et al. Differential ventricular entrainment: a maneuver to differentiate AV node reentrant tachycardia from orthodromic reciprocating tachycardia. *Heart Rhythm.* 2009;6:493-500.)

The comparison of HA interval during tachycardia and during entrainment from the RV apex or near the His bundle to obtain a recordable retrograde His has also been used for differentiation of AVNRT from AVRT. Positive ΔHA (HA during entrainment – HA during SVT) indicates AVNRT, whereas negative ΔHA indicates the presence of an accessory pathway (Fig. 10.29).[62] This technique is limited by the requirement of His bundle activation recording during entrainment.

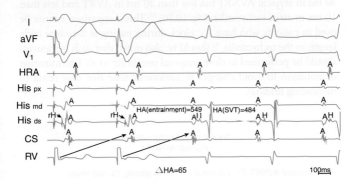

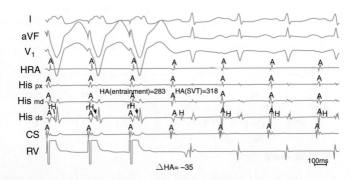

FIG. 10.29. Tachycardia entrainment. The interval ΔHA (HA[entrainment] – HA[SVT]) is considered. A positive ΔHA indicates AVNRT, and a negative one AVRT. *AVNRT,* Atrioventricular nodal reentrant tachycardia; *AVRT,* atrioventricular reentrant tachycardia; *SVT,* supraventricular tachycardia.
(Ho RT, Mark GE, Rhim ES, et al. Differentiating atrioventricular nodal reentrant tachycardia from atrioventricular reentrant tachycardia by DeltaHA values during entrainment from the ventricle. *Heart Rhythm.* 2008;5:83-88.)

Atrial Pacing During Sinus Rhythm

A comparison of the AH interval during tachycardia with the AH interval during atrial pacing at the same CL as the tachycardia is helpful for the diagnosis of a long-RP tachycardia. The difference in the AH interval during atrial pacing and during tachycardia is more than 40 ms in atypical AVNRT but less than 20 ms in AVRT and less than 10 ms in atrial tachycardia (Fig. 10.30).[63] This comparison cannot be used in patients who have AV block during pacing at the same cycle length as the tachycardia. It should be also noted that such maneuvers should be performed in close temporal proximity to SVT termination or initiation to avoid changes in autonomic tone that may result in misleading findings.

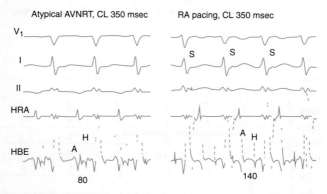

AH *pacing*-AH *tachy* > 40ms
Atypical AVNRT

Atypical AVNRT, CL 350 msec   RA pacing, CL 350 msec

V_1

I

II

HRA

HBE

80   140

FIG. 10.30, cont'd

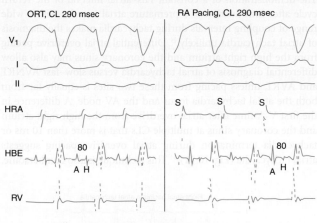

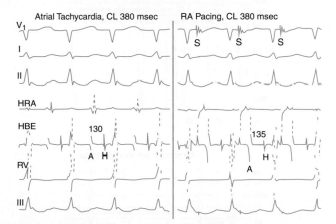

FIG. 10.30 Atrial pacing during SR. The AH intervals during tachycardia and pacing are considered.

(Man KC, Niebauer M, Daoud E, et al. Comparison of atrial-His intervals during tachycardia and atrial pacing in patients with long RP tachycardia. *J Cardiovasc Electrophysiol.* 1995;6:700-710.)

Atrial Pacing During Tachycardia

The demonstration of a constant His–atrial interval of the return cycle after introduction of a premature atrial impulse with a wide range of coupling intervals during tachycardia makes the diagnosis of atrial tachycardia unlikely.[44] Differential atrial overdrive pacing from the high right atrium and the coronary sinus may also allow differential diagnosis of atrial tachycardia versus slow–fast AVNRT and AVRT, unless pacing from these two sites is equally far from both the atrial tachycardia focus and the AV node. A difference in the first V-A time after atrial overdrive from the high right atrium and the coronary sinus at multiple CLs that is more than 10 ms or tachycardia termination during atrial overdrive pacing suggests atrial tachycardia (Fig. 10.31).[64] This technique is also cumbersome.

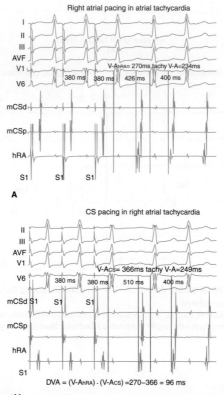

FIG. 10.31, cont'd

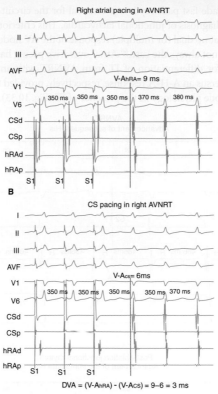

FIG. 10.31 Atrial pacing during tachycardia: differential RA and CS pacing.
A: Example of atrial differential pacing and measurement of the ΔVA interval in atrial tachycardia (s >10 ms). *B:* Example of atrial differential pacing and measurement of the ΔVA interval in atrioventricular nodal reentrant tachycardia (<10 ms).
CS, Coronary sinus; *RA,* right atrium. (Sarkozy A, Richter S, Chierchia GB, et al. A novel pacing manoeuvre to diagnose atrial tachycardia. *Europace.* 2008;10(4):459-466.)

The use of premature atrial stimuli can also be used for differential diagnosis of slow–fast AVNRT and nonreentrant junctional tachycardia (JT) (Fig. 10.32).[65] An atrial premature complex that is timed to His refractoriness and advances the His depolarization of the second ventricular depolarization after the atrial stimulus indicates that antero-grade slow pathway conduction is involved and establishes the diagnosis of AVNRT. An atrial extrastimulus that advances the His potential immediately after it without terminating the tachycardia indicates that the retrograde fast pathway is not essential for the circuit and establishes the diagnosis of junctional tachycardia. This criterion, however, requires that no dual (or multiple) response of the AV node is present, and this is not always the case.[66] Atrial overdrive pacing has also been proposed for differentiation of JT from AVNRT with an A-H-H-A response versus an A-H-A response, respectively, provided there is not dual AV node physiology in the presence of JT (Fig. 10.33).[67]

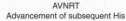

AVNRT
Advancement of subsequent His

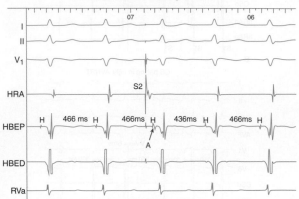

Post-ablation junctional rhythm
Adancement of the immediate His

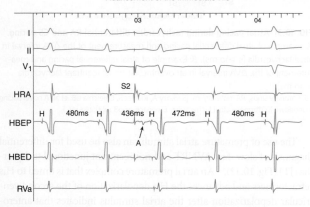

FIG. 10.32. His-synchronous atrial extrastimuli during tachycardia.
(Padanilam BJ, Ahmed AS, Clark BA, et al. Differentiating junctional tachycardia and atrioventricular node re-entry tachycardia based on response to atrial extrastimulus pacing. *J Am Coll Cardiol.* 2008;52:1711-1717.)

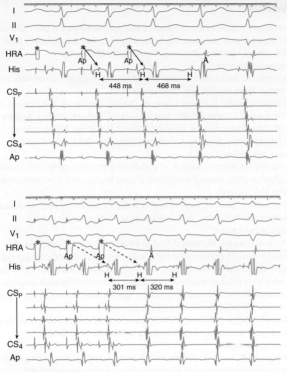

FIG. 10.33. Atrial overdrive pacing. *Upper panel:* Junctional tachycardia. A-H-HA response after cessation of pacing. *Lower panel:* Atrioventricular nodal reentrant tachycardia. A-H-A response after cessation of pacing.

(Fan R, Tardos JG, Almasry I, et al. Novel use of atrial overdrive pacing to rapidly differentiate junctional tachycardia from atrioventricular nodal reentrant tachycardia. *Heart Rhythm.* 2011;8: 840-844.)

All diagnostic maneuvers often cannot be used for all SVTs. The electrophysiologist should be familiar with multiple diagnostic criteria to be able to selectively apply the appropriate maneuvers needed to establish a diagnosis.

IRREGULAR NARROW-QRS (≤120 ms) TACHYCARDIAS

The most common irregular, narrow-QRS tachycardia is AF. However, focal atrial tachycardia, atrial flutter, and multifocal atrial tachycardia with varying AV block may also present as irregular rhythms. Junctional ectopic tachycardia may also be irregular, but it is a rare arrhythmia in adults.

References

1. Michowitz Y, Tovia-Brodie O, Heusler I, et al. Differentiating the QRS morphology of posterior fascicular ventricular tachycardia from right bundle branch block and left anterior hemiblock aberrancy. *Circ Arrhythm Electrophysiol.* 2017;10(9):e005074.

2. Katritsis DG, Josephson ME. Differential diagnosis of regular, narrow-QRS tachycardias. *Heart Rhythm.* 2015;12(7):1667-1676.

3. Garcia-Fernandez FJ, Ibanez Criado JL, Quesada Dorador A, collaborators of the Spanish Catheter Ablation Registry. Spanish Catheter Ablation Registry. 17th Official Report of the Spanish Society of Cardiology Working Group on Electrophysiology and Arrhythmias (2017). *Rev Esp Cardiol (Engl Ed).* 2018;71(11):941-951.

4. Hosseini SM, Rozen G, Saleh A, et al. Catheter ablation for cardiac arrhythmias: utilization and in-hospital complications, 2000 to 2013. *JACC Clin Electrophysiol.* 2017;3(11):1240-1248.

5. Holmqvist F, Kesek M, Englund A, et al. A decade of catheter ablation of cardiac arrhythmias in Sweden: ablation practices and outcomes. *Eur Heart J.* 2019;40(10):820-830.

6. Porter MJ, Morton JB, Denman R, et al. Influence of age and gender on the mechanism of supraventricular tachycardia. *Heart Rhythm.* 2004;1(4):393-396.

7. Gonzalez-Torrecilla E, Almendral J, Arenal A, et al. Combined evaluation of bedside clinical variables and the electrocardiogram for the differential diagnosis of paroxysmal atrioventricular reciprocating tachycardias in patients without pre-excitation. *J Am Coll Cardiol.* 2009;53(25):2353-2358.

8. Liuba I, Jönsson A, Säfström K, Walfridsson H. Gender-related differences in patients with atrioventricular nodal reentry tachycardia. *Am J Cardiol.* 2006;97(3):384-388.

9. Rosano GMC, Leonardo F, Rosano GMC, et al. Cyclical variation in paroxysmal supraventricular tachycardia in women. *Lancet.* 1996;347(9004):786-788.

10. Chang SH, Kuo CF, Chou IJ, et al. Outcomes associated with paroxysmal supraventricular tachycardia during pregnancy. *Circulation.* 2017;135(6):616-618.

11. Thavendiranathan P, Bagai A, Khoo C, Dorian P, Choudhry NK. Does this patient with palpitations have a cardiac arrhythmia? *JAMA.* 2009;302(19):2135-2143.

12. Gürsoy S, Steurer G, Brugada J, Andries E, Brugada P. The hemodynamic mechanism of pounding in the neck in atrioventricular nodal reentrant tachycardia. *N Engl J Med.* 1992;327(11):772-774.

13. Contreras-Valdes FM, Josephson ME. "Frog Sign" in atrioventricular nodal reentrant tachycardia. *N Engl J Med.* 2016;374(15):e17.

14. Brugada J, Katritsis DG, Arbelo E, et al. 2019 ESC Guidelines for the management of patients with supraventricular tachycardia. *Eur Heart J.* 2020;41(5):655-720.

15. Katritsis DG, Josephson ME. Differential diagnosis of regular, narrow-QRS tachycardias. *Heart Rhythm.* 2015;12(7):1667-1676.

16. Roberts-Thomson KC, Kistler PM, Kalman JM. Focal atrial tachycardia I: clinical features, diagnosis, mechanisms, and anatomic location. *Pacing Clin Electrophysiol.* 2006;29(6):643-652.

17. Bogossian H, Ninios I, Frommeyer G, et al. U Wave during supraventricular tachycardia: simulation of a long RP tachycardia and hiding the common type AVNRT. *Ann Noninvasive Electrocardiol.* 2015;20(3):292-295.

18. Nagashima K, Watanabe I, Okumura Y, et al. Ventriculoatrial Intervals ≤70 ms in orthodromic atrioventricular reciprocating tachycardia. *Pacing Clin Electrophysiol.* 2016;39(10):1108-1115.

19. Letsas KP, Weber R, Siklody CH, et al. Electrocardiographic differentiation of common type atrioventricular nodal reentrant tachycardia from atrioventricular reciprocating tachycardia via a concealed accessory pathway. *Acta Cardiol.* 2010;65(2):171-176.

20. Kalbfleisch SJ, el-Atassi R, Calkins H, Langberg JJ, Morady F. Differentiation of paroxysmal narrow QRS complex tachycardias using the 12-lead electrocardiogram. *J Am Coll Cardiol.* 1993;21(1):85-89.

21. Tai CT, Chen SA, Chiang CE, et al. A new electrocardiographic algorithm using retrograde P waves for differentiating atrioventricular node reentrant tachycardia from atrioventricular reciprocating tachycardia mediated by concealed accessory pathway. *J Am Coll Cardiol.* 1997;29(2):394-402.

22. Di Toro D, Hadid C, López C, Fuselli J, Luis V, Labadet C. Utility of the aVL lead in the electrocardiographic diagnosis of atrioventricular node re-entrant tachycardia. *Europace.* 2009;11(7):944-948.

23. Haghjoo M, Bahramali E, Sharifkazemi M, Shahrzad S, Peighambari M. Value of the aVR lead in differential diagnosis of atrioventricular nodal reentrant tachycardia. *Europace.* 2012;14(11):1624-1628.

24. Knight BP, Ebinger M, Oral H, et al. Diagnostic value of tachycardia features and pacing maneuvers during paroxysmal supraventricular tachycardia. *J Am Coll Cardiol.* 2000;36(2):574-582.

25. Katritsis DG, Becker A. The atrioventricular nodal reentrant tachycardia circuit: a proposal. *Heart Rhythm.* 2007;4(10):1354-1360.

26. Jaïs P, Matsuo S, Knecht S, et al. A deductive mapping strategy for atrial tachycardia following atrial fibrillation ablation: importance of localized reentry. *J Cardiovasc Electrophysiol.* 2009;20(5):480-491.

27. Green M, Heddle B, Dassen W, et al. Value of QRS alteration in determining the site of origin of narrow QRS supraventricular tachycardia. *Circulation.* 1983;68(2):368-373.

28. Chen SA, Tai CT, Chiang CE, Chang MS. Role of the surface electrocardiogram in the diagnosis of patients with supraventricular tachycardia. *Cardiol Clin.* 1997;15(4):539-565.

29. Morady F. Significance of QRS alternans during narrow QRS tachycardias. *Pacing Clin Electrophysiol.* 1991;14(12):2193-2198.

30. Crawford TC, Mukerji S, Good E, et al. Utility of atrial and ventricular cycle length variability in determining the mechanism of paroxysmal supraventricular tachycardia. *J Cardiovasc Electrophysiol.* 2007;18(7):698-703.

31. Markowitz SM, Stein KM, Mittal S, Slotwiner DJ, Lerman BB. Differential effects of adenosine on focal and macroreentrant atrial tachycardia. *J Cardiovasc Electrophysiol.* 1999;10(4):489-502.

32. Alzand BS, Manusama R, Gorgels AP, Wellens HJ. An "almost wide" QRS tachycardia. *Circ Arrhythm Electrophysiol.* 2009;2(2):e1-e3.

33. Katritsis DG, Boriani G, Cosio FG, et al. European Heart Rhythm Association (EHRA) consensus document on the management of supraventricular arrhythmias, endorsed by Heart Rhythm Society (HRS), Asia-Pacific Heart Rhythm Society (APHRS), and Sociedad Latinoamericana de Estimulacion Cardiaca y Electrofisiologia (SOLAECE). *Europace.* 2017;19(3):465-511.

34. Katritsis DG, Ellenbogen KA, Becker AE. Atrial activation during atrioventricular nodal reentrant tachycardia: studies on retrograde fast pathway conduction. *Heart Rhythm.* 2006;3(9):993-1000.

35. Katritsis DG, Ellenbogen KA, Becker AE, Camm AJ. Retrograde slow pathway conduction in patients with atrioventricular nodal re-entrant tachycardia. *Europace.* 2007;9(7):458-465.

36. Katritsis DG, Josephson ME. Classification of electrophysiological types of atrioventricular nodal re-entrant tachycardia: a reappraisal. *Europace.* 2013;15(9):1231-1240.

37. Vijayaraman P, Kok LC, Rhee B, Ellenbogen KA. Unusual variant of atrioventricular nodal reentrant tachycardia. *Heart Rhythm.* 2005;2(1):100-102.

38. Katritsis DG, Marine JE, Latchamsetty R, et al. Coexistent types of atrioventricular nodal re-entrant tachycardia: implications for the tachycardia circuit. *Circ Arrhythm Electrophysiol.* 2015;8(5):1189-1193.

39. Crozier I, Wafa S, Ward D, Camm J. Diagnostic value of comparison of ventriculoatrial interval during junctional tachycardia and right ventricular apical pacing. *Pacing Clin Electrophysiol.* 1989;12(6):942-953.

40. Tai CT, Chen SA, Chiang CE, Chang MS. Characteristics and radiofrequency catheter ablation of septal accessory atrioventricular pathways. *Pacing Clin Electrophysiol.* 1999;22(3):500-511.

41. Martinez-Alday JD, Almendral J, Arenal A, et al. Identification of concealed posteroseptal Kent pathways by comparison of ventriculoatrial intervals from apical and posterobasal right ventricular sites. *Circulation.* 1994;89(3):1060-1067.

42. Miller JM, Rosenthal ME, Gottlieb CD, Vassallo JA, Josephson ME. Usefulness of the delta HA interval to accurately distinguish atrioventricular nodal reentry from orthodromic septal bypass tract tachycardias. *Am J Cardiol.* 1991;68(10):1037-1044.

43. Hirao K, Otomo K, Wang X, et al. Para-Hisian pacing. A new method for differentiating retrograde conduction over an accessory AV pathway from conduction over the AV node. *Circulation.* 1996;94(5):1027-1035.

44. Kadish AH, Morady F. The response of paroxysmal supraventricular tachycardia to overdrive atrial and ventricular pacing: can it help determine the tachycardia mechanism? *J Cardiovasc Electrophysiol.* 1993;4(3):239-252.

45. Katritsis DG, Becker AE, Ellenbogen KA, Giazitzoglou E, Korovesis S, Camm AJ. Effect of slow pathway ablation in atrioventricular nodal reentrant tachycardia on the electrophysiologic characteristics of the inferior atrial inputs to the human atrioventricular node. *Am J Cardiol.* 2006;97(6):860-865.

46. Padanilam BJ, Ahmed AS, Clark BA, et al. Differentiating atrioventricular reentry tachycardia and atrioventricular node reentry tachycardia using premature his bundle complexes. *Circ Arrhythm Electrophysiol.* 2020;13(1):e007796.

47. Miles WM, Yee R, Klein GJ, Zipes DP, Prystowsky EN. The preexcitation index: an aid in determining the mechanism of supraventricular tachycardia and localizing accessory pathways. *Circulation.* 1986;74(3):493-500.

48. Knight BP, Zivin A, Souza J, et al. A technique for the rapid diagnosis of atrial tachycardia in the electrophysiology laboratory. *J Am Coll Cardiol.* 1999;33(3): 775-781.

49. Vijayaraman P, Kok LC, Rhee B, Ellenbogen KA. Wide complex tachycardia: what is the mechanism? *Heart Rhythm.* 2005;2(1).107-109.

50. Crawford TC, Morady F, Pelosi F, Jr. A long R-P paroxysmal supraventricular tachycardia: What is the mechanism? *Heart Rhythm.* 2007;4(10):1364-1365.

51. Kalra D, Morady F. Supraventricular tachycardia: what is the mechanism? *Heart Rhythm.* 2008;5(8):1219-1220.

52. Kaneko Y, Nakajima T, Irie T, Ota M, Iijima T, Kurabayashi M. V-A-A-V activation sequence at the onset of a long RP tachycardia: what is the mechanism? *J Cardiovasc Electrophysiol.* 2015;26(1):101-103.

53. Ormaetxe JM, Almendral J, Arenal A, et al. Ventricular fusion during resetting and entrainment of orthodromic supraventricular tachycardia involving septal accessory pathways. Implications for the differential diagnosis with atrioventricular nodal reentry. *Circulation.* 1993;88(6):2623-2631.

54. Nagashima K, Kumar S, Stevenson WG, et al. Anterograde conduction to the His bundle during right ventricular overdrive pacing distinguishes septal pathway atrioventricular reentry from atypical atrioventricular nodal reentrant tachycardia. *Heart Rhythm.* 2015;12(4):735-743.

55. AlMahameed ST, Buxton AE, Michaud GF. New criteria during right ventricular pacing to determine the mechanism of supraventricular tachycardia. *Circ Arrhythm Electrophysiol.* 2010;3(6):578-584.

56. Dandamudi G, Mokabberi R, Assal C, et al. A novel approach to differentiating orthodromic reciprocating tachycardia from atrioventricular nodal reentrant tachycardia. *Heart Rhythm.* 2010;7(9):1326-1329.

57. Rosman JZ, John RM, Stevenson WG, et al. Resetting criteria during ventricular overdrive pacing successfully differentiate orthodromic reentrant tachycardia from atrioventricular nodal reentrant tachycardia despite interobserver disagreement concerning QRS fusion. *Heart Rhythm.* 2011;8(1):2-7.

58. Michaud GF, Tada H, Chough S, et al. Differentiation of atypical atrioventricular node re-entrant tachycardia from orthodromic reciprocating tachycardia using a septal accessory pathway by the response to ventricular pacing. *J Am Coll Cardiol.* 2001;38(4):1163-1167.

59. Gonzalez-Torrecilla E, Arenal A, Atienza F, et al. First postpacing interval after tachycardia entrainment with correction for atrioventricular node delay: a simple maneuver for differential diagnosis of atrioventricular nodal reentrant tachycardias versus orthodromic reciprocating tachycardias. *Heart Rhythm.* 2006;3(6): 674-679.

60. Bennett MT, Leong-Sit P, Gula LJ, et al. Entrainment for distinguishing atypical atrioventricular node reentrant tachycardia from atrioventricular reentrant tachycardia over septal accessory pathways with long-RP [corrected] tachycardia. *Circ Arrhythm Electrophysiol.* 2011;4(4):506-509.

61. Segal OR, Gula LJ, Skanes AC, Krahn AD, Yee R, Klein GJ. Differential ventricular entrainment: a maneuver to differentiate AV node reentrant tachycardia from orthodromic reciprocating tachycardia. *Heart Rhythm.* 2009;6(4):493-500.

62. Ho RT, Mark GE, Rhim ES, Pavri BB, Greenspon AJ. Differentiating atrioventricular nodal reentrant tachycardia from atrioventricular reentrant tachycardia by DeltaHA values during entrainment from the ventricle. *Heart Rhythm.* 2008;5(1): 83-88.

63. Man KC, Niebauer M, Daoud E, et al. Comparison of atrial-His intervals during tachycardia and atrial pacing in patients with long RP tachycardia. *J Cardiovasc Electrophysiol.* 1995;6(9):700-710.

64. Sarkozy A, Richter S, Chierchia GB, et al. A novel pacing manoeuvre to diagnose atrial tachycardia. *Europace.* 2008;10(4):459-466.

65. Padanilam BJ, Manfredi JA, Steinberg LA, Olson JA, Fogel RI, Prystowsky EN. Differentiating junctional tachycardia and atrioventricular node re-entry tachycardia based on response to atrial extrastimulus pacing. *J Am Coll Cardiol.* 2008;52(21):1711-1717.

66. Chen H, Shehata M, Cingolani E, Chugh SS, Chen M, Wang X. Differentiating atrioventricular nodal re-entrant tachycardia from junctional tachycardia: conflicting reponses? *Circ Arrhythm Electrophysiol.* 2015;8(1):232-235.

67. Fan R, Tardos JG, Almasry I, Barbera S, Rashba EJ, Iwai S. Novel use of atrial overdrive pacing to rapidly differentiate junctional tachycardia from atrioventricular nodal reentrant tachycardia. *Heart Rhythm.* 2011;8(6):840-844.

11

Differential Diagnosis of Wide-QRS (>120 ms) Tachycardias

Wide-QRS tachycardias can be ventricular tachycardia (VT), supraventricular tachycardia (SVT) conducting with bundle branch block (BBB) aberration or through a bystander accessory pathway (AP), or an AP-mediated tachycardia, with reported proportions of 80%, 15%, and 5%, respectively.[1,2] The correct diagnosis of VT is critical to management because misdiagnosis and administration of drugs usually used for SVT can be harmful for patients in VT.[3] *Therefore the default diagnosis should be VT until proven otherwise.* The differential diagnosis includes the following (Box 11.1):

1. SVT with BBB. This may arise as a result of preexisting BBB or the development of aberrancy during tachycardia (so-called phase 3 block), which is more commonly a right bundle branch block (RBBB) pattern, because of the longer RP of the right bundle branch.

2. SVT with antegrade conduction over an AP ("preexcited SVT") that participates in the circuit (antidromic atrioventricular reentrant tachycardia [AVRT]) or is a bystander during atrial fibrillation (AF), focal atrial tachycardia/flutter (AT/AFL), atrioventricular nodal reentrant tachycardia (AVNRT).

3. SVT with widening of QRS interval induced by drugs or electrolyte disturbances. Class IC and IA drugs cause use-dependent slowing of conduction, and class III drugs prolong refractoriness at His-Purkinje tissue more than in the ventricular myocardium. They can both result in atypical BBB morphologies during SVT that mimics VT.

4. Pacemaker-related endless loop tachycardia and artifacts can also mimic VT.

Box 11.1 Differential Diagnosis of Wide-QRS Tachycardias

WIDE-QRS (>120 ms) TACHYCARDIAS

Regular

- Ventricular tachycardia/flutter
- Ventricular paced rhythm
- Antidromic AV reentrant tachycardia
- Supraventricular tachycardias with aberration/bundle branch block (preexisting or rate-dependent during tachycardia)
- Atrial or junctional tachycardia with preexcitation/bystander AP
- Supraventricular tachycardia with QRS widening caused by electrolyte disturbance or antiarrhythmic drugs

Irregular

- AF or atrial flutter or focal AT with varying AV block conducted with aberration
- Antidromic AV reentrant tachycardia caused by a nodoventricular/fascicular AP with variable VA conduction
- Preexcited AF
- Polymorphic VT
- Torsades de pointes
- Ventricular fibrillation

AF, Atrial fibrillation; *AP,* accessory pathway; *AV,* atrioventricular; *VA,* ventriculoatrial; *VT,* ventricular tachycardia.

REGULAR WIDE-QRS (>120 ms) TACHYCARDIAS
ELECTROCARDIOGRAPHIC DIFFERENTIAL DIAGNOSIS

If the QRS morphology is identical during sinus rhythm and tachycardia, then this is most likely not a VT. However, bundle branch reentrant VTs and high septal VTs exiting close to the conduction system can have similar morphologies to sinus rhythm. The presence of a contralateral BBB pattern in sinus rhythm is more indicative of VT.

AV Dissociation

The presence of either atrioventricular (AV) dissociation or capture/fusion beats in the 12-lead electrocardiogram (ECG) during tachycardia is a key diagnostic feature of VT (Table 11.1 and Fig. 11.1). AV dissociation may be difficult to recognize because P waves are often hidden by wide QRS and T waves during a wide-QRS tachycardia. P waves are usually more prominent in inferior leads and modified chest lead placement (Lewis lead).[1] The relation between atrial and ventricular events is 1:1 or greater (more atrial than ventricular beats) in most SVTs. AVNRT can be associated with 2:1 conduction,[4] but this is rare. Although ventriculo-atrial conduction can be found in up to 50% of patients with VT and a 1:1 relation is possible, most VTs have a relation less than 1:1 (more QRS complexes than P waves).

Table 11.1 Summary of Key ECG Criteria That Suggest VT Rather Than SVT in Wide-Complex Tachycardia

AV dissociation	Ventricular rate > atrial rate
Fusion/capture beats	Different QRS morphology from that of tachycardia
Chest lead negative concordance	All precordial chest leads negative
RS in precordial leads	Absence of RS in precordial leads
	RS > 100 ms in any lead*
QRS complex in aVR	Initial R wave
	Initial R or Q wave > 40 ms
	Presence of a notch of a predominantly negative complex
QRS axis −90 degrees to ±180 degrees	Both in the presence of RBBB and LBBB morphology
R-wave peak time in lead II	R-wave peak time ≥ 50 ms
RBBB morphology	*Lead V1:* Monophasic R, Rsr', biphasic qR complex, broad R (>40 ms), and a double-peaked R wave with the left peak taller than the right (the so-called rabbit ear sign)
	Lead V6: R/S ratio < 1 (rS, QS patterns)
LBBB morphology	*Lead V1:* Broad R wave, slurred or notched down stroke of the S wave, and delayed nadir of S wave
	Lead V6: Q or QS wave

*RS: beginning of R to deepest part of S.
AV, Atrioventricular; *ECG,* electrocardiogram; *LBBB,* left bundle branch block; *RBBB,* right bundle branch block; *SVT,* supraventricular tachycardia; *VT,* ventricular tachycardia.
Brugada J, Katritsis DG, Arbelo E, et al. 2019 ESC Guidelines for the management of patients with supraventriculartachycardia Eur Heart J. 2020;41(5):655-720.

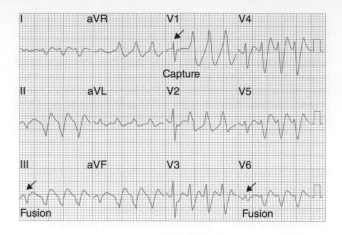

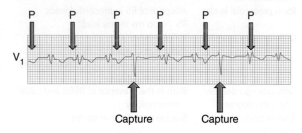

FIG. 11.1. **Fusion and capture beats.**

QRS Duration

A QRS duration greater than 140 ms with RBBB or greater than 160 ms with left BBB (LBBB) pattern suggests VT. These criteria are not helpful for differentiating VT from SVT in specific settings, such as preexcited SVT or when class IC or class IA antiarrhythmic drugs are administered.[5]

QRS Axis

Because VT circuits (especially after myocardial infarction [MI] or in cardiomyopathies) often lie outside the normal His-Purkinje network, significant axis shifts are likely to occur, enabling diagnosis.

Therefore in SVT patients with aberrancy the QRS axis is confined between –60 degrees and +120 degrees. Extreme axis deviation (axis from - 90 degrees to ±180 degrees) in particular is strongly indicative of VT in the presence of both RBBB and LBBB.[2]

Chest Lead Concordance

The presence of negative chest lead concordance (all QRS complexes negative V1–V6) is almost diagnostic of VT with a specificity of more than 90% but only present in 20% of VTs (Fig. 11.2). Positive concordance can be indicative of VT or an antidromic tachycardia using a left posterior or left lateral AP.[6]

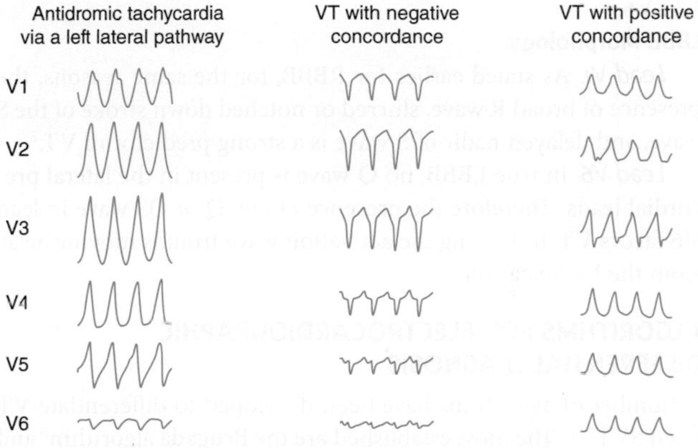

Antidromic tachycardia via a left lateral pathway	VT with negative concordance	VT with positive concordance
V1		
V2		
V3		
V4		
V5		
V6		

FIG. 11.2. **Negative and positive QRS concordance.** *VT*, Ventricular tachycardia.

RBBB Morphology.

Lead V1. Typical RBBB aberrancy has a small initial r′ because in RBBB the high septum is activated primarily from the left septal bundle. Therefore the following patterns are evident: rSR′, rSr′, or rR′ in lead V1. However, in VT the activation wave front progresses from the left ventricle (LV) to the right precordial lead V1, in a way that a prominent R wave (monophasic R, Rsr′, biphasic qR complex, or broad R > 40 ms) will be more commonly seen in lead V1.[7] Additionally, a double-peaked R wave (M pattern) in lead V1 favors VT if the left peak is taller than the right peak (the so-called *rabbit ear* sign). A taller right rabbit ear characterizes the RBBB aberrancy but does not exclude VT.

Lead V6. A small amount of normal right ventricular (RV) voltage is directed away from V6. Because this is a small vector in RBBB aberrancy, the R/S ratio is greater than 1. In VT, all the RV voltage, and some of the left, is directed away from V6, leading to an R/S ratio less than 1 (rS, QS patterns). An RBBB morphology with an R/S ratio in V6 of less than 1 is seen rarely in SVT with aberrancy, mainly when the patient has a left axis deviation during sinus rhythm.

Differentiating fascicular VT from SVT with bifascicular block (RBBB and left anterior hemiblock) is very challenging. Features that indicate SVT in this context include QRS greater than 140 ms, r′ in V1, overall negative QRS in aVR, and R/S ratio greater than 1 in V6.

LBBB Morphology.

Lead V1. As stated earlier for RBBB, for the same reasons, the presence of broad R wave, slurred or notched down stroke of the S wave, and delayed nadir of S wave is a strong predictor of VT.[7]

Lead V6. In true LBBB, no Q wave is present in the lateral precordial leads. Therefore the presence of any Q or QS wave in lead V6 favors VT, indicating the activation wave front is moving away from the LV apical site.

ALGORITHMS FOR ELECTROCARDIOGRAPHIC DIFFERENTIAL DIAGNOSIS

A number of algorithms have been developed to differentiate VT from SVT.[8-10] The most established are the Brugada algorithm[8] and the Vereckei algorithm,[9] which uses a single lead aVR.[11]

RS Interval in Precordial Leads

The absence of RS complex in precordial leads (only R and S complexes are seen on ECG) is only found in VTs (Fig. 11.3). An RS complex is found in all SVTs and in 74% of VTs. The longest interval from the onset of the R wave to the deepest part of the S wave longer than 100 ms, irrespective of the morphology of the tachycardia, is not observed in any SVT with aberrant conduction. About half of the VTs have an RS interval of 100 ms or less and the other half have an RS interval of more than 100 ms. The Brugada et al.[8] algorithm has a sensitivity and specificity of 98.7% and 96.5%, respectively.

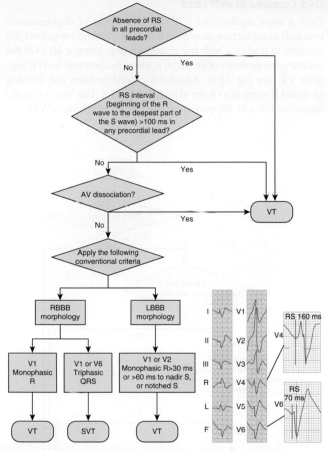

FIG. 11.3. Differential diagnosis of wide QRS tachycardia using the Brugada et al.[8] algorithm. The RS interval measures 160 ms in lead V_4, and 70 ms in lead V_6. Thus the longest RS interval is more than 100 ms and diagnostic of ventricular tachycardia.

AV, Atrioventricular; *LBBB,* left bundle branch block; *RBBB,* right bundle branch block. (Katritsis DG, Boriani G, Cosio F, et al. European Heart Rhythm Association (EHRA) consensus document on the management of supraventricular arrhythmias, endorsed by Heart Rhythm Society (HRS), Asia-Pacific Heart Rhythm Society (APHRS), and Sociedad Latinoamericana de Estimulación Cardiaca y Electrofisiología (SOLAECE). *Europace.* 2017;19:465-511.)

QRS Complex in aVR Lead

During sinus rhythm and SVT, the wave front of depolarization proceeds in a direction away from lead aVR, yielding a negative QRS complex in lead aVR with few exceptions (e.g., inferior MI). On the contrary, the presence of an initial R wave (Rs complex) in aVR suggests VT (see Fig. 11.5). Additional criteria in cases not showing an initial R wave in aVR are shown in Fig. 11.4. The Vereckei et al.[9] algorithm has a 91.5% overall accuracy in the diagnosis of VTs.

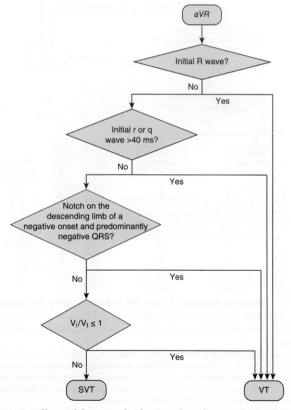

FIG. 11.4. Differential diagnosis of wide-QRS tachycardia using the Vereckei et al.[9] algorithm. In the lower panel the crossing points of the *vertical lines* with the QRS contour in lead aVR show the onset and end of the QRS complex in lead aVR.

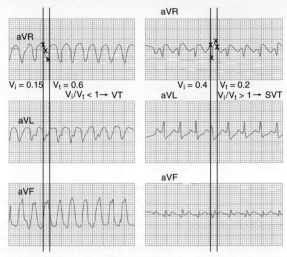

FIG. 11.4, cont'd The crossing points and initial and terminal 40 ms of the chosen QRS complex are marked by *small crosses*; v_i/v_t is the ventricular activation velocity ratio determined by measuring the vertical excursion in mV recorded on the electrocardiogram during the initial (v_i) and terminal (v_t) 40 ms of the QRS complex. *Left:* During the initial 40 ms of the QRS, the depolarization progressed vertically 0.15 mV; therefore v_i = 0.15. During the terminal 40 ms of the QRS, the depolarization progressed vertically 0.6 mV; therefore v_t = 0.6. Thus $v_i/v_t < 1$ yields a diagnosis of VT. *Right:* Determined the same way as in the left panel, v_i = 0.4 and v_t = 0.2; thus $v_i/v_t > 1$ suggests a diagnosis of SVT.

SVT, Supraventricular tachycardia; *VT,* ventricular tachycardia. (Katritsis DG, Boriani G, Cosio F, et al. European Heart Rhythm Association (EHRA) consensus document on the management of supraventricular arrhythmias, endorsed by Heart Rhythm Society (HRS), Asia-Pacific Heart Rhythm Society (APHRS), and Sociedad Latinoamericana de Estimulación Cardiaca y Electrofisiologia (SOLAECE). *Europace.* 2017;19:465-511.)

R-Wave Peak Time at Lead II ≥50 ms

This criterion has the potential advantage that lead II is a lead easy to obtain and it almost always is present on ECG rhythm strips recorded in different settings (e.g., ECG monitoring in emergency departments and intensive care units). The R-wave peak time at lead II 50 ms or greater, independent of whether the complex is positive or negative, has been reported to have a sensitivity of 93% and a specificity of 99% for identifying VT (Fig. 11.5),[10] but these results were not verified in the first large external application of this criterion.[12]

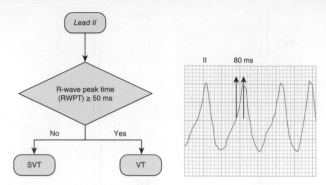

FIG. 11.5. Measurement of the R-wave peak time (RWPT) in lead II. R-wave peak time (RWPT) measured from the isoelectric line to the point of first change in polarity was greater than 50 ms (80 ms).

SVT, Supraventricular tachycardia; *VT*, ventricular tachycardia. (Katritsis DG, Boriani G, Cosio F, et al. European Heart Rhythm Association (EHRA) consensus document on the management of supraventricular arrhythmias, endorsed by Heart Rhythm Society (HRS), Asia-Pacific Heart Rhythm Society (APHRS), and Sociedad Latinoamericana de Estimulación Cardiaca y Electrofisiologia (SOLAECE). *Europace.* 2017;19:465-511.)

All these criteria have limitations. Conditions like bundle branch reentrant tachycardia, fascicular VT, VT with exit site close to the His-Purkinje system, and wide-QRS tachycardia occurring during antiarrhythmic drug treatment are difficult to diagnose by using mentioned morphologic criteria. This is most pronounced in VT originating from septal sites, particularly Purkinje sites and the septal outflow tract regions.[13] Left posterior fascicular VT, the most common form of idiopathic left ventricular VT, is often misdiagnosed as SVT with RBBB and left anterior hemiblock (LAH) aberration (Fig. 11.6).[14]

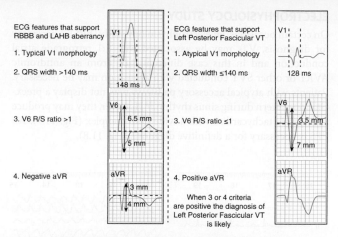

ECG features that support RBBB and LAHB aberrancy	ECG features that support Left Posterior Fascicular VT
1. Typical V1 morphology	1. Atypical V1 morphology
2. QRS width >140 ms	2. QRS width ≤140 ms
3. V6 R/S ratio >1	3. V6 R/S ratio ≤1
4. Negative aVR	4. Positive aVR

When 3 or 4 criteria are positive the diagnosis of Left Posterior Fascicular VT is likely

FIG. 11.6. Differentiating posterior fascicular ventricular tachycardia from right bundle branch block (RBBB) and left anterior hemiblock aberrancy.
ECG, Electrocardiogram; *LAHB*, left anterior hemiblock aberrancy. (Michowitz Y, Tovia-Brodie O, Heusler I, et al. Differentiating the QRS morphology of posterior fascicular ventricular tachycardia from right bundle branch block and left anterior hemiblock aberrancy. *Circ Arrhythm Electrophysiol.* 2017;10(9):e005074.)

Differentiation between VT and antidromic AVRT can be difficult because the QRS morphology in antidromic AVRT can be similar to that of a VT that arises near the mitral annulus, where an AP would insert. A diagnostic algorithm has been developed based on the analysis of 267 wide-QRS tachycardias that were either VT or antidromic AVRT. The derived criteria were found to have a sensitivity of 75% and specificity of 100%,[15] and the algorithm was also validated in another study,[16] but experience is still limited.

Several other studies have found that various ECG-based algorithms have specificities of 40% to 80% and accuracies of approximately 75%.[6,14,17-20] Indeed, a similar diagnostic accuracy of approximately 75% would be achieved effortlessly by considering every wide-QRS tachycardia to be a VT, because only 25% to 30% are SVTs. Therefore emerging approaches to integrate these algorithms to provide more accurate scoring systems are being evaluated.[21]

ELECTROPHYSIOLOGY STUDY

On certain occasions, an electrophysiology study (EPS) is necessary for diagnosis. VTs may be associated with 1:1 retrograde atrial conduction and in this case differentiation from an antidromic AVRT or other SVT conducted with aberration may be necessary. Patients with atypical accessory pathways may not display a preexcitation pattern during sinus rhythm.[22] However, they may produce antidromic tachycardias with a wide QRS complex (Fig. 11.7). An EPS is necessary for a definitive diagnosis (Fig. 11.8).

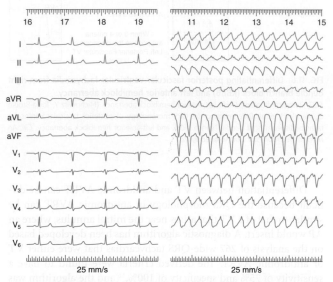

FIG. 11.7. Twelve-lead electrocardiograms (ECGs) during sinus rhythm *(left panel)* **and a wide QRS tachycardia** *(right panel)* **in a patient with an atypical atriofascicular pathway.** The tachycardia represents antidromic atrioventricular reentrant tachycardia.

I, II, II, aVR, aVL, aVF, V1 to V6, Surface ECG leads. (From Katritsis DG, Wellens HJ, Josephson ME. Mahaim accessory pathways. *Arrhythm Electrophysiol Rev.* 2017;6:29-32.)

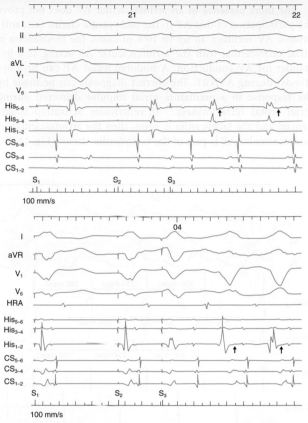

FIG. 11.8 Induction of tachycardia by atrial and ventricular pacing (same patient as in Fig. 11.7). *Upper panel:* During constant atrial pacing at a cycle length of 500 ms the surface electrocardiogram (ECG) is preexcited. The last extrastimulus at 320 ms induces maximum preexcitation and thus indicates conduction along the Mahaim fiber. The impulse activates the His retrogradely *(arrows)* through the right bundle branch and then through the slow pathway of the atrioventricular (AV) node is conducted to the atria. *Lower panel:* During constant atrial pacing at a cycle length of 500 ms retrograde atrial activation is concentric through the AV node. The last extrastimulus at 260 ms results in prolonged retrograde conduction that returns antegradely via the Mahaim pathway. The next beat is a typical antidromic reentry beat with the His bundle *(arrow)* being activated retrogradely through the right bundle branch and then through the slow pathway of the AV node (as indicated by the prolonged activation time) to the atria.

I, II, III, aVL, aVR, V1, and *V6,* Surface ECG leads; *CS,* coronary sinus; *His,* His bundle; *HRA,* high right atrium. (Katritsis DG, Wellens HJ, Josephson ME. Mahaim accessory pathways. *Arrhythm Electrophysiol Rev.* 2017;6:29-32.)

The mere presence of an atriofascicular AP does not prove the participation of that AP in the tachycardia circuit (i.e., antidromic AV reentry). In up to 10% of cases, the mechanism is atrial tachycardia, with the atriofascicular AP acting as a bystander for AV conduction. A nodofascicular AP can be a bystander during AVNRT. The correct diagnosis can be made by the response to a premature atrial impulse delivered during atrial septal refractoriness.[23] If ventricular activation is advanced and the tachycardia is reset, then the atriofascicular or nodofascicular AP is part of the tachycardia circuit (Fig. 11.9).

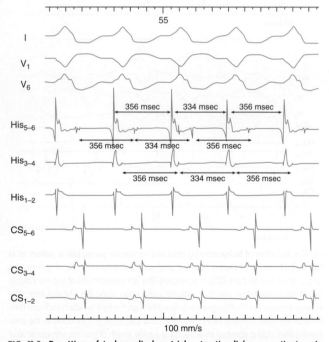

FIG. 11.9. Resetting of tachycardia by atrial extrastimuli (same patient as in Fig. 11.7). Note advancement of the ventricular, retrograde His, and atrial electrograms by 22 ms without a change in retrograde activation sequence.

I, V1, and *V6,* Surface ECG leads; *CS,* coronary sinus; *His,* His bundle. (Katritsis DG, Wellens HJ, Josephson ME. Mahaim accessory pathways. *Arrhythm Electrophysiol Rev.* 2017;6:29-32.)

Entrainment maneuvers, as described in Chapter 10 for narrow-QRS tachycardias, may also be employed. Fig. 11.10 demonstrates overdrive V pacing during a wide-QRS tachycardia.[24] The postpacing interval is within 55 ms of the tachycardia cycle length (TCL), indicating that the right ventricular apex is close to the tachycardia circuit, which excludes the diagnosis of AVNRT. The stimulus-to-atrial electrogram (SA) interval during pacing is within 50 ms of the VA interval during tachycardia, which also is inconsistent with AVNRT (see Chapter 10). The diagnosis is antidromic AVRT caused by an atriofascicular accessory pathway.

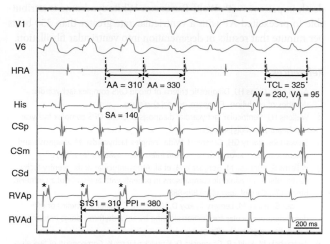

FIG. 11.10. Overdrive pacing from the right ventricular apex during left bundle branch block tachycardia. The tachycardia cycle length (TCL) was 325 ms, with atrioventricular (AV) and ventriculoatrial (VA) intervals as indicated. The last three beats of overdrive pacing are shown (asterisks), with acceleration of the AA interval to the pacing rate, followed by continuation of the tachycardia. The postpacing interval (PPI) exceeded the TCL by 55 ms, and the stimulus-to-atrial (SA) interval exceeded the VA interval by 45 ms.

I, aVF, V1, and V6, Electrocardiogram leads; *CSp, CSm, CSd,* proximal, mid, and distal coronary sinus; *His,* His bundle; *HRA,* high right atrium; *RVAd,* distal ventricular apex; *RVAp,* proximal right ventricular apex. (Quinn FR, Mitchell LB, Mardell A, et al. Overdrive ventricular pacing to clarify the diagnosis of a left bundle branch block morphology tachycardia. *Heart Rhythm.* 2008;5(10):1479-1481.)

IRREGULAR WIDE-QRS (>120 ms) TACHYCARDIAS

The differential diagnosis of an irregular wide QRS tachycardia is either preexcited AF or polymorphic VT or atrial tachycardias with variable block in the context of aberrancy. Preexcited AF manifests itself by irregularity, a varying QRS morphology, and a rapid ventricular rate (as a result of the short RP of the AP). The changing QRS morphology results from varying degrees of fusion caused by activation over both the AP and the AV node, which also results in variation in the width of the delta wave. Another cause of variable QRS morphology during preexcited AF is the presence of more than one anterogradely conducting AP with variable fusion. The ventricular rate generally is high in preexcited AF.[25] The increased risk of sudden death in patients with Wolff-Parkinson-White syndrome is attributable to preexcited AF with a ventricular rate greater than 350 beats per minute that results in degeneration into ventricular fibrillation.

References

1. Alzand BS, Crijns HJ. Diagnostic criteria of broad QRS complex tachycardia: decades of evolution. *Europace*. 2011;13(4):465-472.
2. Wellens HJ. Ventricular tachycardia: diagnosis of broad QRS complex tachycardia. *Heart*. 2001;86(5):579-585.
3. Stewart RB, Bardy GH, Greene H. Wide complex tachycardia: Misdiagnosis and outcome after emergent therapy. *Ann Intern Med*. 1986;104(6):766-771.
4. Willems S, Shenasa M, Borggrefe M, et al. Atrioventricular nodal reentry tachycardia: electrophysiologic comparisons in patients with and without 2:1 infra-His block. *Clin Cardiol*. 1993;16(12):883-888.
5. Ranger S, Talajic M, Lemery R, Roy D, Villemaire C, Nattel S. Kinetics of use-dependent ventricular conduction slowing by antiarrhythmic drugs in humans. *Circulation*. 1991;83(6):1987-1994.
6. Jastrzebski M, Kukla P, Czarnecka D, Kawecka-Jaszcz K. Comparison of five electrocardiographic methods for differentiation of wide QRS-complex tachycardias. *Europace*. 2012;14(8):1165-1171.
7. Kindwall KE, Brown J, Josephson ME. Electrocardiographic criteria for ventricular tachycardia in wide complex left bundle branch block morphology tachycardias. *Am J Cardiol*. 1988;61(15):1279-1283.
8. Brugada P, Brugada J, Mont L, Smeets J, Andries EW. A new approach to the differential diagnosis of a regular tachycardia with a wide QRS complex. *Circulation*. 1991;83(5):1649-1659.
9. Vereckei A, Duray G, Szénási G, Altemose GT, Miller JM. New algorithm using only lead aVR for differential diagnosis of wide QRS complex tachycardia. *Heart Rhythm*. 2008;5(1):89-98.
10. Pava LF, Perafán P, Badiel M, et al. R-wave peak time at DII: A new criterion for differentiating between wide complex QRS tachycardias. *Heart Rhythm*. 2010;7(7):922-926.

11. Katritsis DG, Boriani G, Cosio FG, et al. European Heart Rhythm Association (EHRA) consensus document on the management of supraventricular arrhythmias, endorsed by Heart Rhythm Society (HRS), Asia-Pacific Heart Rhythm Society (APHRS), and Sociedad Latinoamericana de Estimulación Cardiaca y Electrofisiologia (SOLAECE). *Eur Heart J.* 2018;39(16):1442-1445.

12. Jastrzebski M, Kukla P, Czarnecka D, Kawecka-Jaszcz K. Comparison of five electrocardiographic methods for differentiation of wide QRS-complex tachycardias. *Europace.* 2012;14(8):1165-1171.

13. Yadav AV, Nazer B, Drew BJ, et al. Utility of conventional electrocardiographic criteria in patients with idiopathic ventricular tachycardia. *JACC Clin Electrophysiol.* 2017;3(7):669-677.

14. Michowitz Y, Tovia-Brodie O, Heusler I, et al. Differentiating the QRS morphology of posterior fascicular ventricular tachycardia from right bundle branch block and left anterior hemiblock aberrancy. *Circ Arrhythm Electrophysiol.* 2017;10(9):e005074.

15. Steurer G, Gursoy S, Frey B, et al. The differential diagnosis on the electrocardiogram between ventricular tachycardia and preexcited tachycardia. *Clin Cardiol.* 1994;17(6):306-308.

16. Jastrzebski M, Moskal P, Kukla P, Fijorek K, Kisiel R, Czarnecka D. Specificity of wide QRS complex tachycardia criteria and algorithms in patients with ventricular preexcitation. *Ann Noninvasive Electrocardiol.* 2018;23(2):e12493.

17. Ceresnak SR, Liberman L, Avasarala K, Tanel R, Motonaga KS, Dubin AM. Are wide complex tachycardia algorithms applicable in children and patients with congenital heart disease? *J Electrocardiol.* 2010;43(6):694-700.

18. Jastrzebski M, Kukla P, Czarnecka D, Kawecka-Jaszcz K. Specificity of the wide QRS complex tachycardia algorithms in recipients of cardiac resynchronization therapy. *J Electrocardiol.* 2012;45(3):319-326.

19. Lau EW, Ng GA. Comparison of the performance of three diagnostic algorithms for regular broad complex tachycardia in practical application. *Pacing Clin Electrophysiol.* 2002;25(5):822-827.

20. Baxi RP, Hart KW, Vereckei A, et al. Vereckei criteria as a diagnostic tool amongst emergency medicine residents to distinguish between ventricular tachycardia and supra-ventricular tachycardia with aberrancy. *J Cardiol.* 2012;59(3):307-312.

21. Jastrzebski M, Sasaki K, Kukla P, Fijorek K, Stec S, Czarnecka D. The ventricular tachycardia score: a novel approach to electrocardiographic diagnosis of ventricular tachycardia. *Europace.* 2016;18(4):578-584.

22. Katritsis DG, Wellens HJ, Josephson ME. Mahaim accessory pathways. *Arrhythm Electrophysiol Rev.* 2017;6:29-32.

23. Tchou P, Lehmann MH, Jazayeri M, Akhtar M. Atriofascicular connection or a nodoventricular Mahaim fiber? Electrophysiologic elucidation of the pathway and associated reentrant circuit. *Circulation.* 1988;77(4):837-848.

24. Quinn FR, Mitchell LB, Mardell A, Veenhuyzen GD. Overdrive ventricular pacing to clarify the diagnosis of a left bundle branch block morphology tachycardia. *Heart Rhythm.* 2008;5(10):1479-1481.

25. Jolobe OM. Caveats in preexcitation-related atrial fibrillation. *Am J Emerg Med.* 2010;28(2):252-253.

12

Atrial Tachycardias

ATRIAL PREMATURE BEATS

An atrial premature beat (APB) is characterized by a nonsinus P wave that occurs before the next anticipated sinus beat. Several electrocardiographic leads may be needed to distinguish P waves originating in the sinus node versus an ectopic focus. In the rare case of sinus nodal premature beats, the P wave will be identical.[1] The postextrasystolic cycle length is typically less than compensatory because of penetration and resetting of the sinus node by the premature depolarization, but suppression of sinus node automaticity may also occur and result in pauses equal to or longer than the sinus cycle. Intraventricular conduction may be normal or aberrant, whereas the PR interval can be longer than that of the normal sinus beat because of atrioventricular nodal delay. This especially occurs in the rare case of interpolated APBs, which do not depolarize the sinus node and do not affect the sinus rate. Blocked premature beats may masquerade as pauses or bradycardias when P waves are not seen. The T wave of those beats that precede a pause should be carefully inspected to detect any "hidden" premature P wave. Nonconducted APBs are a common cause of unexpected pauses. They can arise anywhere in the atria, including the sinus node.

PHYSIOLOGIC SINUS TACHYCARDIA

Sinus tachycardia is defined as a nonparoxysmal increase in sinus rate to more than 100 beats per minute (bpm) in keeping with the level of physical, emotional, pathologic, or pharmacologic stress.[2,3]

It is due to physiologic influences on individual pacemaker cells and from an anatomic shift in the site of origin of atrial depolarization superiorly within the sinus node.

In normal sinus rhythm, the P wave on a 12-lead electrocardiogram (ECG) in adults is positive in leads I, II, and aVF and V_3 to V_6. It is negative in aVR and V_1 and V_2. In sinus tachycardia P waves have a normal contour, but a larger amplitude may develop and the wave may become peaked.

INAPPROPRIATE SINUS TACHYCARDIA

Inappropriate sinus tachycardia (IST) is a fast sinus rhythm (>100 bpm) at rest or minimal activity that is out of proportion with the level of physical, emotional, pathologic, or pharmacologic stress. The syndrome of inappropriate sinus tachycardia is also defined as a sinus heart rate greater than 100 bpm at rest (with a mean 24-hour heart rate >90 bpm not a result of primary causes) and is associated with distressing symptoms of palpitations.[4,5]

The underlying mechanism of IST remains poorly understood and is likely to be multifactorial (dysautonomia, neurohormonal dysregulation, intrinsic sinus node hyperactivity). A gain-of-function mutation of the pacemaker hyperpolarization-activated cyclic nucleotide-gated *(HCN) 4* channel has been reported in a familial form of IST.[6] There is also evolving evidence that immunoglobulin G anti-β receptor antibodies are found in IST.[7]

Diagnosis

Diagnosis is based on the following:

- The presence of a persistent sinus tachycardia, greater than 100 bpm at rest or greater than 90 bpm on average over 24 hours, during the day with excessive rate increase in response to activity and nocturnal normalization of rate.
- The tachycardia and associated symptoms are usually nonparoxysmal with P-wave morphology and endocardial activation identical to sinus rhythm.
- Exclusion of a secondary systemic cause (e.g., hyperthyroidism, physical deconditioning), and postural orthostatic tachycardia syndrome (POTS).

Catheter Ablation

The limited and disappointing experience with catheter ablation reported in small observational studies suggests that catheter ablation should not be considered as part of the routine management of most patients with IST.[8-14] It may be considered in very symptomatic patients who do not respond to therapy with both a beta blocker and ivabradine.[3] It is aimed at modifying the sinus node with an unavoidable, concomitant risk of iatrogenic sinus nodal disease and the need for permanent pacing. Catheter modification of the sinus node is moderately effective (60%), but the benefits may be short term and can be complicated by the need of permanent pacing in 10% of the patients. Narrowing of the superior vena cava and phrenic nerve palsy may also occur.

SINUS NODAL REENTRANT TACHYCARDIA

Sinus nodal reentrant tachycardia arises from a reentry circuit involving the sinus node and, in contrast to IST, is characterized by paroxysmal episodes of tachycardia.[15] On the ECG, the polarity and configuration of the P waves are similar to the configuration of sinus P waves.[16]

It is unclear whether the reentrant circuit is completely confined to the sinus node or if surrounding atrial tissue is involved.

Diagnosis

Diagnosis is based on the following:

- The tachycardia is paroxysmal.
- P-wave morphology is almost identical to sinus rhythm.
- Endocardial atrial activation is similar to that of sinus rhythm.
- Induction and/or termination of the arrhythmia occurs with premature atrial stimuli.
- Termination occurs with vagal maneuvers or adenosine.
- Induction of the arrhythmia is independent of atrial or atrioventricular (AV) nodal conduction time.

Catheter Ablation

Catheter ablation should be considered in symptomatic patients who do not respond to drug therapy.[17-19] The earliest atrial activation is the site of radiofrequency (RF) current applications, and results have been much better than those with IST, but clinical experience is limited.[17-19]

POSTURAL ORTHOSTATIC TACHYCARDIA SYNDROME

POTS is defined as a clinical syndrome usually characterized by an increase in heart rate of 30 bpm or more when standing for more than 30 seconds (or $\geq$40 bpm in individuals aged 12 to 19 years), and absence of orthostatic hypotension (>20 mm Hg drop in systolic blood pressure).[4,20]

A number of mechanisms have been described, including autonomic nervous system dysfunction, peripheral autonomic denervation, hypovolemia, hyperadrenergic stimulation, diabetic neuropathy, deconditioning, anxiety, and hypervigilance.[20-23]

POTS is diagnosed during a 10-minute active stand test or head-up tilt test with noninvasive beat-to-beat hemodynamic monitoring.[4,20]

FOCAL ATRIAL TACHYCARDIA

Focal atrial tachycardia (AT) is defined as an organized atrial rhythm 100 bpm or greater initiated from a discrete origin and spreading over both atria in a centrifugal pattern. The ventricular rate varies, depending on AV nodal conduction. In asymptomatic young people (younger than age 50 years) the prevalence of focal AT has been reported to be as low as 0.34%, with an increased prevalence of 0.46% in symptomatic arrhythmia patients.[24]

Atrial activation originates from a discrete focus (<1 cm in diameter) with centrifugal spread. Focal AT accounts for up to 10% of SVT referred for ablation.[25] Microreentry, abnormal automaticity, and triggered activity are the possible mechanisms. Focal AT is usually not associated with underlying heart disease, with a prognosis that is benign unless a tachycardia-induced cardiomyopathy develops.

Diagnosis

The P waves during focal AT are distinct, with intervening isoelectric intervals, in contrast to a continuous undulation typical of macroreentrant atrial tachycardia (MRAT). However, an isoelectric interval may not be present during very rapid rates and/or in the presence of atrial disease resulting in slowing of conduction.

Focal AT is characterized by a change in P-wave morphology and by 1:1 AV conduction or second-degree AV block. Most focal ATs arise in the right atrium, usually along the crista terminalis, and less commonly at sites along the tricuspid annulus. Other possible sites of origin include the coronary sinus ostium, mitral annulus, perinodal or para-Hisian region, ostia of the pulmonary veins, left atrial septum, and near the aortic coronary cusps. The morphology of the P wave assists in identifying the tachycardia origin.[26-28] Foci arising from the superior crista terminalis display a negative or positive–negative P wave in lead V1. The P wave may be indistinguishable from that during sinus rhythm. A positive or negative–positive biphasic P wave in V1 and negative P wave in lead I indicates a left atrial focus, whereas a negative or positive–negative P wave indicates a right atrial focus (Figs. 12.1 and 12.2).

The distinction between focal AT and AV nodal reentrant tachycardia or AV reentrant tachycardia can be made by analyzing the R-P relationship on the surface ECG. A variable R-P relationship strongly favors AT.

The diagnosis of focal AT at times can only be established with certainty in the electrophysiology laboratory (see Fig. 12.2).

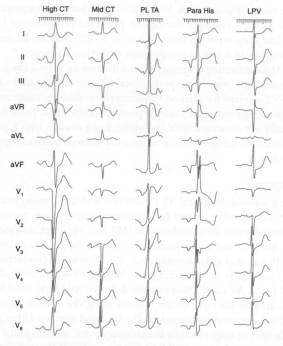

| | High CT | Mid CT | PL TA | Para His | LPV |

FIG. 12.1. P-morphologies of focal atrial tachycardia.
CT, Crista terminalis; *LPV,* left pulmonary vein; *PL,* posterolateral; *TA,* tricuspid annulus. (Markowitz SM, Thomas G, Liu CF, et al. Atrial tachycardias and atypical atrial flutters: mechanisms and approaches to ablation. *Arrhythm Electrophysiol Rev.* 2019;8:131-137.)

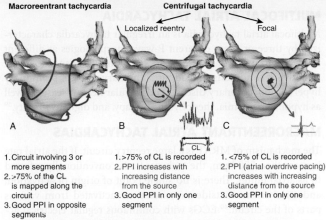

Macroreentrant tachycardia **Centrifugal tachycardia**

Localized reentry   Focal

A   B   C

CL

1. Circuit involving 3 or more segments
2. >75% of the CL is mapped along the circuit
3. Good PPI in opposite segments

1. >75% of CL is recorded
2. PPI increases with increasing distance from the source
3. Good PPI in only one segment

1. <75% of CL is recorded
2. PPI (atrial overdrive pacing) increases with increasing distance from the source
3. Good PPI in only one segment

FIG. 12.2. Different mechanisms of atrial tachycardias. In localized reentry fractionation is present and accounts for a significant part of the cycle length (CL), while in truly focal AT the electrogram at the earliest site is much narrower, with sometimes a preceding sharp activity.

(Katritsis DG, Boriani G, Cosio FG, et al. European Heart Rhythm Association (EHRA) consensus document on the management of supraventricular arrhythmias, endorsed by Heart Rhythm Society (HRS), Asia-Pacific Heart Rhythm Society (APHRS), and Sociedad Latinoamericana de Estimulacion Cardiaca y Electrofisiologia (SOLAECE). *Europace.* 2017;19(3):465-511.)

Catheter Ablation

Catheter ablation is the treatment of choice for recurrent focal AT, especially when the AT is incessant and has caused or may cause a tachycardia-induced cardiomyopathy.[29] Distinguishing macroreentrant ATs from focal ATs is critical for the ablation strategy. Focal ATs display a centrifugal activation pattern that spreads throughout the atria. Mapping and ablation of focal ATs is based on determining the earliest activation site. In pulmonary vein (PV)–related AT, focal ablation may be performed but electrical isolation of both the culprit PV along with other PVs may be preferred. In contemporary studies, catheter ablation is reported to have average acute success rate 85% with a 20% recurrence rate; 1.4% of patients experiencing complications such as vascular complications, AV block, and pericardial effusion; and approximately 0.1% mortality.[30-38]

MULTIFOCAL ATRIAL TACHYCARDIA

Multifocal atrial tachycardia is an irregular tachycardia character-ized by three or more different P-wave morphologies at different rates. Multifocal atrial tachycardia is commonly associated with underlying conditions, including pulmonary disease, pulmonary hypertension, coronary disease, and valvular heart disease, as well as hypomagnesaemia, theophylline therapy, and digitalis toxicity.[39]

MACROREENTRANT ATRIAL TACHYCARDIAS

The mechanism of MRAT is a large reentry circuit. If the atrial rate is more than 250 bpm, the tachycardia is conventionally referred to as atrial flutter. There is no single point of origin of activation, and atrial tissues outside the circuit are activated from various parts of the circuit.[40] ECGs with continuous regular electrical ac-tivity, most commonly but not invariably of the sawtooth pattern, mostly are due to macroreentrant atrial circuits, but microreentry is also possible. However, macroreentrant tachycardias with a sig-nificant part of the activation of the circuit in protected areas may display a focal AT pattern, with discrete P waves.[40]

CAVOTRICUSPID ISTHMUS–DEPENDENT FLUTTER (TYPICAL FLUTTER)

Definitions. Atrial flutter has an atrial rate of 250 to 330 bpm. Cavotricuspid isthmus (CTI)–dependent flutter represents a mac-roreentry circuit around the tricuspid annulus using the CTI as a critical passage at the inferior boundary.[41] The crista terminalis and eustachian ridge are the functional posterior barriers, and the tricuspid annulus the anterior barrier (Fig. 12.3).[42] In typical counterclockwise atrial flutter, activation goes downward along the right atrium (RA) free wall, through the CTI, and upward along the right atrial septum. Activation of the left atrium (LA) is passive (Fig. 12.4). The upper part of the circuit may be anterior or posterior to the superior vena cava. The activation pattern is counterclockwise (or anticlockwise) when viewed from a caudal left anterior oblique perspective.

Counterclockwise (common or typical) isthmus-dependent flutter is characterized electrocardiographically by a sawtooth pattern in the inferior leads and a positive flutter deflection in lead V1 with transition to a negative deflection at some point between V2 and V6. A less common pattern (10%) involves clockwise rotation around the tricuspid annulus.[40] **Clockwise (reverse) isthmus-dependent flutter** shows the opposite pattern (see Fig. 12.4)—that is, positive flutter waves in the inferior leads and wide, negative flutter waves in lead V1, transitioning to positive waves in lead V6).

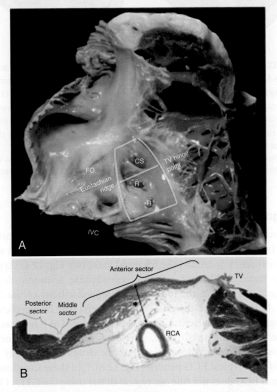

FIG. 12.3. Anatomy of the cavotricuspid isthmus. (A) Heart specimen with area of interest is highlighted. (B) Histologic section of the inferolateral isthmus of an illustrative case. The three sectors of the cavotricuspid isthmus (posterior, middle, and anterior) are indicated. Myocardial thickness is measured at these three levels. The minimal distance between the adventitia of the right coronary artery and the endocardiumis also assessed *(asterisks)*.
(Baccillieri MS, Rizzo S, De Gaspari M, et al. Anatomy of the cavotricuspid isthmus for radio-frequency ablation in typical atrial flutter. *Heart Rhythm.* 2019;116(11):1611-1618.)

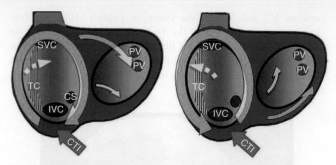

FIG. 12.4. Circuits of CTI-dependent flutter, common (anti-clockwise) and reverse (clockwise). *Left panel:* Common (anticlockwise) flutter. The schema on the right displays the atria in a left anterior oblique view. Mitral and tricuspid rings are enlarged to show the posterior walls. The terminal crest (TC) is shown as a *vertically dashed area* reaching from the superior vena cava (SVC) to the inferior vena cava (IVC). *Right panel:* Reverse (clockwise) flutter. The circular arrow shows typical counterclockwise reentrant activation.

CS, Coronary sinus ostium; *CTI,* cavotricuspid isthmus; *PV,* left pulmonary veins ostia. (Cosio FG. Atrial flutter, typical and atypical: a review. *Arrhythm Electrophysiol Rev.* 2017;6:55-62.)

Diagnosis

The most common patterns of CTI-dependent atrial flutter include a tachycardia showing a counterclockwise rotation in the left anterior oblique view around the tricuspid valve (see Fig. 12.4). Typical atrial flutter (AFL) has a strong reproducible anatomic dependence,[43] resulting in the morphologic reproducibility of the ECG (Fig. 12.5). However, the classic ECG pattern may be significantly changed when atrial activation has been modified as it is in cardiac surgery involving atrial tissue, after extensive RF ablation, or advanced atrial disease.[44,45] Antiarrhythmic drugs (AADs) may also modify the typical ECG pattern (Fig. 12.6).[46] In these situations an atypical ECG does not rule out typical flutter using the CTI.[47] Often there is 2:1 AV conduction with a resultant ventricular rate of approximately 150 bpm. Varying block produces an irregular rhythm, whereas 1:1 conduction may lead to hemodynamic instability. In some cases presenting with 2:1 AV block, the diagnosis of AFL may not be obvious on the ECG. In these situations intravenous adenosine increases the degree of AV block and reveals the typical ECG pattern. However, adenosine can produce a rebound increase in AV conduction to 1:1 and may also precipitate AF.[48,49]

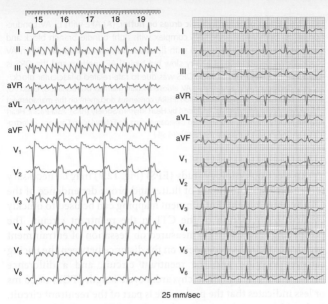

25 mm/sec

FIG. 12.5. A 12-lead electrocardiogram of common and reverse atrial flutter. *Left panel:* In common or typical (anticlockwise) flutter, atrial activity in leads II and III is a continuous undulation with a negative initial deflection and terminal positive deflection (sawtooth pattern). There is a biphasic flutter wave in V1. *Right panel:* In reverse flutter, note the dominant positive deflections in the flutter waves and the W-shaped deflection in lead V1.

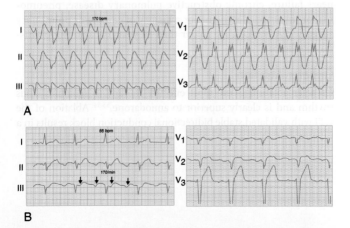

FIG. 12.6. Effect of antiarrhythmic drugs on flutter. (A) AFL with 1:1 AV conduction at 170 bpm and a wide QRS complex with right bundle branch block and superior axis in a patient treated with flecainide for paroxysmal AF. (B) 2:1 AV block allows recognition of a very slow but typical AFL pattern and the QRS is narrow, indicating that the wide QRS was due to rate-related bifascicular block. *AF,* atrial fibrillation; *AFL,* atrial flutter; *AV,* atrioventricular. (Katritsis DG, Boriani G, Cosio FG, et al. European Heart Rhythm Association (EHRA) consensus document on the management of supraventricular arrhythmias, endorsed by Heart Rhythm Society (HRS), Asia-Pacific Heart Rhythm Society (APHRS), and Sociedad Latinoamericana de Estimulacion Cardiaca y Electrofisiologia (SOLAECE). *Europace.* 2017;19(3):465-511.)

An electrophysiology study (EPS) (Fig. 12.7) may be necessary to demonstrate the circuit of flutter and prove dependence of the CTI by entrainment. Entrainment mapping can be used to quickly confirm participation of the CTI in the reentrant circuit. The postpacing interval (PPI) measured on cessation of entrainment overdrive pacing is dependent on the distance between the pacing catheter location and the reentrant circuit, and a difference between the PPI and the tachycardia cycle length (TCL) of 20 ms or less indicates that the pacing site is part of the reentrant circuit. It should be noted, however, that a long PPI may be due to delayed conduction and does not exclude isthmus-dependent flutter (Figs. 12.8 and 12.9).[50] Localized capture without consistent advancement of the other atrial electrograms should be differentiated from true entrainment.

In the majority of patients there is underlying disease, such as heart failure, chronic obstructive pulmonary disease, pneumonia, or myocardial ischemia or a history of cardiac or pulmonary surgery.[51] Advanced age (older than 80 years) is a strong predisposing factor.[52]

Catheter Ablation

Catheter ablation is the most effective therapy to maintain sinus rhythm and is clearly superior to amiodarone.[53,54] Ablation of the CTI with validated stable bidirectional conduction block results in a

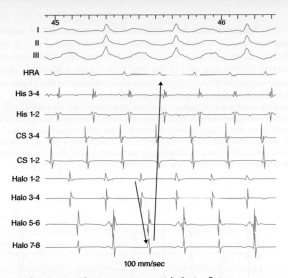

FIG. 12.7. Electrograms during common, anticlockwise flutter.
I, II, III, ECG leads; *HRA,* high right atrium; *His,* His bundle electrogram; *Halo,* Halo multipolar catheter.

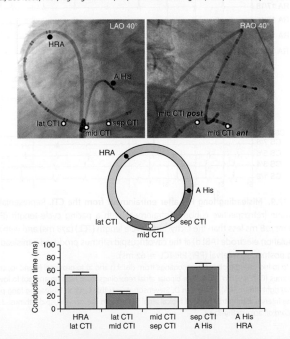

FIG. 12.8. Instrumentation for entrainment and measurement of segmental conduction times. The *white dots* indicate entrainment pacing sites at the cavotricuspid isthmus. *(Top)* Catheter position on fluoroscopy. *(Middle)* Schematic illustrating the five segments of the atrial flutter circuit (LAO view). *(Bottom)* Baseline segmental atrial conduction times during atrial flutter (mean values with standard error, data from the prospective study).

A His, Atrial signal at the His position; *HRA,* high right atrium; *LAO,* left anterior oblique; *lat CTI,* lateral cavotricuspid isthmus; *mid CTI ant,* anterior mid cavotricuspid isthmus (close to the tricuspid valve); *mid CTI post,* posterior mid cavotricuspid isthmus (close to the inferior vena cava); *RAO,* right anterior oblique view; *sep CTI,* septal cavotricuspid isthmus. (Vollmann D, Stevenson WG, Luthje L, et al. Misleading long post-pacing interval after entrainment of typical atrial flutter from the cavotricuspid isthmus. *J Am Coll Cardiol.* 2012;59:819-824.)

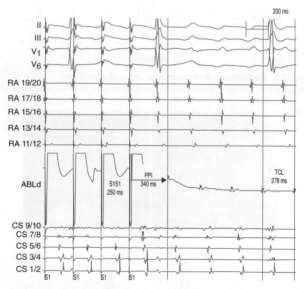

FIG. 12.9. Misleading long PPI after entrainment from the CTI. Representative example (retrospective cohort). Entrainment with a pacing cycle length (PCL) (250 ms) 28 ms less than the tachycardia cycle length (TCL) (278 ms) and with the stimulation electrode (ABLd) at the cavotricuspid isthmus produced a misleading long postpacing interval (PPI; PPI-TCL = 62 ms).

CS 1 to 10 indicates bipolar atrial recordings from distal (1 and 2) to proximal (9 and 10) coronary sinus (CS); *RA 11 to 20* indicate bipolar atrial recordings from high (19 and 20) to low (11 and 12) right atrium (RA). (Vollmann D, Stevenson WG, Luthje L, et al. Misleading long postpacing interval after entrainment of typical atrial flutter from the cavotricuspid isthmus. *J Am Coll Cardiol.* 2012;59:819-824.)

recurrence rate less than 10%.[55] However, the incidence of AF is high in the long term.[56] When typical CTI-dependent AFL ensues during antiarrhythmic drug therapy (class IC or amiodarone) for AF, CTI ablation is an acceptable choice to ensure that an AAD can be continued for AF control.[53,54]

On completion of the ablation line, complete bidirectional block should be confirmed to avoid recurrences of the flutter. This can be achieved by noting reversal of conduction along a duo-decapolar Halo catheter positioned around the tricuspid annulus and along the CTI, during coronary sinus, and mid-Halo pacing. Instead of from pairs 1–2 toward 9–10, the activation sequence is earlier at 9–10 and latest at 1–2, and vice versa, respectively (Figs. 12.10 and 12.11).[57]

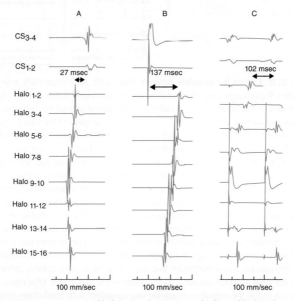

FIG. 12.10. **Demonstration of bidirectional cavotricuspid isthmus block with pacing maneuvers.** The Halo catheter is positioned around the tricuspid annulus, with electrodes 1–2 close to the ablation line on the cavotricuspid isthmus. (A) Normal activation during sinus rhythm before ablation. (B) After ablation, CS pacing demonstrates absence of conduction across the isthmus, with activation of atrial electrograms recorded by the Halo complete isthmus being consistent with conduction only in the counterclockwise direction. (C) After ablation, right lateral atrial pacing through the Halo demonstrates absence of conduction across the isthmus, with conduction only in the clockwise direction and delayed activation of the CS. *CS,* Coronary sinus; *Halo,* Halo multipolar catheter.

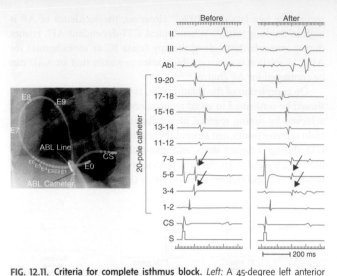

FIG. 12.11. Criteria for complete isthmus block. *Left:* A 45-degree left anterior oblique fluoroscopic view of catheter positions during atrial flutter ablation (ABL) is shown. A duo-decapolar halo catheter is positioned around the tricuspid annulus and along the cavotricuspid isthmus. Electrode pairs of the halo catheter are labeled E1 to E9. Note that E1 and E2 are positioned just lateral to the intended ABL line. A quadripolar electrode catheter is positioned within the coronary sinus (CS) for pacing. The ABL catheter is positioned at the intended ABL line. *Right:* Shown are leads II and III, a recording obtained with the ablation catheter *(Abl)* positioned on the ablation line in the cavotricuspid isthmus, recordings from the 20-pole catheter, a coronary sinus electrogram *(CS)*, and a stimulus channel *(S)*. Electrodes 3–4 and 5–6 were positioned just lateral to the ablation line. The recordings were obtained during coronary sinus pacing. Before complete isthmus block, the atrial activation pattern recorded with the 20-pole catheter was consistent with conduction across the cavotricuspid isthmus, the initial electrogram polarity was positive at electrodes 3–4 and 5–6 of the 20-pole catheter *(arrows)*, and the atrial potential recorded on the ablation line was single. After complete isthmus block, the activation sequence was consistent with conduction only in the counterclockwise direction around the tricuspid annulus, the initial electrogram polarity became negative at electrodes 3–4 and 5–6, and there was a double potential with an interval of 125 ms between the two components at this site along the ablation line.

(Tada H, Oral H, Ozaydin M, et al. Randomized comparison of anatomic and electrogram mapping approaches to ablation of typical atrial flutter. *J Cardiovasc Electrophysiol.* 2002;13:662-666.)

Double potentials have also been considered a reliable criterion of CTI block in patients undergoing RF ablation of typical atrial flutter. An interval separating the two components of double potentials greater than 110 ms along the entire ablation line was always associated with complete block (Fig. 12.12).[58]

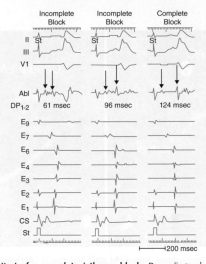

FIG. 12.12. Criteria for complete isthmus block. Recordings during coronary sinus (CS) pacing before (*left* and *middle*) and after (*right*) complete isthmus block are shown. Displayed are leads II, III, and V1, electrograms recorded by the ablation catheter (Abl), electrograms recorded at E9 through E1 of the halo catheter, an electrogram recorded in the CS and the stimulus (St) channel. The *arrows* in the electrograms recorded by the Abl point to the components of the double potentials (DPs). The Abl was positioned at exactly the same site in all three panels. *(Left)* After several applications of radiofrequency energy along the ablation line, the interval separating the two components of DPs (DP1–2) is 61 ms, and there is incomplete block. *(Middle)* After an additional application of radiofrequency energy, the DP1–2 interval increases to 96 ms, but isthmus block is still incomplete. *(Right)* After a final application of radiofrequency energy, the DP1–2 interval lengthens to 124 ms, and now there is complete block, based on both the atrial activation sequence in E1 to E9 and a change in the initial polarity of E1 and E2 from positive to negative. Note that when the DP1–2 interval was 96 ms, the segment separating the two components of the DP was not isoelectric, providing further evidence that there was a persistent gap in the ablation line. On the transition to complete block, the segment with the DP became isoelectric. (Tada H, Oral H, Sticherling C, et al. Double potentials along the ablation line as a guide to radiofrequency ablation of typical atrial flutter. *J Am Coll Cardiol.* 2001;38:750-755.)

When a Halo catheter is not used, demonstration of block can be accomplished by pacing from both sides of the isthmus ablation line (Figs. 12.13–12.18). Electroanatomic activation mapping during pacing at both sides of the ablation line also can be used to verify complete block, but this is unnecessarily time consuming.

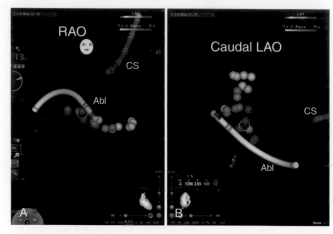

FIG. 12.13. Electroanatomic images of RAO and caudal LAO views of the ablation catheter *(Abl)* positioned just lateral to the ablation line created in the cavotricuspid isthmus. The ablation tags vary in color depending on the contact force. A decapolar catheter within the coronary sinus (CS) is partially seen. *LAO,* Left anterior oblique; *RAO,* right anterior oblique.

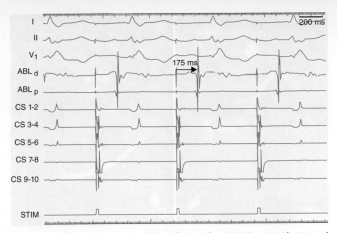

FIG. 12.14. Pacing at 600 ms from the mid-CS as shown in Fig. 12.13. The interval between the pacing stimulus and the electrogram recorded just lateral to the ablation line is 175 ms.

I, II, and V1, Electrocardiogram leads; *ABL p,* proximal pair of electrodes of the ablation catheter; *ABL d,* distal pair of electrodes of the ablation catheter; *CS,* coronary sinus; *STIM,* stimulus channel.

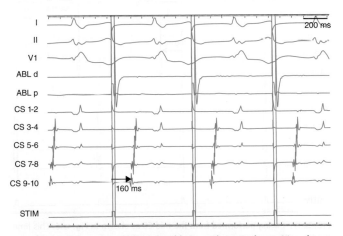

FIG. 12.15. Pacing performed from the ablation catheter at the position shown in Fig. 12.13. The interval between the stimulus and the proximal CS atrial electrogram is 160 ms. (See Fig. 12.14 for abbreviations.)

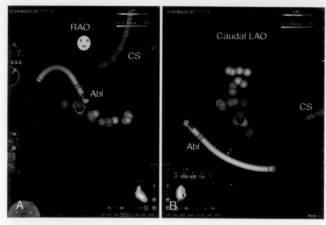

FIG. 12.16. The ablation catheter has been repositioned and is now approximately 2 cm lateral to its initial position in Fig. 12.13.

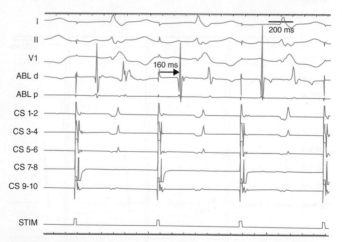

FIG. 12.17. Pacing performed from the mid-CS as shown in Fig. 12.6. This time the interval between the pacing stimulus and the electrogram recorded by the ablation is 160 ms, indicative of complete block across the cavotricuspid isthmus in the clockwise direction. (See Fig. 12.14 for abbreviations.)

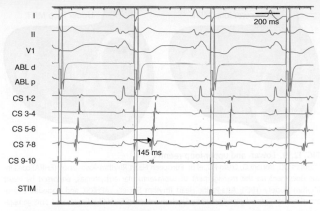

FIG. 12.18. Pacing performed from the ablation catheter at the position shown in **Fig. 12.16.** The interval between the pacing stimulus and the proximal CS atrial electrogram has shortened to 145 ms, indicative of complete block across the cavotricuspid isthmus in the counter-clockwise direction. (See Fig. 12.14 for abbreviations.)

In 2017 and 2018, studies a mortality rate of 0.2% to 0.34% and a stroke rate 0.19% to 0.5% were reported.[34,37] In a 2018 registry, ablation for flutter had a higher mortality than that for AF (0.3% vs 0.05%), but this was most probably because of comorbidities or advanced age of patients referred for flutter ablation.[35] Overall average acute success rate is 95% with a 10% recurrence rate and complications such as vascular complications, stroke, myocardial infarction, and pericardial effusion occurring in approximately 2% of cases.[30-38]

OTHER CTI-DEPENDENT FLUTTERS

An atypical ECG does not exclude CTI-dependent flutter, especially after extensive left atrial ablation.[59] **Lower-loop reentry** refers to a circuit rotating around the inferior vena cava instead of around the tricuspid annulus (Fig. 12.19). It may be clockwise or counterclockwise.[60] When rotating counterclockwise, it might be considered a variant of typical counterclockwise flutter with a caudal shift of the cranial turning point posterior to the entry of the superior vena cava, resulting in a similar ECG appearance. **Figure-of-8 double-loop reentry** may also occur around the inferior vena cava and tricuspid annulus and mimic typical clockwise atrial flutter.[60] Other circuits using part of the CTI or even restricted to the CTI can have a similar ECG appearance to typical common flutter.[61,62]

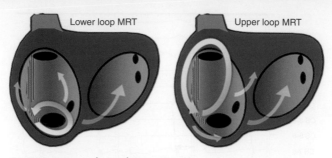

FIG. 12.19. Lower- and upper-loop reentry.
(Katritsis DG, Boriani G, Cosio FG, et al. European Heart Rhythm Association (EHRA) consensus document on the management of supraventricular arrhythmias, endorsed by Heart Rhythm Society (HRS), Asia-Pacific Heart Rhythm Society (APHRS), and Sociedad Latinoamericana de Estimulación Cardiaca y Electrofisiologia (SOLAECE). *Eur Heart J.* 2018;39:1442-1445.)

NON–CTI-DEPENDENT (ATYPICAL) FLUTTERS/MRAT

The terms *non–CTI-dependent MRAT* and *atypical flutter* are used interchangeably, and describe flutter waves in the ECG not suggestive of typical flutter. However, an atypical ECG appearance can be present when typical circuits develop in diseased atria, most often after surgery or extensive ablation, or because of the effects of antiarrhythmic drugs. An EPS is usually required to determine the location of the reentry circuit. **Upper-loop reentry** may mimic a typical flutter ECG pattern without being CTI dependent (see Fig. 12.19).[59] Atypical atrial flutter/MRAT could also arise from upper loop reentry in the RA with conduction through the gap in the crista terminalis.[63] Figure-8 double-loop reentry tachycardias mimicking the ECG pattern of a common atrial flutter may also occur after surgical atriotomy.[64,65] As in other reentrant tachycardias, the difference between PPI and TCL (PPI-TCL) during entrainment mapping is a function of the distance from the pacing site to the reentry circuit. Sites exhibiting negative PPI-TCL values are more commonly located within a narrow isthmus and exhibit slower local conduction velocity compared with sites with classically accepted dPPI values (0 to 30 ms) (Fig. 12.20).[65]

Atypical atrial flutter/MRAT often is scar related and is fairly common in patients who have undergone extensive left atrial ablation for atrial fibrillation or who have an incisional scar in the right atrium after open heart surgery.

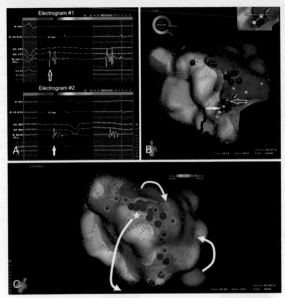

FIG. 12.20. Narrow slow-conducting isthmus and ablation by a complete linear lesion. (A) and (B) Measurement of the local conduction velocity. In this example of a counterclockwise perimitral flutter, conduction velocity is measured around the large black tag indicating a postpacing interval (PPI) of 252 ms (difference between PPI and tachycardia cycle length [TCL; dPPI] = −10 ms). Two representative electrograms are selected on the electroanatomic map along an axis parallel to the path of the wave front (*empty* and *filled arrows*, B). The respective raw electrograms are displayed (A, *empty* and *filled arrows*) to measure the time delay between them (17 ms). The distance is then measured on the electroanatomic map (6.61 mm, *inset top right corner*). *White tags* indicate the path of the leading wave front. *Small black tags* indicate lines of conduction block (before ablation). (C) Final lesion set *(red tags)* consisting of a line between the mitral annulus and the right superior pulmonary vein. Of note, the critical isthmus with dPPI = −10 ms pointed out in (B) was targeted first, resulting in a sustained TCL increase from 262 to 340 ms because of a secondary counterclockwise perimitral flutter with conduction cranially to the anterior left atrial (LA) wall scar. The tachycardia was subsequently terminated by completion of the line from the anterior mitral annulus to the right superior pulmonary vein. LA activation map during right atrial (RA) pacing confirmed the complete line of block by showing posteroanterior activation of the roof and appendage regions in *blue*, delayed compared with LA breakthrough *(star in red area)*. Differential pacing (not shown) was also performed to confirm bidirectional block. *CS*, Coronary sinus.

(Johner N, Shah DC, Jousset F, et al. Electrophysiological and anatomical correlates of sites with postpacing intervals shorter than tachycardia cycle length in atypical atrial flutter. *Circ Arrhythm Electrophysiol.* 2019;12:e006955.)

Right Atrial MRAT

Atrial sutures and patches used for complex congenital heart disease surgery together with progressive atrial damage create multiple obstacles and protected isthmuses that constitute the substrate for complex and multiple MRAT.[66,67] This usually happens around RA free wall scars (Figs. 12.21 and 12.22). However, in patients with complex congenital heart disease, the presence of extensive atrial scars hinders the differential diagnosis of focal or MRATs.[68]

Right atrial MRAT may also occur in the absence of previous intervention. Most of these are sustained around areas of "electrical silence" in the RA free wall, probably as a result of fibrosis.[45,69]

RF ablation of the critical isthmuses of the reentry circuits is the most effective treatment. Circuits around scars of longitudinal atriotomy can be mapped and ablated with good long-term results.[70]

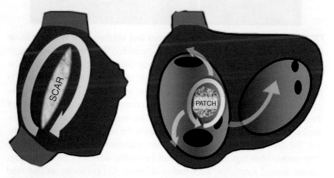

FIG. 12.21. Atrial macroreentry around postoperative scars.
(Katritsis DG, Boriani G, Cosio FG, et al. European Heart Rhythm Association (EHRA) consensus document on the management of supraventricular arrhythmias, endorsed by Heart Rhythm Society (HRS), Asia-Pacific Heart Rhythm Society (APHRS), and Sociedad Latinoamericana de Estimulación Cardiaca y Electrofisiologia (SOLAECE). *European Heart Journal.* 2018;39:1442-1445.)

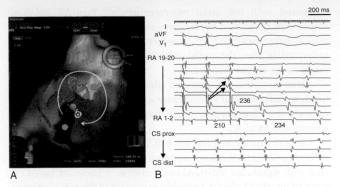

FIG. 12.22. Right atrial MRAT. (A) High-density electroanatomic map generated by the Rhythmia system demonstrates reentry around a line of conduction block (indicated by *blue tags*) in the lateral right atrium (RA). (B) Entrainment from poles 7–8 of a multipolar catheter loop in the lateral RA shows a postpacing interval nearly identical to the tachycardia cycle length. Note that electrograms on more proximal poles RA 11–12 and 13–14, which are activated earlier, are entrained orthodromically with delay. This is an example of downstream overdrive pacing seen with reentrant arrhythmias. *CS,* Coronary sinus.
(Markowitz SM, Thomas G, Liu CF. Atrial tachycardias and atypical atrial flutters: mechanisms and approaches to ablation. *Arrhythm Electrophysiol Rev.* 2019;8:131-137.)

Left Atrial MRAT

Circuits sustaining left atrial MRAT are most commonly caused by electrically silent areas of abnormal tissue after medical interventions or progressive atrial degeneration/fibrosis.[71] Anatomic obstacles such as the ostia of PVs and mitral annulus are often involved.

Because of its widespread use, AF ablation is the procedure that often causes the lesions able to sustain reentry circuits, usually after linear ablation or extensive defragmentation. Localized segmental PVs disconnection may cause focal tachycardias,[72] and circumferential antral ablation may also create MRAT because of gaps in the lines.[65,73-76] AT caused by a small reentrant circuit after ablation of atrial fibrillation often can be distinguished from macroreentry by a shorter P wave duration. Right atrial MRATs have a higher incidence of negative P waves in at least one precordial lead compared with left atrial macroreentry.[77,78] Post-AF ablation MRAT can be ablated by deployment of a stable line of block at critical isthmuses.[56,73,74,79,80] However, intervention to treat these tachycardias after the initial AF ablation should be delayed, if possible, for at least 3 months.[81]

Atrial circuits are also created after *surgery* for different conditions, including mitral valve disease, and are related to incisions or cannulation.[82] Surgery to treat AF may also result in macroreentry circuits and focal AT.[83]

Circuits causing atypical left MRAT may also occur in the LA without prior intervention, commonly, but not invariably, associated with significant left-sided heart disease.[84] These are based on areas of electrical silence, probably as a result of fibrosis, engaging anatomic obstacles such as the ostia of the PVs or the mitral annulus, and may be ablated by interrupting critical isthmuses.[85] Circuits may also happen in the LA septum as a result of slow conduction caused by atrial disease or antiarrhythmic drugs.[86]

References

1. Katritsis DG, Boriani G, Cosio FG, et al. European Heart Rhythm Association (EHRA) consensus document on the management of supraventricular arrhythmias, endorsed by Heart Rhythm Society (HRS), Asia-Pacific Heart Rhythm Society (APHRS), and Sociedad Latinoamericana de Estimulacion Cardiaca y Electrofisiologia (SOLAECE). *Europace.* 2016.

2. Page RL, Joglar JA, Caldwell MA, et al. 2015 ACC/AHA/HRS guideline for the management of adult patients with supraventricular tachycardia: executive summary: A Report of the American College of Cardiology/American Heart Association Task Force on Clinical Practice Guidelines and the Heart Rhythm Society. *J Am Coll Cardiol.* 2016;67(13):1575-1623.

3. Brugada J, Katritsis DG, Arbelo E, et al. 2019 ESC Guidelines for the management of supraventricular tachycardias. *Eur Heart J.* 2020;41(5):655-720.

4. Sheldon RS, Grubb BP, Olshansky B, et al. 2015 heart rhythm society expert consensus statement on the diagnosis and treatment of postural tachycardia syndrome, inappropriate sinus tachycardia, and vasovagal syncope. *Heart Rhythm.* 2015;12(6):e41-e63.

5. Olshansky B, Sullivan RM. Inappropriate sinus tachycardia. *Europace.* 2019;21(2):194-207.

6. Baruscotti M, Bucchi A, Milanesi R, et al. A gain-of-function mutation in the cardiac pacemaker HCN4 channel increasing cAMP sensitivity is associated with familial Inappropriate Sinus Tachycardia. *Eur Heart J.* 2017;38(4):280-288.

7. Ruzieh M, Moustafa A, Sabbagh E, Karim MM, Karim S. Challenges in treatment of inappropriate sinus tachycardia. *Curr Cardiol Rev.* 2018;14(1):42-44.

8. Man KC, Knight B, Tse HF, et al. Radiofrequency catheter ablation of inappropriate sinus tachycardia guided by activation mapping. *J Am Coll Cardiol.* 2000;35(2):451-457.

9. Marrouche NF, Beheiry S, Tomassoni G, et al. Three-dimensional nonfluoroscopic mapping and ablation of inappropriate sinus tachycardia: Procedural strategies and long-term outcome. *J Am Coll Cardiol.* 2002;39(6):1046-1054.

10. Callans DJ, Ren JF, Schwartzman D, Gottlieb CD, Chaudhry FA, Marchlinski FE. Narrowing of the superior vena cava–right atrium junction during radiofrequency catheter ablation for inappropriate sinus tachycardia: analysis with intracardiac echocardiography. *J Am Coll Cardiol.* 1999;33(6):1667-1670.

11. Takemoto M, Mukai Y, Inoue S, et al. Usefulness of non-contact mapping for radiofrequency catheter ablation of inappropriate sinus tachycardia: new procedural strategy and long-term clinical outcome. *Intern Med.* 2012;51(4):357-362.

12. Koplan BA, Parkash R, Couper G, Stevenson WG. Combined epicardial-endocardial approach to ablation of inappropriate sinus tachycardia. *J Cardiovasc Electrophysiol.* 2004;15(2):237-240.

13. Jacobson JT, Kraus A, Lee R, Goldberger JJ. Epicardial/endocardial sinus node ablation after failed endocardial ablation for the treatment of inappropriate sinus tachycardia. *J Cardiovasc Electrophysiol.* 2014;25(3):236-241.

14. Rodriguez-Manero M, Kreidieh B, Al Rifai M, et al. Ablation of inappropriate sinus tachycardia: a systematic review of the literature. *JACC Clin Electrophysiol.* 2017;3(3):253-265.

15. Glukhov AV, Hage LT, Hansen BJ, et al. Sinoatrial node reentry in a canine chronic left ventricular infarct model: role of intranodal fibrosis and heterogeneity of refractoriness. *Circ Arrhythm Electrophysiol.* 2013;6(5):984-994.

16. Gomes JA, Hariman RJ, Kang PS, Chowdry IH. Sustained symptomatic sinus node reentrant tachycardia: Incidence, clinical significance, electrophysiologic observations and the effects of antiarrhythmic agents. *J Am Coll Cardiol.* 1985;5(1):45-57.

17. Malik AK, Ching CK, Liew R, Chong DT, Teo WS. Successful ablation of sinus node reentrant tachycardia using remote magnetic navigation system. *Europace.* 2012;14(3):455-456.

18. Cossu SF, Steinberg JS. Supraventricular tachyarrhythmias involving the sinus node: clinical and electrophysiologic characteristics. *Prog Cardiovasc Dis.* 1998;41(1):51-63.

19. Sanders Jr WE, Sorrentino RA, Greenfield RA, Shenasa H, Hamer ME, Wharton JM. Catheter ablation of sinoatrial node reentrant tachycardia. *J Am Coll Cardiol.* 1994;23(4):926-934.

20. Bryarly M, Phillips LT, Fu Q, Vernino S, Levine BD. Postural orthostatic tachycardia syndrome: JACC foucus seminar. *J Am Coll Cardiol.* 2019;73(10):1207-1228.

21. Benarroch EE. Postural tachycardia syndrome: a heterogeneous and multifactorial disorder. *Mayo Clin Proc.* 2012;87(12):1214-1225.

22. Tomichi Y, Kawano H, Mukaino A, et al. Postural orthostatic tachycardia in a patient with type 2 diabetes with diabetic neuropathy. *Int Heart J.* 2018;59(6):1488-1490.

23. Low PA, Sandroni P, Joyner M, Shen WK. Postural tachycardia syndrome (POTS). *J Cardiovasc Electrophysiol.* 2009;20(3):352-358.

24. Poutiainen AM, Koistinen MJ, Airaksinen KE, et al. Prevalence and natural course of ectopic atrial tachycardia. *Eur Heart J.* 1999;20(9):694-700.

25. Porter MJ, Morton JB, Denman R, et al. Influence of age and gender on the mechanism of supraventricular tachycardia. *Heart Rhythm.* 2004;1(4):393-396.

26. Gonzalez-Torrecilla E, Arenal A, Atienza F, et al. EGC diagnosis of paroxysmal supraventricular tachycardias in patients without preexcitation. *Ann Noninvasive Electrocardiol.* 2011;16(1):85-95.

27. Kistler PM, Roberts-Thomson KC, Haqqani HM, et al. P-wave morphology in focal atrial tachycardia: development of an algorithm to predict the anatomic site of origin. *J Am Coll Cardiol.* 2006;48(5):1010-1017.

28. Markowitz SM, Thomas G, Liu CF, Cheung JW, Ip JE, Lerman BB. Atrial tachycardias and atypical atrial flutters: mechanisms and approaches to ablation. *Arrhythm Electrophysiol Rev.* 2019;8(2):131-137.

29. Medi C, Kalman JM, Haqqani H, et al. Tachycardia-mediated cardiomyopathy secondary to focal atrial tachycardia: long-term outcome after catheter ablation. *J Am Coll Cardiol.* 2009;53(19):1791-1797.

30. Garcia-Fernandez FJ, Ibanez Criado JL, Quesada Dorador A, collaborators of the Spanish Catheter Ablation R, Registry C. Spanish Catheter Ablation Registry. 17th Official Report of the Spanish Society of Cardiology Working Group on Electrophysiology and Arrhythmias (2017). *Rev Esp Cardiol (Engl Ed).* 2018;71(11):941-951.

31. Spector P, Reynolds MR, Calkins H, et al. Meta-analysis of ablation of atrial flutter and supraventricular tachycardia. *Am J Cardiol.* 2009;104(5):671-677.

32. Bohnen M, Stevenson WG, Tedrow UB, et al. Incidence and predictors of major complications from contemporary catheter ablation to treat cardiac arrhythmias. *Heart Rhythm.* 2011;8(11):1661-1666.

33. Keegan R, Aguinaga L, Fenelon G, et al. The first Latin American Catheter Ablation Registry. *Europace.* 2015;17(5):794-800.

34. Steinbeck G, Sinner MF, Lutz M, Muller-Nurasyid M, Kaab S, Reinecke H. Incidence of complications related to catheter ablation of atrial fibrillation and atrial flutter: a nationwide in-hospital analysis of administrative data for Germany in 2014. *Eur Heart J.* 2018;39(45):4020-4029.

35. Konig S, Ueberham L, Schuler E, et al. In-hospital mortality of patients with atrial arrhythmias: insights from the German-wide Helios hospital network of 161 502 patients and 34 025 arrhythmia-related procedures. *Eur Heart J.* 2018;39(44):3947-3957.

36. Katritsis DG, Zografos T, Siontis KC, et al. Endpoints for successful slow pathway catheter ablation in typical and atypical atrioventricular nodal re-entrant tachycardia: a contemporary, multicenter study. *JACC Clin Electrophysiol.* 2019;5(1):113-119.

37. Hosseini SM, Rozen G, Saleh A, et al. Catheter ablation for cardiac arrhythmias: utilization and in-hospital complications, 2000 to 2013. *JACC Clin Electrophysiol.* 2017;3(11):1240-1248.

38. Holmqvist F, Kesek M, Englund A, et al. A decade of catheter ablation of cardiac arrhythmias in Sweden: ablation practices and outcomes. *Eur Heart J.* 2019;40(10):820-830.

39. Kastor JA. Multifocal atrial tachycardia. *N Engl J Med.* 1990;322(24):1713-1717.

40. Saoudi N, Cosio F, Waldo A, et al. Classification of atrial flutter and regular atrial tachycardia according to electrophysiologic mechanism and anatomic bases: a statement from a joint Expert Group from the Working Group of Arrhythmias of the European Society of Cardiology and the North American Society of Pacing and Electrophysiology. *J Cardiovasc Electrophysiol.* 2001;12(7):852-866.

41. Cosio FG. Atrial flutter, typical and atypical: a review. *Arrhythm Electrophysiol Rev.* 2017;6(2):55-62.

42. Baccillieri MS, Rizzo S, De Gaspari M, et al. Anatomy of the cavotricuspid isthmus for radiofrequency ablation in typical atrial flutter. *Heart Rhythm.* 2019;16(11):1611-1618.

43. Olgin JE, Kalman JM, Fitzpatrick AP, Lesh MD. Role of right atrial endocardial structures as barriers to conduction during human type i atrial flutter: activation and entrainment mapping guided by intracardiac echocardiography. *Circulation.* 1995;92(7):1839-1848.

44. Chugh A, Latchamsetty R, Oral H, et al. Characteristics of cavotricuspid isthmus-dependent atrial flutter after left atrial ablation of atrial fibrillation. *Circulation.* 2006;113(5):609-615.

45. Stevenson IH, Kistler PM, Spence SJ, et al. Scar-related right atrial macroreentrant tachycardia in patients without prior atrial surgery: electroanatomic characterization and ablation outcome. *Heart Rhythm.* 2005;2(6):594-601.

46. Havránek S, Simek J, Stovícek P, Wichterle D. Distribution of mean cycle length in cavo-tricuspid isthmus dependent atrial flutter. *Physiol Res.* 2012;61(1):43-51.

47. Barbato G, Carinci V, Tomasi C, Frassineti V, Margheri M, Di Pasquale G. Is electrocardiography a reliable tool for identifying patients with isthmus-dependent atrial flutter? *Europace.* 2009;11(8):1071-1076.

48. Brodsky MA, Allen BJ, Grimes JA, Gold C. Enhanced atrioventricular conduction during atrial flutter after intravenous adenosine. *N Engl J Med.* 1994;330(4). 288-289.

49. Strickberger SA, Man KC, Daoud EG, et al. Adenosine-induced atrial arrhythmia: a prospective analysis. *Ann Intern Med.* 1997;127(6):417-422.

50. Vollmann D, Stevenson WG, Luthje L, et al. Misleading long post-pacing interval after entrainment of typical atrial flutter from the cavotricuspid isthmus. *J Am Coll Cardiol.* 2012;59(9):819-824.

51. Granada J, Uribe W, Chyou PH, et al. Incidence and predictors of atrial flutter in the general population. *J Am Coll Cardiol.* 2000;36(7):2242-2246.

52. Curtis AB, Karki R, Hattoum A, Sharma UC. Arrhythmias in Patients ≥80 years of age: pathophysiology, management, and outcomes. *J Am Coll Cardiol.* 2018;71(18):2041-2057.

53. Natale A, Newby KH, Pisanó E, et al. Prospective randomized comparison of antiarrhythmic therapy versus first-line radiofrequency ablation in patients with atrial flutter. *J Am Coll Cardiol.* 2000;35(7):1898-1904.

54. Da Costa A, Thévenin J, Roche F, et al. Results from the Loire-Ardèche-Drôme-Isère-Puy-de-Dôme (LADIP) trial on atrial flutter, a multicentric prospective randomized study comparing amiodarone and radiofrequency ablation

after the first episode of symptomatic atrial flutter. *Circulation*. 2006;114(16): 1676-1681.

55. Schwartzman D, Callans DJ, Gottlieb CD, Dillon SM, Movsowitz C, Marchlinski FE. Conduction block in the inferior vena caval-tricuspid valve isthmus: association with outcome of radiofrequency ablation of type I atrial flutter. *J Am Coll Cardiol*. 1996;28(6):1519-1531.

56. De Bortoli A, Shi LB, Ohm OJ, et al. Incidence and clinical predictors of subsequent atrial fibrillation requiring additional ablation after cavotricuspid isthmus ablation for typical atrial flutter. *Scand Cardiovasc J*. 2017;51(3):123-128.

57. Tada H, Oral H, Ozaydin M, et al. Randomized comparison of anatomic and electrogram mapping approaches to ablation of typical atrial flutter. *J Cardiovasc Electrophysiol*. 2002;13(7):662-666.

58. Tada H, Oral H, Sticherling C, et al. Double potentials along the ablation line as a guide to radiofrequency ablation of typical atrial flutter. *J Am Coll Cardiol*. 2001;38(3):750-755.

59. Bochoeyer A, Yang Y, Cheng J, et al. Surface Electrocardiographic characteristics of right and left atrial flutter. *Circulation*. 2003;108(1):60-66.

60. Zhang S, Younis G, Hariharan R, et al. Lower loop reentry as a mechanism of clockwise right atrial flutter. *Circulation*. 2004;109(13):1630-1635.

61. Yang Y, Cheng J, Bochoeyer A, et al. Atypical right atrial flutter patterns. *Circulation*. 2001;103(25):3092-3098.

62. Yang Y, Varma N, Badhwar N, et al. Prospective observations in the clinical and electrophysiological characteristics of intra-isthmus reentry. *J Cardiovasc Electrophysiol*. 2010;21(10):1099-1106.

63. Tai CT, Huang JL, Lin YK, et al. Noncontact three-dimensional mapping and ablation of upper loop re-entry originating in the right atrium. *J Am Coll Cardiol*. 2002;40(4):746-753.

64. Shah D, Jais P, Takahashi A, et al. Dual-loop intra-atrial reentry in humans. *Circulation*. 2000;101(6):631-639.

65. Johner N, Shah DC, Jousset F, Dall'Aglio PB, Namdar M. Electrophysiological and anatomical correlates of sites with postpacing intervals shorter than tachycardia cycle length in atypical atrial flutter. *Circ Arrhythm Electrophysiol*. 2019;12(3):e006955.

66. Zrenner B, Dong JUN, Schreieck J, et al. Delineation of intra-atrial reentrant tachycardia circuits after mustard operation for transposition of the great arteries using biatrial electroanatomic mapping and entrainment mapping. *J Cardiovasc Electrophysiol*. 2003;14(12):1302-1310.

67. Ueda A, Suman-Horduna I, Mantziari L, et al. Contemporary outcomes of supraventricular tachycardia ablation in congenital heart disease: a single-center experience in 116 patients. *Circ Arrhythm Electrophysiol*. 2013;6(3):606-613.

68. Akca F, Bauernfeind T, De Groot NMS, Shalganov T, Schwagten B, Szili-Torok T. The presence of extensive atrial scars hinders the differential diagnosis of focal or macroreentrant atrial tachycardias in patients with complex congenital heart disease. *Europace*. 2014;16(6):893-898.

69. Satomi K, Chun KRJ, Tilz R, et al. Catheter ablation of multiple unstable macro-reentrant tachycardia within the right atrium free wall in patients without previous cardiac surgery. *Circ Arrhythm Electrophysiol.* 2010;3(1):24-31.

70. Scaglione M, Caponi D, Ebrille E, et al. Very long-term results of electroanatomic-guided radiofrequency ablation of atrial arrhythmias in patients with surgically corrected atrial septal defect. *Europace.* 2014;16(12):1800-1807.

71. Ouyang F, Ernst S, Vogtmann T, et al. Characterization of reentrant circuits in left atrial macroreentrant tachycardia: critical isthmus block can prevent atrial tachycardia recurrence. *Circulation.* 2002;105(16):1934-1942.

72. Gerstenfeld EP, Callans DJ, Dixit S, et al. Mechanisms of organized left atrial tachycardias occurring after pulmonary vein isolation. *Circulation.* 2004;110(11):1351-1357.

73. Wasmer K, Mönnig G, Bittner A, et al. Incidence, characteristics, and outcome of left atrial tachycardias after circumferential antral ablation of atrial fibrillation. *Heart Rhythm.* 2012;9(10):1660-1666.

74. Satomi K, Bänsch D, Tilz R, et al. Left atrial and pulmonary vein macroreentrant tachycardia associated with double conduction gaps: a novel type of man-made tachycardia after circumferential pulmonary vein isolation. *Heart Rhythm.* 2008;5(1):43-51.

75. Katritsis D, Wood MA, Shepard RK, Giazitzoglou E, Kourlaba G, Ellenbogen KA. Atrial arrhythmias following ostial or circumferential pulmonary vein ablation. *J Interv Card Electrophysiol.* 2006;16(2):123-130.

76. Barbhaiya CR, Baldinger SH, Kumar S, et al. Downstream overdrive pacing and intracardiac concealed fusion to guide rapid identification of atrial tachycardia after atrial fibrillation ablation. *Europace.* 2018;20(4):596-603.

77. Yokokawa M, Latchamsetty R, Ghanbari H, et al. Characteristics of atrial tachycardia due to small vs large reentrant circuits after ablation of persistent atrial fibrillation. *Heart Rhythm.* 2013;10(4):469-476

78. Chang SL, Tsao HM, Lin YJ, et al. Differentiating macroreentrant from focal atrial tachycardias occurred after circumferential pulmonary vein isolation. *J Cardiovasc Electrophysiol.* 2011;22(7):748-755.

79. Miyazaki S, Shah AJ, Hocini M, Haïssaguerre M, Jaïs P. Recurrent spontaneous clinical perimitral atrial tachycardia in the context of atrial fibrillation ablation. *Heart Rhythm.* 2015;12(1):104-110.

80. Ammar S, Luik A, Hessling G, et al. Ablation of perimitral flutter: acute and long-term success of the modified anterior line. *Europace.* 2015;17(3):447-452.

81. Chugh A, Oral H, Lemola K, et al. Prevalence, mechanisms, and clinical significance of macroreentrant atrial tachycardia during and following left atrial ablation for atrial fibrillation. *Heart Rhythm.* 2005;2(5):464-471.

82. Markowitz SM, Brodman RF, Stein KM, et al. Lesional tachycardias related to mitral valve surgery. *J Am Coll Cardiol.* 2002;39(12):1973-1983.

83. Takahashi K, Miyauchi Y, Hayashi M, et al. Mechanisms of postoperative atrial tachycardia following biatrial surgical ablation of atrial fibrillation in relation to the surgical lesion sets. *Heart Rhythm.* 2016;13(5):1059-1065.

84. Zhang J, Tang C, Zhang Y, Han H, Li Z, Su XI. Electroanatomic characterization and ablation outcome of nonlesion related left atrial macroreentrant tachycardia in patients without obvious structural heart disease. *J Cardiovasc Electrophysiol.* 2013;24(1):53-59.

85. Fukamizu S, Sakurada H, Hayashi T, et al. Macroreentrant atrial tachycardia in patients without previous atrial surgery or catheter ablation: clinical and electrophysiological characteristics of scar-related left atrial anterior wall reentry. *J Cardiovasc Electrophysiol.* 2013;24(4):404-412.

86. Marrouche NF, Natale A, Wazni OM, et al. Left septal atrial flutter: electrophysiology, anatomy, and results of ablation. *Circulation.* 2004;109(20):2440-2447.

13

Atrial Fibrillation

DEFINITIONS AND CLASSIFICATION

Atrial fibrillation (AF) is characterized by uncoordinated atrial activation without effective atrial contraction.[1-4] On the electrocardiogram (ECG), AF is characterized by rapid oscillations or fibrillatory waves that vary in amplitude, shape, and timing; that usually have a cycle length less than 200 ms; and that are associated with an irregular ventricular response. QRS complexes may also be of variable amplitude. Regular R-R intervals are possible in the presence of atrioventricular (AV) block, junctional rhythm, ventricular pacing, or ventricular tachycardia.

Paroxysmal AF is defined as AF that terminates spontaneously or with intervention within 7 days of onset. Episodes typically convert back to sinus rhythm within 48 hours. Up to 8% of patients per year with paroxysmal AF progress to persistent AF.[5]

Persistent AF is continuous AF that is sustained beyond 7 days.

Long-standing persistent AF is AF that has lasted for 1 year or longer.

Permanent AF refers to the situation when the presence of the arrhythmia is accepted by the patient and physician. Hence, rhythm control interventions are, by definition, not pursued in patients with permanent AF. However, the "permanent" label does not preclude the option of rhythm control by catheter ablation.

223

Lone (idiopathic) AF has been variously defined but generally applies to young individuals (younger than 60 years) without clinical or echocardiographic evidence of cardiopulmonary disease, including hypertension. Increasing knowledge about the pathophysiology of AF suggests that in almost every patient a cause is present.

Nonvalvular AF is defined by the American Heart Association, American College of Cardiology, and Heart Rhythm Society (AHA/ACC/HRS) as AF in the absence of rheumatic mitral stenosis, a mechanical or bioprosthetic heart valve, or mitral valve repair.[1] The European Society of Cardiology (ESC) has defined nonvalvular AF as AF not related to rheumatic valvular disease (predominantly mitral stenosis) or prosthetic heart valves.[3]

AF can be vagally mediated (e.g., nocturnal, postprandial) and also can be associated with sympathetic overactivity. The terms **vagal** and **adrenergic** AF are oversimplifications because the balance between sympathetic and parasympathetic influences is as important as absolute tone.

ELECTROPHYSIOLOGIC MECHANISMS

Structural remodeling of the atria as a result of heart disease, atrial wall stretch, genetic causes, or other nonidentified mechanisms results in electrical dissociation between muscle bundles and local conduction heterogeneities that facilitate the initiation and perpetuation of AF.[6] Structural atrial abnormalities consist of areas of patchy fibrosis, enhanced connective tissue deposits juxtaposed with normal atrial fibers, inflammatory changes, intracellular substrate accumulation, and disruption of cell coupling at gap junctions with remodeling of connexins (i.e., transmembrane ion channel proteins in the gap junctions).[7] Connexin gene variants are associated with AF, and connexin gene transfer in animal studies has prevented AF.[8] Fibrosis and inflammatory changes, identified by biopsy and delayed enhancement magnetic resonance, have also been documented in patients with lone AF.[9,10]

After the onset of AF, changes of atrial electrophysiologic properties and mechanical function occur within days (>24 hours). Shortening of the atrial effective refractory period results from abbreviation of the atrial action potential duration, which is caused by a decrease in the calcium channel current (I_{Ca}) and an increase in the potassium channel current (I_{K1}) and the constitutively active acetylcholine-sensitive current (I_{KACh}).[8] Increased diastolic sarcoplasmic reticulum Ca^{2+} leak and related delayed after-depolarizations/triggered activity promote cellular arrhythmogenesis.[11] Ryanodine receptor type 2–mediated sarcoplasmic reticulum calcium leak also drives AF progression.[12] Downregulation of the Ca^{2+} inward current and impaired release of Ca^{2+} from intracellular Ca^{2+} stores cause loss of contractility and increased compliance with subsequent atrial dilation. Electrical remodeling of the atria is therefore perpetuated by AF itself in a way that "AF begets AF."[13] Restoration of sinus rhythm results in recovery of normal atrial refractoriness within a few days. LA structure and function are increasingly abnormal with a greater electrical burden of AF, and LA dysfunction may be present despite normal LA size and sinus rhythm.[14]

The initiation and perpetuation of AF requires both triggers for its onset and a substrate for its maintenance (Fig. 13.1).

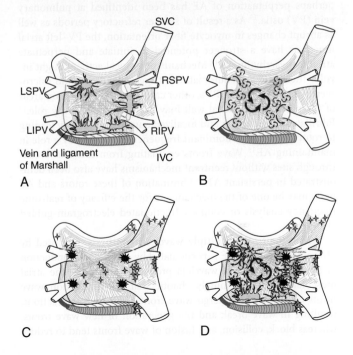

FIG. 13.1. Structure and mechanisms of atrial fibrillation. (A) Schematic drawing of the left and right atria as viewed from the posterior. The extension of muscular fibers onto the pulmonary veins (PVs) can be appreciated. Shown in yellow are the four major left atrial (LA) autonomic ganglionic plexi and axons (superior left, inferior left, anterior right, and inferior right). Shown in blue is the coronary sinus, which is enveloped by muscular fibers that have connections to the atria. Also shown in blue is the vein and ligament of Marshall, which travels from the coronary sinus to the region between the left superior PV and the LA appendage. (B) Large and small reentrant wavelets that play a role in initiating and sustaining atrial fibrillation (AF). (C) Common locations of PV (red) and also the common sites of origin of non-PV triggers (shown in green). (D) Composite of the anatomic and arrhythmic mechanisms of AF.

(Calkins H, Hindricks G, Cappato R, et al. 2017 HRS/EHRA/ECAS/APHRS/SOLAECE expert consensus statement on catheter and surgical ablation of atrial fibrillation. *Europace.* 2018;201:e1-e160.)

Focal electrical activity contributing to the initiation and perhaps perpetuation of AF has been identified at pulmonary vein (PV) ostia.[15] As a result of shorter refractory periods as well as abrupt changes in myocyte fiber orientation, the PV–left atrial junctions have a stronger potential to initiate and perpetuate atrial tachyarrhythmias.[16] Mechanisms of focal activity might involve increased local automaticity, triggered activity, and microreentry. Apart from the PVs, other cardiac veins and certain areas of the posterior left atrial wall may have a profibrillatory role.[17] Fibrillatory conduction and localized anisotropic reentry leading to rotors with a high dominant frequency may also play a role in maintaining AF.[18] Wave fronts emanating from foci and breakthrough sites without reentrant mechanisms have also been demonstrated in persistent AF.[19] Elimination of these rotors and AF nests may be one of the mechanisms for the efficacy of real-time frequency analysis or complex fractionated electrogram-guided ablation.

According to the **multiple wavelet hypothesis**, proposed by Moe and colleagues, AF is perpetuated by continuous conduction of several independent wavelets propagating through the atrial musculature in a seemingly chaotic manner. Fibrillation wave fronts continuously undergo wave front–wave back interactions, resulting in wave break and the generation of new wave fronts, whereas block, collision, and fusion of wave fronts tend to reduce their number. As long as the number of wave fronts does not decline below a critical level, the multiple wavelets will sustain the arrhythmia.

Areas rich in **autonomic innervation** may be the source of activity that triggers AF.[20] Ganglionated plexi that can be identified around the circumference of the left atrial–PV junction may also contribute to induction and perpetuation of AF.[17] These plexi are usually located 1 to 2 cm outside the PV ostia, they mediate both sympathetic and parasympathetic activity, and their ablation (autonomic denervation) has been found efficacious when added to antral PV isolation.[21]

These mechanisms are not mutually exclusive and may coexist at various times. Although in most patients with paroxysmal AF localized sources of the arrhythmia can be identified, such attempts are often not successful in patients with persistent or permanent AF. This can be interpreted within the context of the multifactorial etiology of AF. Mechanisms of AF initiation and perpetuation, particularly in patients with persistent AF, are complex and heterogeneous.[22]

DIAGNOSIS

Patients may present with palpitations or otherwise unexplained fatigue or effort intolerance, or the arrhythmia may be an incidental finding.[23] The cause of stroke remains unexplained in 20% to 40% of cases. Among these unexplained strokes, 10% to 30% may be caused by AF that has eluded detection.[24] Discovery of subclinical AF with **implantable devices** and **wearable monitors** is common, especially in populations known to have an increased risk of stroke (or recurrent stroke).[24] Opportunistic screening for AF in patients 65 years and older is reasonable, and several methods and devices are now available for screening.[24-26] *Wrist-worn*, optically based heart rate monitors are user friendly, but appropriate validation of the device used is imperative.[27] In mechanocardiography, mechanical cardiac activity is recorded with accelerometers and gyroscopes, standard components of modern *smartphones*. High sensitivity and specificity of this method for AF detection with the use of smartphones has been reported.[28] Smartphone technologies have been developed that can assess heart rate and rhythm using either photoplethysmography or single-lead ECG but usually provide only a brief rhythm assessment without information on AF duration or burden.[29-31] In a 2019 comparison, an Food and Drug Administration–cleared AF-sensing watch (*Apple Watch with KardiaBand*) that allows a patient to record a 30-second lead I rhythm strip was found highly sensitive for detection of AF and assessment of AF duration in an ambulatory population compared with an insertable cardiac monitor (*Reveal*).[32] In an evaluation of an Apple Watch Application study, the probability of receiving an irregular pulse notification was low. Among participants who received notification of an irregular pulse, 34% had atrial fibrillation on subsequent ECG patch readings and 84% of notifications were concordant with atrial fibrillation.[33]

Frequent atrial ectopy, atrial tachycardia, and atrial flutter may present with rapid irregular RR intervals and mimic AF. Most atrial tachycardias and flutters show longer atrial cycle lengths 200 ms and greater, but patients on antiarrhythmic drugs may have slower atrial cycle lengths during AF. When the ventricular rate is fast, atrioventricular nodal blockade during the Valsalva maneuver, carotid massage, or intravenous adenosine administration can help to unmask atrial activity. Extremely rapid ventricular rates (>200 beats per minute) suggest the presence of an accessory pathway or ventricular tachycardia.

In the absence of a history of the arrhythmia, AF can be detected by ECG monitoring in approximately one-quarter of all patients with acute ischemic stroke by routine monitoring followed by an intensified or prolonged AF search. Patients with ischemic stroke or transient ischemic attack (TIA) should have continuous ECG monitoring after a stroke for at least 72 hours.[34]

CATHETER ABLATION

Rationale

Randomized controlled drug trials have failed to detect significant mortality and cardiovascular morbidity differences between patients with rate (i.e., controlling ventricular response with the patient in AF) versus rhythm (i.e., maintenance of sinus rhythm [SR]) control achieved with antiarrhythmic medication.[35-43] This is rather surprising in view of the deleterious effects of AF and has been mainly attributed to the *proarrhythmic effects of drugs*, which may negate any benefits conferred by maintenance of SR.[44,45] Assessment of quality of life was also rather inadequate in most trials. In the J-RHYTHM trial, fewer patients requested changes of assigned treatment strategy in the rhythm control versus the rate control group, which was accompanied by improvement in AF-specific quality of life scores.[39] Maintenance of SR also improved quality of life in the SAFE-T trial.[46] Finally, follow-up of most trials was relatively short. However, improved survival with maintenance of sinus rhythm was detected in the CHF-STAT trial (amiodarone in heart failure patients). [47] In an extensive population-based, observational trial, rhythm control therapy was associated with lower rates of stroke/TIA compared to rate control, particularly among patients with moderate and high risk of stroke.[48] In the ATHENA trial, cardiovascular mortality was reduced by dronedarone (3.9% vs 2.7%, $P = .003$).[49] However, dronedarone has resulted in increased mortality in patients with heart failure,[50] and with permanent AF.[51] In a recent meta-analysis of RCTs comparing drugs for rate vs rhythm control, and drugs vs ablation for rhythm control in patients with AF and heart failure, currently available antiarrhythmic drugs for rhythm control did not offer additional benefit in reducing hard endpoints because of the poor efficacy in restoring sinus rhythm and potential toxic effects.[52] In the EAST-AFNET 4 RCT, early rhythm control with either antiarrhythmic drugs or catheter ablation was associated with a lower risk of adverse cardiovascular outcomes than usual care during adequate rate control therapy among patients with early AF and cardiovascular conditions.[53]

Left atrial catheter ablation offers improved rates of SR maintenance compared with antiarrhythmic therapy, being more beneficial in *younger patients and men*. Data mainly from registries and observational studies indicate that average success rates after AF (paroxysmal in 70%) ablation are 57% and 71% after a single and multiple procedures, respectively, with an average follow-up of 14 months, compared with 52% with antiarrhythmic drug therapy.[54] In the MANTRA-PAF randomized trial, 85% of ablated patients versus 71% of medically treated patients with paroxysmal atrial fibrillation (PAF) were free of AF in 2 years ($P = .004$), but the cumulative burden of AF during that time was not significantly different on an intention-to-treat analysis (36% of patients initially assigned to medication eventually had ablation).[55] However, at 5-year follow-up there was a significantly higher rate of AF-free patients in the ablation group.[56] In the RAAFT-2 randomized clinical trial, 45% of patients with PAF were free of arrhythmia 2 years after ablation, compared with 28% of patients on antiarrhythmic therapy.[57] In the SARA randomized trial on patients with persistent AF, 70% of patients were free of arrhythmia at 1 year after ablation, compared with 44% on patients treated with drugs. However, no symptomatic improvement was detected.[58] The CABANA trial randomly allocated 2204 patients to catheter ablation or drug therapy (87.2% received rhythm control). Of the 2204 patients randomized (42.9% had paroxysmal AF and 57.1% had persistent AF), 89.3% completed the trial. Of the patients assigned to catheter ablation, 1006 (90.8%) underwent the procedure. Of the patients assigned to drug therapy, 301 (27.5%) ultimately received catheter ablation. In the intention-to-treat analysis, over a median follow-up of 48.5 months, catheter ablation did not significantly reduce the primary composite end point of death, disabling stroke, serious bleeding, or cardiac arrest that occurred in 8.0% of patients ($n = 89$) in the ablation group versus 9.2% of patients ($n = 101$) in the drug therapy group (hazard ratio [HR], 0.86 [95% confidence interval, 0.65–1.15]; $P = .30$).[59,60] The main problem in interpreting this trial is the high rate of treatment crossovers.[61] This, together with the lower-than-expected event rates, suggests that in clinical practice a reduction in the composite endpoint of all-cause mortality, stroke, major bleeding, or cardiac arrest by catheter ablation may be seen in patients who meet the CABANA eligibility criteria but not in lower-risk patients.[62] Nevertheless, over 5 years of follow-up, AF recurrence was reduced by approximately 50% in catheter ablation patients compared with drug therapy, regardless of their baseline AF type.[63] Cryoballoon ablation has resulted in a significantly lower rate of AF recurrence than antiarrhythmic drug therapy over a follow-up period of one year in two recent randomized trials (EARLY-AF, and STOP-AF).[64,65]

Atrial kick contributes up to 30% of stroke volume, and in patients with *heart failure and AF* catheter ablation is associated with improved left ventricular function and reduced hospitalizations and mortality compared to antiarrhythmic therapy in patients with AF and heart failure with reduced ejection fraction.[52,66] Restoration of sinus rhythm with catheter ablation, however, has been shown to result in significant improvements in ventricular function (CAMFAT trial),[67] particularly in the absence of ventricular fibrosis on cardiac magnetic resonance (CAMERA-MRI trial).[68] Catheter ablation is also superior to amiodarone in achieving freedom from AF at long-term follow-up and reducing unplanned hospitalization and mortality in patients with heart failure and persistent AF (AATAC trial).[69] In the CASTEL-AF trial, catheter ablation was associated with a significantly lower rate of a composite end point of death from any cause or hospitalization for worsening heart failure compared with medical therapy.[70] However, in patients with AF and significantly reduced LVEF ($\leq 35\%$), no benefit of catheter ablation was demonstrated in the AMICA trial.[71] This mainly was due to the fact that at 1 year, LVEF had increased in ablation patients to a similar extent as in medical therapy patients, despite the fact that at any time during follow-up, ablation-group patients more often had SR and a lower AF burden than medical therapy patients.

Both pulmonary vein isolation,[72] and AV nodal modification[73] improve LV function, but PV isolation has been found superior to AV nodal ablation and biventricular pacing in this respect.[74] When the tachycardia itself cannot be ablated, AV nodal modification with biventricular pacing is appropriate. Specific His bundle pacing may offer comparable, or even better results than CRT pacing.[75]

Techniques

Current catheter ablation strategies fall into two broad categories: PV isolation to prevent AF initiation and atrial substrate modification to impede AF perpetuation.[17] Anatomic drawings of the heart relevant to AF ablation are presented in Fig. 13.2.

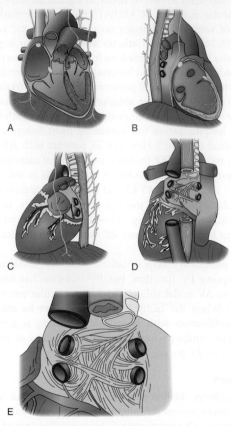

FIG. 13.2. Anatomic drawings of the heart relevant to atrial fibrillation (AF) ablation. This series of drawings shows the heart and associated relevant structures from four different perspectives relevant to AF ablation. This drawing includes the phrenic nerves and the esophagus. (A) The heart viewed from the anterior perspective. (B) The heart viewed from the right lateral perspective. (C) The heart viewed from the left lateral perspective. (D) The heart viewed from the posterior perspective. (E) The left atrium viewed from the posterior perspective. (Calkins H, Hindricks G, Cappato R, et al. 2017 HRS/EHRA/ECAS/APHRS/SOLAECE expert consensus statement on catheter and surgical ablation of atrial fibrillation. *Europace.* 2018;201:e1-e160.)

PV isolation. PV isolation is achieved using radiofrequency (RF) energy by circumferential PV antral ablation assisted by circular multielectrode catheters and electroanatomic mapping systems. Bidirectional PV isolation verified with the use of a circular mapping catheter positioned at the PV–LA junction is the established ablation endpoint. Bidirectional PV isolation is defined by the absence of conduction into the PV from the left atrium (LA–PV entry block) and in the opposite direction (PV–LA exit block) and is an established endpoint of PV ablation (Figs. 13.3 and 13.4). However, usually demonstration of entry block also implies exit block.[76]

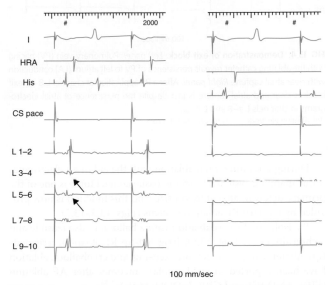

100 mm/sec

FIG. 13.3. Demonstration of entry block. *Left panel:* Mapping of the left superior pulmonary vein during distal coronary sinus pacing. Pulmonary vein (PV) potentials are separated from atrial electrograms. *Right panel:* After successful disconnection no PV potentials are recorded during distal coronary sinus pacing. *Abl,* Ablation electrode; *CS,* coronary sinus; *L,* lasso.

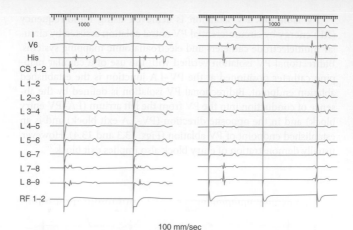

100 mm/sec

FIG. 13.4. Demonstration of exit block. *Left panel:* Pulmonary vein (PV) pacing with the ablating catheter reveals persistence of PV to left atrium (LA) conduction with clear atrial capture. *Right panel:* After a RF application at channel L 8–9, exit block is clear and atrial capture is lost despite the persistence of atrial electrograms in channels L 7–8 and L 8–9.

Abl, Ablation electrode; *CS,* coronary sinus; *L,* lasso.

During circumferential ablation with the aid of an electroanatomic mapping system, electrode–tissue contact force is one of the primary determinants of lesion size, and this function is now provided by modern RF ablation systems (Figs. 13.5–13.7).

PV isolation by cryoablation with a balloon is also feasible and technically easier (Fig. 13.8). Irrigated-tip RF ablation, irrigated-tip catheter using a contact force sensing, and cryoballoon ablation have been reported to yield similar outcomes after AF ablation (FIRE AND ICE and CIRCA-DOSE trials).[77,78]

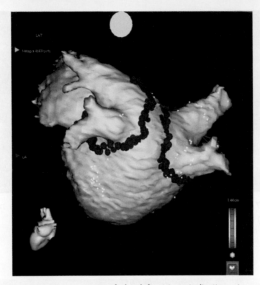

FIG. 13.5. CARTO-Merge image of the left atrium indicating circumferential radiofrequency ablation of the pulmonary veins as seen in the posteroanterior projection.

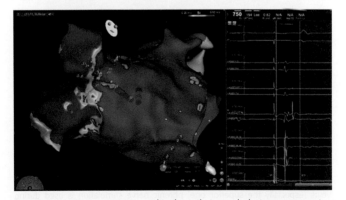

FIG. 13.6. CARTO map using a multipolar catheter and electrogram mapping showing pulmonary vein potentials in the right pulmonary veins.
(Andronache M, Drca N, Viola G. High-resolution mapping in patients with persistent AF. *Arrhythm Electrophysiol Rev.* 2019;8:111-115.)

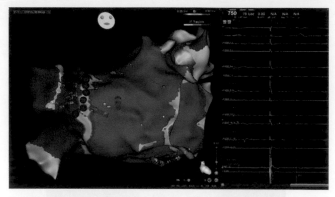

FIG. 13.7. CARTO map using a multipolar catheter and electrogram mapping showing isolation of the right superior pulmonary vein.
(Courtesy of Dr. Nikola Drca.)

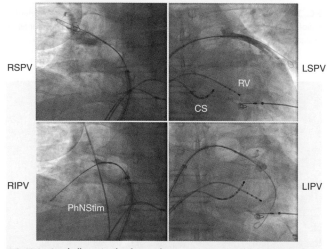

FIG. 13.8. Cryoballoon in the four pulmonary veins. For the right pulmonary veins (especially the superior one) phrenic nerve stimulation is used during cryoablation to detect phrenic nerve damage.
CS, Coronary sinus catheter; *LIPV,* left inferior pulmonary vein; *LSPV,* left superior pulmonary vein; *PhNStim,* catheter for phrenic nerve stimulation; *RIPV,* right inferior pulmonary vein; *RSPV,* right superior pulmonary vein; *RV,* right ventricular apex catheter.

Novel techniques with the use of radiofrequency balloon, laser balloon, or nonthermal pulsed electric field energy (electroporation) for PV isolation[79-81] are also under study.

Non-PV triggers. Non-PV triggers, either in the left or the right atrium may also be sought and ablated, especially in case of recurrence after PV isolation (Fig. 13.9).[20,82]

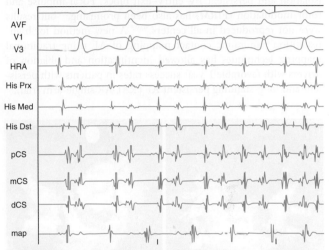

FIG. 13.9. Spontaneous atrial ectopy from the ligament of Marshall induces atrial fibrillation.
CS, Coronary sinus; His, His bundle; HRA, high right atrium; map, transseptally introduced catheter below the os of the left superior pulmonary vein and oriented toward the coronary sinus catheter. (Katritsis D, Ioannidis JP, Anagnostopoulos CE, et al. Identification and catheter ablation of extracardiac and intracardiac components of ligament of Marshall tissue for treatment of paroxysmal atrial fibrillation. J Cardiovasc Electrophysiol. 2001;12:750-758.)

Substrate modification. This approach entails linear lesions along the roof of the left atrium connecting the superior aspects of the left and right upper PV isolation lesions, along the region between the mitral annulus and the left inferior PV (mitral isthmus) and the intervenous ridge, or posterior wall isolation. These approaches, however, carry a potentially increased risk of complications or proarrhythmia, and their value is not established in patients with paroxysmal or persistent AF.[4,83-88]

Other Approaches. Techniques of ablation of *complex fractionated electrograms, rotational activity*, and *autonomic denervation* by targeting areas of the major *ganglionated autonomic plexi* (GP) have also been proposed, but their value is still not established.[21,89-91] In a randomized comparison, however, adding GP ablation to PV isolation produced favorable results (Fig. 13.10).[22] This approach might be useful in cases of recurrences after PV isolation and persistent PV entry–exit block. Focal impulse and rotor modulation (*FIRM*) has also been promising,[92] but results were not reproduced in all centers.[80,93] A new method for high-resolution panoramic contact mapping of AF using traditional mapping techniques has allowed identification and ablation of drivers with favorable 1-year success rates in patients with persistent and long-standing persistent AF (RADAR single-arm trial).[94]

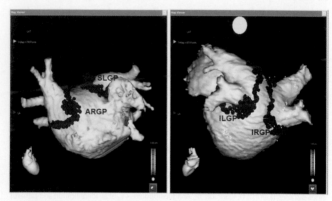

FIG. 13.10. Ganglionated plexi ablation. Pulmonary vein isolation with extension of lesions at the anatomic area of ganglionated plexi.

SLGP, superior left gaglionated plexi; *ARGP,* anterior right gaglionated plexi; *ILGP,* inferior left gaglionated plexi; *IRGP,* inferior right gaglionated plexi. (Katritsis DG, Pokushalov E, Romanov A, et al. Autonomic denervation added to pulmonary vein isolation for paroxysmal atrial fibrillation: a randomized clinical trial. *J Am Coll Cardiol.* 2013;62:2318-2325.)

Other Procedural Issues

Oral amiodarone treatment for 2 months after ablation reduces atrial arrhythmia–related hospitalization and cardioversion rates during the blanking period but does not significantly reduce recurrence of atrial tachyarrhythmias at the 6-month follow-up.[95]

Performance of AF ablation without interruption of warfarin (with an international normalized ratio of 2 to 3) or a direct oral anticoagulant (DOAC) and with additional use of unfractionated heparin (UFH) is well tolerated and associated with fewer thrombotic complications, without increasing the risk of pericardial effusion or other major bleeding events.[96-99] A single- or double-dose skipped approach is also well tolerated with DOACs.[100] A minimally interrupted strategy with cessation of the DOAC 24 hours before the procedure, use of heparin during the procedure, and resumption 4 hours after achieving hemostasis is also reasonable.[101] Warfarin or a DOAC is recommended for all patients for at least 2 to 3 months after an AF ablation procedure. A decision on long-term anticoagulation should be based on the patient's risk factors for stroke and not on the presence or type of AF. Discontinuation of anticoagulation therapy after ablation is generally not recommended in patients who have a CHADS score of 2 or greater. After ablation, aggressive control of weight, blood pressure, lipids, blood sugar, and sleep apnea is important for a favorable outcome.[102]

Success Rates

Long-term (>= 10 years) success rates range from 39 to 80% in patients with paroxysmal AF following one to four procedures, in experienced centres.[103-107] Success rates are lower in patients with permanent AF. According to data from the Danish Register, over the last 8 years, the risk of recurrent AF after ablation has almost halved. Hypertension, female sex, cardioversion 1 year prior to ablation, and AF duration for more than 2 years all increased the associated risk of recurrent AF. Obesity and untreated obstructive sleep apnea also are associated with a higher risk of recurrent post-ablation AF. Patients with diabetes, chronic kidney disease, AF duration over 2 years, and patients with heart failure all experienced no improvement in risk of recurrent AF over time.[108]

Catheter ablation improves quality of life compared to antiar-rhythmic drugs.[109] Ablation may decrease thromboembolic events and, possibly, mortality in patients at high thromboembolic risk.[110] However, certain ablation methods may increase periprocedural stroke,[111] and the effect on mortality is still controversial.[109]

Complications

Complications of catheter ablation occur in 3.5% to 9% of cases and are mainly dependent on the operators experience (<25 procedures per year), age of the patient (>80 years), female gender, $CHADS_2$ score of 2 or greater, and the technique being used (Table 13.1).[4,112-115] The reported in-hospital mortality with AF ablation is 0.06% to 0.4% and mainly is due to tamponade or atrioesophageal fistulae, stroke, and massive pneumonia. Tamponade occurs in 0.67% (in men) to 1.24% (in women) of patients, 16% of whom require surgical intervention.[116] Asymptomatic cerebral emboli may be detected in up to 25% of patients,[99] and stroke and TIA in 0% to 2%.[4] Pulmonary vein stenosis occurs with ostial ablation (1% incidence of stenosis that requires intervention[56]) but not with antral or circumferential lesions. It has decreased with modern techniques to less than 1%, and severe cases are treated with stenting.[117] Esophageal lesions may occur in up to 40% of patients subjected to RF ablation, but atrioesophageal fistulae occur in approximately 0.2% of all patients.[118] They usually occur after extensive ablation of the posterior atrial wall with achieved temperatures greater than 40°C and carry an approximately 50% mortality despite surgical repair.[119,120] Use of irrigated-tip catheters with continuous fluid administration through catheter sheaths, meticulous anticoagulation with UFH without interruption of oral anticoagulation therapy, avoidance of contiguous lesions, restricting energy to less than 25 W, and avoidance of excessive esophageal heating (>1°) during posterior wall ablation are necessary to eliminate the risk of stroke and esophageal damage.[121] Although rarely, circumflex coronary artery injury may result after extensive ablation near the distal coronary sinus and the base of the left atrial appendage as well as in the anterior left atrium. This can result in ventricular fibrillation or sinus node dysfunction requiring permanent pacing.[122]

Iatrogenic arrhythmias occur in 4% to 20% of cases, being more prevalent with linear or fractionated electrogram ablation techniques.[123,124] Usually they are macroreentrant (perimitral or roof dependent) and rarely focal and respond to catheter ablation, although they do not always require repeat ablation.[123] Postprocedure neurocognitive dysfunction has also been reported and depends on ablation techniques and anticoagulation strategies.[125] Other complications of radiofrequency ablation are pericardial effusion (0.6%), myocardial infarction (0.1%), and vascular complications (1.2%).[4] Cryoballoon-mediated PV isolation is at least as effective as RF ablation and might reduce thromboembolic complications and ablation-induced atrial tachycardias but is associated with 1.5% to 6% risk of phrenic nerve pulse, which is usually reversible.[78,126-129] An anterosuperior orientation of the right superior PV, lack of early branching, short distance to the superior vena cava, and an obtuse external angle between the right superior PV and right anterolateral wall of the LA on computed tomography are anatomic predictors of phrenic nerve injury.[130] Cough and hemoptysis after bronchial injury are very rare.[131]

TABLE 13.1 Signs and Symptoms After AF Ablation

	Differential	Suggested Evaluation
Signs and Symptoms of Complications Within a Month Postablation		
Back pain	Musculoskeletal, retroperitoneal hematoma	Physical exam, CT imaging
Chest pain	Pericarditis, pericardial effusion, coronary stenosis (ablation related), pulmonary vein stenosis, musculoskeletal (after cardioversion), worsening reflux	Physical exam, chest x-ray, ECG, echocardiogram, stress test, cardiac catheterization, chest CT
Cough	Infectious process, bronchial irritation (mechanical cryoballoon), pulmonary vein stenosis	Physical exam, chest x-ray, chest CT
Dysphagia	Esophageal irritation (related to transesophageal echocardiography), atrioesophageal fistula	Physical exam, chest CT or MRI

TABLE 13.1 Signs and Symptoms After AF Ablation—cont'd

	Differential	Suggested Evaluation
Early satiety, nausea	Gastric denervation	Physical exam, gastric emptying study
Fever	Infectious process, pericarditis, atrioesophageal fistula	Physical exam, chest x-ray, chest CT, urinalysis, laboratory blood work
Fever, dysphagia, neurologic symptoms	Atrial esophageal fistula	Physical exam, laboratory blood work, chest CT or MRI; avoid endoscopy with air insufflation
Groin pain at site of access	Pseudoaneurysm, AV fistula, hematoma	Ultrasound of the groin, laboratory blood work; consider CT scan if ultrasound negative
Headache	Migraine (related to anesthesia or transseptal access, hemorrhagic stroke), effect of general anesthetic	Physical exam, brain imaging (MRI)
Hypotension	Pericardial effusion/tamponade, bleeding, sepsis, persistent vagal reaction	Echocardiography, laboratory blood work
Hemoptysis	PV stenosis or occlusion, pneumonia	Chest x-ray, chest CT or MR scan, VQ scan
Neurologic symptoms	Cerebral embolic event, atrial esophageal fistula	Physical exam, brain imaging, chest CT or MRI
Shortness of breath	Volume overload, pneumonia, pulmonary vein stenosis, phrenic nerve injury	Physical exam, chest x-ray, chest CT, laboratory blood work

Signs and Symptoms of Complications More Than a Month Postablation

Fever, dysphagia, neurologic symptoms	Atrial esophageal fistula	Physical exam, laboratory blood work, chest CT or MRI; avoid endoscopy with air insufflation

Continued

TABLE 13.1 Signs and Symptoms After AF Ablation—cont'd

	Differential	Suggested Evaluation
Persistent cough, atypical chest pain	Infectious process, pulmonary vein stenosis	Physical exam, laboratory blood work, chest x-ray, chest CT or MRI
Neurologic symptoms	Cerebral embolic event, atrial esophageal fistula	Physical exam, brain imaging, chest CT or MRI
Hemoptysis	PV stenosis or occlusion, pneumonia	CT scan, VQ scan

AF, Atrial fibrillation; *CT,* computed tomography; *ECG,* electrocardiogram; *MRI,* magnetic resonance imaging; *PV,* pulmonary vein; *VQ,* ventilation-perfusion.
Calkins H, Hindricks G, Cappato R, et al. 2017 HRS/EHRA/ECAS/APHRS/SOLAECE expert consensus statement on catheter and surgical ablation of atrial fibrillation. *Europace.* 2018;201: e1-e160.

References

1. January CT, Wann LS, Alpert JS, et al. 2014 AHA/ACC/HRS guideline for the management of patients with atrial fibrillation: a report of the American College of Cardiology/American Heart Association Task Force on practice guidelines and the Heart Rhythm Society. *Circulation.* 2014;130(23):e199-e267.
2. January CT, Wann LS, Calkins H, et al. 2019 AHA/ACC/HRS Focused Update of the 2014 AHA/ACC/HRS Guideline for the Management of Patients With Atrial Fibrillation. *Circulation.* 2019:CIR0000000000000665.
3. Hindricks G, Potpara T, Dagres N, et al. 2020 ESC Guidelines for the diagnosis and management of atrial fibrillation developed in collaboration with the European Association of Cardio-Thoracic Surgery (EACTS). *Eur Heart J.* 2020.10.1093/eurheartj/ehaa612.
4. Calkins H, Hindricks G, Cappato R, et al. 2017 HRS/EHRA/ECAS/APHRS/SOLAECE expert consensus statement on catheter and surgical ablation of atrial fibrillation. *Europace.* 2018;201:e1-e160.
5. Padfield GJ, Steinberg C, Swampillai J, et al. Progression of paroxysmal to persistent atrial fibrillation: 10-year follow-up in the Canadian Registry of Atrial Fibrillation. *Heart Rhythm.* 2017;14(6):801-807.
6. Lau DH, Schotten U, Mahajan R, et al. Novel mechanisms in the pathogenesis of atrial fibrillation: practical applications. *Eur Heart J.* 2016;37(20):1573-1581.
7. Allessie M, Ausma J, Schotten U. Electrical, contractile and structural remodeling during atrial fibrillation. *Cardiovasc Res.* 2002;54(2):230-246.
8. Kato T, Iwasaki YK, Nattel S. Connexins and atrial fibrillation: filling in the gaps. *Circulation.* 2012;125(2):203-206.
9. Gal P, Marrouche NF. Magnetic resonance imaging of atrial fibrosis: redefining atrial fibrillation to a syndrome. *Eur Heart J.* 2017;38(1):14-19.

10. Haemers P, Hamdi H, Guedj K, et al. Atrial fibrillation is associated with the fibrotic remodelling of adipose tissue in the subepicardium of human and sheep atria. *Eur Heart J.* 2017;38(1):53-61.

11. Voigt N, Heijman J, Wang Q, et al. Cellular and molecular mechanisms of atrial arrhythmogenesis in patients with paroxysmal atrial fibrillation. *Circulation.* 2014;129(2):145-156.

12. Li N, Chiang DY, Wang S, et al. Ryanodine receptor-mediated calcium leak drives progressive development of an atrial fibrillation substrate in a transgenic mouse model. *Circulation.* 2014;129(12):1276-1285.

13. Wijffels MC, Kirchhof CJ, Dorland R, Allessie MA. Atrial fibrillation begets atrial fibrillation. A study in awake chronically instrumented goats. *Circulation.* 1995;92(7):1954-1968.

14. Gupta DK, Shah AM, Giugliano RP, et al. Left atrial structure and function in atrial fibrillation: ENGAGE AF-TIMI 48. *Eur Heart J.* 2014;35(22):1457-1465.

15. Haissaguerre M, Jais P, Shah DC, et al. Spontaneous initiation of atrial fibrillation by ectopic beats originating in the pulmonary veins. *N Engl J Med.* 1998;339(10):659-666.

16. Kumagai K, Ogawa M, Noguchi H, Yasuda T, Nakashima H, Saku K. Electrophysiologic properties of pulmonary veins assessed using a multielectrode basket catheter. *J Am Coll Cardiol.* 2004;43(12):2281-2289.

17. Katritsis D, Merchant FM, Mela T, Singh JP, Heist EK, Armoundas AA. Catheter ablation of atrial fibrillation the search for substrate-driven end points. *J Am Coll Cardiol.* 2010;55(21):2293-2298.

18. Mandapati R, Skanes A, Chen J, Berenfeld O, Jalife J. Stable microreentrant sources as a mechanism of atrial fibrillation in the isolated sheep heart. *Circulation.* 2000;101(2):194-199.

19. Lee S, Sahadevan J, Khrestian CM, Cakulev I, Markowitz A, Waldo AL. Simultaneous biatrial high-density (510-512 Electrodes) epicardial mapping of persistent and long-standing persistent atrial fibrillation in patients: new insights into the mechanism of its maintenance. *Circulation.* 2015;132(22):2108-2117.

20. Katritsis D, Ioannidis JP, Anagnostopoulos CE, et al. Identification and catheter ablation of extracardiac and intracardiac components of ligament of Marshall tissue for treatment of paroxysmal atrial fibrillation. *J Cardiovasc Electrophysiol.* 2001;12(7):750-758.

21. Katritsis DG, Pokushalov E, Romanov A, et al. Autonomic denervation added to pulmonary vein isolation for paroxysmal atrial fibrillation: a randomized clinical trial. *J Am Coll Cardiol.* 2013;62(24):2318-2325.

22. Latchamsetty R, Morady F. Source determination in atrial fibrillation. *Arrhythm Electrophysiol Rev.* 2018;7(3):165-168.

23. Freedman B, Camm J, Calkins H, et al. Screening for atrial fibrillation: a report of the AF-SCREEN International Collaboration. *Circulation.* 2017;135(19):1851-1867.

24. Noseworthy PA, Kaufman ES, Chen LY, et al. Subclinical and device-detected atrial fibrillation: pondering the knowledge gap: a scientific statement from the American Heart Association. *Circulation.* 2019;140(25):e944-e963.

25. Mairesse GH, al. e. Screening for atrial fibrillation: a European Heart Rhythm Association (EHRA) consensus document endorsed by the Heart Rhythm Society (HRS),

Asia Pacific Heart Rhythm Society (APHRS), and Sociedad Latinoamericana de Estimulacion Card iaca y Electrofisiologia (SOLAECE). *Europace.* 2017;19:1589-1623.

26. Sana F, Isselbacher EM, Singh JP, et al. Wearable devices for ambulatory cardiac monitoring. *J Am Coll Cardiol.* 2020;75(13):1582-1592.

27. Wang R, Blackburn G, Desai M, et al. Accuracy of wrist-worn heart rate monitors. *JAMA Cardiol.* 2016.

28. Jaakkola J, Jaakkola S, Lahdenoja O, et al. Mobile phone detection of atrial fibrillation with mechanocardiography. The MODE-AF Study (Mobile Phone Detection of Atrial Fibrillation). *Circulation.* 2018;137(14):1524-1527.

29. Krivoshei L, Weber S, Burkard T, et al. Smart detection of atrial fibrillationdagger. *Europace.* 2017;19(5):753-757.

30. Tison GH, Sanchez JM, Ballinger B, et al. Passive detection of atrial fibrillation using a commercially available smartwatch. *JAMA Cardiol.* 2018;3(5):409-416.

31. Guo Y, Lane DA, Wang L, et al. Mobile health technology to improve care for patients with atrial fibrillation. *J Am Coll Cardiol.* 2020;75(13):1523-1534.

32. Wasserlauf J, You C, Patel R, Valys A, Albert D, Passman R. Smartwatch performance for the detection and quantification of atrial fibrillation. *Circ Arrhythm Electrophysiol.* 2019;12(6):e006834.

33. Perez MV, Mahaffey KW, Hedlin H, et al. Large-scale assessment of a smartwatch to identify atrial fibrillation. *N Engl J Med.* 2019;381(20):1909-1917.

34. Schnabel RB, Haeusler KG, Healey JS, et al. Searching for atrial fibrillation post-stroke: A White Paper of the AF-SCREEN International Collaboration. *Circulation.* 2019;140(22):1834-1850.

35. Wyse DG, Waldo AL, DiMarco JP, et al. A comparison of rate control and rhythm control in patients with atrial fibrillation. *N Engl J Med.* 2002;347(23):1825-1833.

36. Hohnloser SH, Kuck KH, Lilienthal J. Rhythm or rate control in atrial fibrillation—Pharmacological Intervention in Atrial Fibrillation (PIAF): a randomised trial. *Lancet.* 2000;356(9244).1789-1794.

37. Carlsson J, Miketic S, Windeler J, et al. Randomized trial of rate-control versus rhythm-control in persistent atrial fibrillation: the Strategies of Treatment of Atrial Fibrillation (STAF) study. *J Am Coll Cardiol.* 2003;41(10):1690-1696.

38. Van Gelder IC, Hagens VE, Bosker HA, et al. A comparison of rate control and rhythm control in patients with recurrent persistent atrial fibrillation. *N Engl J Med.* 2002;347(23):1834-1840.

39. Ogawa S, Yamashita T, Yamazaki T, et al. Optimal treatment strategy for patients with paroxysmal atrial fibrillation: J-RHYTHM Study. *Circ J.* 2009;73(2): 242-248.

40. Opolski G, Torbicki A, Kosior DA, et al. Rate control vs rhythm control in patients with nonvalvular persistent atrial fibrillation: the results of the Polish How to Treat Chronic Atrial Fibrillation (HOT CAFE) Study. *Chest.* 2004;126(2):476-486.

41. Roy D, Talajic M, Nattel S, et al. Rhythm control versus rate control for atrial fibrillation and heart failure. *N Engl J Med.* 2008;358(25):2667-2677.

42. Gillinov AM, Bagiella E, Moskowitz AJ, et al. Rate control versus rhythm control for atrial fibrillation after cardiac surgery. *N Engl J Med.* 2016;374(20):1911-1921.

43. Katritsis DG, Gersh BJ, Camm AJ. *Clinical Cardiology: Current Practice Guidelines.* Oxford University Press; Oxford, UK 2016.

44. Corley SD, Epstein AE, DiMarco JP, et al. Relationships between sinus rhythm, treatment, and survival in the Atrial Fibrillation Follow-Up Investigation of Rhythm Management (AFFIRM) Study. *Circulation.* 2004;109(12):1509-1513.

45. Lafuente-Lafuente C, Valembois L, Bergmann JF, Belmin J. Antiarrhythmics for maintaining sinus rhythm after cardioversion of atrial fibrillation. *Cochrane Database Syst Rev.* 2015;(3):CD005049.

46. Singh BN, Singh SN, Reda DJ, et al. Amiodarone versus sotalol for atrial fibrillation. *N Engl J Med.* 2005;352(18):1861-1872.

47. Deedwania PC, Singh BN, Ellenbogen K, Fisher S, Fletcher R, Singh SN. Spontaneous conversion and maintenance of sinus rhythm by amiodarone in patients with heart failure and atrial fibrillation: observations from the veterans affairs congestive heart failure survival trial of antiarrhythmic therapy (CHF-STAT). The Department of Veterans Affairs CHF-STAT Investigators. *Circulation.* 1998;98(23): 2574-2579.

48. Tsadok MA, Jackevicius CA, Essebag V, et al. Rhythm versus rate control therapy and subsequent stroke or transient ischemic attack in patients with atrial fibrillation. *Circulation.* 2012;126(23):2680-2687.

49. Hohnloser SH, Crijns HJ, van Eickels M, et al. Effect of dronedarone on cardiovascular events in atrial fibrillation. *N Engl J Med.* 2009;360(7):668-678.

50. Kober L, Torp-Pedersen C, McMurray JJ, et al. Increased mortality after dronedarone therapy for severe heart failure. *N Engl J Med.* 2008;358(25):2678-2687.

51. Connolly SJ, Camm AJ, Halperin JL, et al. Dronedarone in high-risk permanent atrial fibrillation. *N Engl J Med.* 2011;365(24):2268-2276.

52. Chen S, Purerfellner H, Meyer C, et al. Rhythm control for patients with atrial fibrillation complicated with heart failure in the contemporary era of catheter ablation: a stratified pooled analysis of randomized data. *Eur Heart J.* 2020;41 (30):2863-2873.

53. Kirchhof P, Camm AJ, Goette A, et al. Early Rhythm-Control Therapy in Patients with Atrial Fibrillation. *N Engl J Med.* 2020;383(14):1305-1316.

54. Calkins H, Reynolds MR, Spector P, et al. Treatment of atrial fibrillation with antiarrhythmic drugs or radiofrequency ablation: two systematic literature reviews and meta-analyses. *Circ Arrhythm Electrophysiol.* 2009;2(4):349-361.

55. Cosedis Nielsen J, Johannessen A, Raatikainen P, et al. Radiofrequency ablation as initial therapy in paroxysmal atrial fibrillation. *N Engl J Med.* 2012;367(17): 1587-1595.

56. Nielsen JC, Johannessen A, Raatikainen P, et al. Long-term efficacy of catheter ablation as first-line therapy for paroxysmal atrial fibrillation: 5-year outcome in a randomised clinical trial. *Heart.* 2017;103(5):368-376.

57. Morillo CA, Verma A, Connolly SJ, et al. Radiofrequency ablation vs antiarrhythmic drugs as first-line treatment of paroxysmal atrial fibrillation (RAAFT-2): a randomized trial. *JAMA.* 2014;311(7):692-700.

58. Mont L, Bisbal F, Hernandez-Madrid A, et al. Catheter ablation vs. antiarrhythmic drug treatment of persistent atrial fibrillation: a multicentre, randomized, controlled trial (SARA study). *Eur Heart J.* 2014;35(8):501-507.

59. Packer DL, Mark DB, Robb RA, et al. Effect of catheter ablation vs antiarrhythmic drug therapy on mortality, stroke, bleeding, and cardiac arrest among patients

with atrial fibrillation: The CABANA Randomized Clinical Trial. *JAMA*. 2019;321(13): 1261-1274.

60. Camm AJ. Left atrial ablation for management of atrial fibrillation: CABANA vs. real-world data. Apples and oranges? *Eur Heart J*. 2019;40(16): 1265-1267.

61. Pocock SJ, Collier TJ. Statistical appraisal of 6 recent clinical trials in cardiology: JACC State-of-the-Art Review. *J Am Coll Cardiol*. 2019;73(21):2740-2755.

62. Noseworthy PA, Gersh BJ, Kent DM, et al. Atrial fibrillation ablation in practice: assessing CABANA generalizability. *Eur Heart J*. 2019;40(16):1257-1264.

63. Poole JE, Bahnson TD, Monahan KH, et al. Recurrence of Atrial Fibrillation After Catheter Ablation or Antiarrhythmic Drug Therapy in the CABANA Trial. *J Am Coll Cardiol*. 2020;75(25):3105-3118.

64. Andrade JG, Wells GA, Deyell MW, et al. Cryoablation or Drug Therapy for Initial Treatment of Atrial Fibrillation. *NEJM*. 2020. DOI: 10.1056/NEJMoa2029980

65. Wazni OM, Dandamudi G, Sood N, et al. Cryoballoon Ablation as Initial Therapy for Atrial Fibrillation. *N Engl J Med*. 2020.

66. Asad ZUA, Yousif A, Khan MS, Al-Khatib SM, Stavrakis S. catheter ablation versus medical therapy for atrial fibrillation. A systematic review and meta-analysis of randomized controlled trials. *Circ Arrhythm Electrophysiol*. 2019;12(9):e007414.

67. Hunter RJ, Berriman TJ, Diab I, et al. A randomized controlled trial of catheter ablation versus medical treatment of atrial fibrillation in heart failure (The CAMTAF trial). *Circ Arrhythm Electrophysiol*. 2014;7:31-38.

68. Prabhu S, Taylor AJ, Costello BT, et al. Catheter ablation versus medical rate control in atrial fibrillation and systolic dysfunction (CAMERA-MRI). *J Am Coll Cardiol*. 2017;70(16):1949-1961.

69. Di Biase L, Mohanty P, Mohanty S, et al. Ablation versus amiodarone for treatment of persistent atrial fibrillation in patients with congestive heart failure and an implanted device: results from the AATAC Multicenter Randomized Trial. *Circulation*. 2016;133(17):1637-1644.

70. Marrouche NF, Brachmann J, Andresen D, et al. Catheter ablation for atrial fibrillation with heart failure. *N Engl J Med*. 2018;378(5):417-427.

71. Kuck KH, Merkely B, Zahn R, et al. Catheter ablation versus best medical therapy in patients with persistent atrial fibrillation and congestive heart failure: The Randomized AMICA Trial. *Circ Arrhythm Electrophysiol*. 2019;12(12):e007731.

72. Hsu LF, Jais P, Sanders P, et al. Catheter ablation for atrial fibrillation in congestive heart failure. *N Engl J Med*. 2004;351(23):2373-2383.

73. Wood MA, Brown-Mahoney C, Kay GN, Ellenbogen KA. Clinical outcomes after ablation and pacing therapy for atrial fibrillation: a meta-analysis. *Circulation*. 2000;101(10):1138-1144.

74. Khan MN, Jais P, Cummings J, et al. Pulmonary-vein isolation for atrial fibrillation in patients with heart failure. *N Engl J Med*. 2008;359(17): 1778-1785.

75. Arnold AD, Whinnett ZI, Vijarayaman P. His–Purkinje Conduction System Pacing: State of the Art in 2020. *Arrhythm Electrophysiol Rev*. DOI: 2020.10.15420/aer. 2020.14

76. Duytschaever M, De Meyer G, Acena M, et al. Lessons from dissociated pulmonary vein potentials: entry block implies exit block. *Europace.* 2013;15(6):805-812.

77. Andrade JG, Champagne J, Dubuc M, et al. Cryoballoon or radiofrequency ablation for atrial fibrillation assessed by continuous monitoring: A Randomized Clinical Trial. *Circulation.* 2019;140(22):1779-1788.

78. Kuck KH, Brugada J, Furnkranz A, et al. Cryoballoon or radiofrequency ablation for paroxysmal atrial fibrillation. *N Engl J Med.* 2016;374(23):2235-2245.

79. Reddy VY, Neuzil P, Koruth JS, et al. Pulsed field ablation for pulmonary vein isolation in atrial fibrillation. *J Am Coll Cardiol.* 2019;74(3):315-326.

80. Schmidt B, Neuzil P, Luik A, et al. Laser balloon or wide-area circumferential irrigated radiofrequency ablation for persistent atrial fibrillation: A Multicenter Prospective Randomized Study. *Circ Arrhythm Electrophysiol.* 2017;10(12):e005767.

81. Reddy VY, Anic A, Koruth J, et al. Pulsed field ablation in patients with persistent atrial fibrillation. *J Am Coll Cardiol.* 2020;76(9):1068-1080.

82. Higa S, Lo LW, Chen SA. Catheter ablation of paroxysmal atrial fibrillation originating from non-pulmonary vein areas. *Arrhythm Electrophysiol Rev.* 2018;7(4): 273-281.

83. Verma A, Jiang CY, Betts TR, et al. Approaches to catheter ablation for persistent atrial fibrillation. *N Engl J Med.* 2015;372(19):1812-1822.

84. Vogler J, Willems S, Sultan A, et al. Pulmonary vein isolation versus defragmentation: The CHASE-AF Clinical Trial. *J Am Coll Cardiol.* 2015;66(24):2743-2752.

85. McLellan AJ, Ling LH, Azzopardi S, et al. A minimal or maximal ablation strategy to achieve pulmonary vein isolation for paroxysmal atrial fibrillation: a prospective multi-centre randomized controlled trial (the Minimax study). *Eur Heart J.* 2015;36(28):1812-1821.

86. Providencia R, Lambiase PD, Srinivasan N, et al. Is There still a role for complex fractionated atrial electrogram ablation in addition to pulmonary vein isolation in patients with paroxysmal and persistent atrial fibrillation? Meta-analysis of 1415 Patients. *Circ Arrhythm Electrophysiol.* 2015;8(5):1017-1029.

87. Mohanty S, Gianni C, Mohanty P, et al. Impact of rotor ablation in nonparoxysmal atrial fibrillation patients: results from the Randomized OASIS Trial. *J Am Coll Cardiol.* 2016;68(3):274-282.

88. Fink T, Schluter M, Heeger CH, et al. Stand-alone pulmonary vein isolation versus pulmonary vein isolation with additional substrate modification as index ablation procedures in patients with persistent and long-standing persistent atrial fibrillation: The Randomized Alster-Lost-AF Trial (Ablation at St. Georg Hospital for Long-Standing Persistent Atrial Fibrillation). *Circ Arrhythm Electrophysiol.* 2017;10(7):e005114.

89. Katritsis DG, Giazitzoglou E, Zografos T, Pokushalov E, Po SS, Camm AJ. Rapid pulmonary vein isolation combined with autonomic ganglia modification: a randomized study. *Heart Rhythm.* 2011;8(5):672-678.

90. Baykaner T, Zaman JAB, Wang PJ, Narayan SM. Ablation of atrial fibrillation drivers. *Arrhythm Electrophysiol Rev.* 2017;6(4):195-201.

91. Baykaner T, Zografos TA, Zaman JAB, et al. Spatial relationship of organized rotational and focal sources in human atrial fibrillation to autonomic ganglionated plexi. *Int J Cardiol.* 2017;240:234-239.

92. Narayan SM, Baykaner T, Clopton P, et al. Ablation of rotor and focal sources reduces late recurrence of atrial fibrillation compared with trigger ablation alone: extended follow-up of the CONFIRM trial (Conventional Ablation for Atrial Fibrillation With or Without Focal Impulse and Rotor Modulation). *J Am Coll Cardiol.* 2014;63(17):1761-1768.

93. Baykaner T, Rogers AJ, Meckler GL, et al. Clinical implications of ablation of drivers for atrial fibrillation: a systematic review and meta-analysis. *Circ Arrhythm Electrophysiol.* 2018;11(5):e006119.

94. Choudry S, Mansour M, Sundaram S, et al. RADAR: a multicenter food and drug administration investigational device exemption clinical trial of persistent atrial fibrillation. *Circ Arrhythm Electrophysiol.* 2020;13(1):e007825.

95. Darkner S, Chen X, Hansen J, et al. Recurrence of arrhythmia following short-term oral AMIOdarone after CATheter ablation for atrial fibrillation: a double-blind, randomized, placebo-controlled study (AMIO-CAT trial). *Eur Heart J.* 2014;35(47):3356-3364.

96. Di Biase L, Burkhardt JD, Santangeli P, et al. Periprocedural stroke and bleeding complications in patients undergoing catheter ablation of atrial fibrillation with different anticoagulation management: results from the Role of Coumadin in Preventing Thromboembolism in Atrial Fibrillation (AF) Patients Undergoing Catheter Ablation (COMPARE) randomized trial. *Circulation.* 2014;129(25):2638-2644.

97. Calkins H, Willems S, Gerstenfeld EP, et al. Uninterrupted dabigatran versus warfarin for ablation in atrial fibrillation. *N Engl J Med.* 2017;376(17):1627-1636.

98. Cappato R, Marchlinski FE, Hohnloser SH, et al. Uninterrupted rivaroxaban vs. uninterrupted vitamin K antagonists for catheter ablation in non-valvular atrial fibrillation. *Eur Heart J.* 2015;36(28):1805-1811.

99. Kirchhof P, Haeusler KG, Blank B, et al. Apixaban in patients at risk of stroke undergoing atrial fibrillation ablation. *Eur Heart J.* 2018;39(32):2942-2955.

100. Yu HT, Shim J, Park J, et al. When is it appropriate to stop non-vitamin K antagonist oral anticoagulants before catheter ablation of atrial fibrillation? A multicentre prospective randomized study. *Eur Heart J.* 2019;40(19):1531-1537.

101. Weitz JI, Healey JS, Skanes AC, Verma A. Periprocedural management of new oral anticoagulants in patients undergoing atrial fibrillation ablation. *Circulation.* 2014;129(16):1688-1694.

102. Pathak RK, Middeldorp ME, Lau DH, et al. Aggressive risk factor reduction study for atrial fibrillation and implications for the outcome of ablation: the ARREST-AF cohort study. *J Am Coll Cardiol.* 2014;64(21):2222-2231.

103. Sorgente A, Tung P, Wylie J, Josephson ME. Six year follow-up after catheter ablation of atrial fibrillation: a palliation more than a true cure. *Am J Cardiol.* 2012;109(8):1179-1186.

104. Gaita F, Scaglione M, Battaglia A, et al. Very long-term outcome following transcatheter ablation of atrial fibrillation. Are results maintained after 10 years of follow up? *Europace.* 2018;20(3):443-450.

105. Ganesan AN, Shipp NJ, Brooks AG, et al. Long-term outcomes of catheter ablation of atrial fibrillation: a systematic review and meta-analysis. *J Am Heart Assoc.* 2013;2(2):e004549.

106. Tilz RR, Heeger CH, Wick A, et al. Ten-year clinical outcome after circumferential pulmonary vein isolation utilizing the hamburg approach in patients with symptomatic drug-refractory paroxysmal atrial fibrillation. *Circ Arrhythm Electrophysiol.* 2018;11(2):e005250.

107. Bertaglia E, Senatore G, De Michieli L, et al. Twelve-year follow-up of catheter ablation for atrial fibrillation: a prospective, multicenter, randomized study. *Heart Rhythm.* 2017;14(4):486-492.

108. Pallisgaard JL, Gislason GH, Hansen J, et al. Temporal trends in atrial fibrillation recurrence rates after ablation between 2005 and 2014: a nationwide Danish cohort study. *Eur Heart J.* 2018;39(6):442-449.

109. Morillo CA. Radiofrequency ablation versus antiarrhythmic drug therapy for atrial fibrillation: meta-analysis of quality of life, morbidity, and mortality. *JACCCEP.* 2016;2(2):170-180.

110. Friberg L, Tabrizi F, Englund A. Catheter ablation for atrial fibrillation is associated with lower incidence of stroke and death: data from Swedish health registries. *Eur Heart J.* 2016;37(31):2478-2487.

111. Siontis KC, Ioannidis JPA, Katritsis GD, et al. Radiofrequency ablation versus antiarrhythmic drug therapy for atrial fibrillation: meta-analysis of quality of life, morbidity, and mortality. *JACC Clin Electrophysiol.* 2016;2(2):170-180.

112. Arbelo E, Brugada J, Hindricks G, et al. The atrial fibrillation ablation pilot study: a European Survey on Methodology and results of catheter ablation for atrial fibrillation conducted by the European Heart Rhythm Association. *Eur Heart J.* 2014;35(22):1466-1478.

113. Deshmukh A, Patel NJ, Pant S, et al. In-hospital complications associated with catheter ablation of atrial fibrillation in the United States between 2000 and 2010: analysis of 93 801 procedures. *Circulation.* 2013;128(19):2104-2112.

114. Gupta A, Perera T, Ganesan A, et al. Complications of catheter ablation of atrial fibrillation: a systematic review. *Circ Arrhythm Electrophysiol.* 2013;6(6):1082-1088.

115. Barbhaiya CR, Kumar S, John RM, et al. Global survey of esophageal and gastric injury in atrial fibrillation ablation: incidence, time to presentation, and outcomes. *J Am Coll Cardiol.* 2015;65(13):1377-1378.

116. Michowitz Y, Rahkovich M, Oral H, et al. Effects of sex on the incidence of cardiac tamponade after catheter ablation of atrial fibrillation: results from a worldwide survey in 34 943 atrial fibrillation ablation procedures. *Circ Arrhythm Electrophysiol.* 2014;7(2):274-280.

117. Fender EA, Widmer RJ, Hodge DO, et al. Severe pulmonary vein stenosis resulting from ablation for atrial fibrillation: presentation, management, and clinical outcomes. *Circulation.* 2016;134(23):1812-1821.

118. Kapur S, Barbhaiya C, Deneke T, Michaud GF. Esophageal injury and atrioesophageal fistula caused by ablation for atrial fibrillation. *Circulation.* 2017;136(13):1247-1255.

119. Singh SM, d'Avila A, Singh SK, et al. Clinical outcomes after repair of left atrial esophageal fistulas occurring after atrial fibrillation ablation procedures. *Heart Rhythm.* 2013;10(11):1591-1597.

120. Halbfass P, Pavlov B, Muller P, et al. Progression from esophageal thermal asymptomatic lesion to perforation complicating atrial fibrillation ablation: a single-center registry. *Circ Arrhythm Electrophysiol.* 2017;10(8):e005233.

121. Martinek M, Meyer C, Hassanein S, et al. Identification of a high-risk population for esophageal injury during radiofrequency catheter ablation of atrial fibrillation: procedural and anatomical considerations. *Heart Rhythm.* 2010;7(9):1224-1230.

122. Chugh A, Makkar A, Yen Ho S, et al. Manifestations of coronary arterial injury during catheter ablation of atrial fibrillation and related arrhythmias. *Heart Rhythm.* 2013;10(11):1638-1645.

123. Katritsis D, Wood MA, Shepard RK, Giazitzoglou E, Kourlaba G, Ellenbogen KA. Atrial arrhythmias following ostial or circumferential pulmonary vein ablation. *J Interv Card Electrophysiol.* 2006;16(2):123-130.

124. Wasmer K, Monnig G, Bittner A, et al. Incidence, characteristics, and outcome of left atrial tachycardias after circumferential antral ablation of atrial fibrillation. *Heart Rhythm.* 2012;9(10):1660-1666.

125. Medi C, Evered L, Silbert B, et al. Subtle post-procedural cognitive dysfunction after atrial fibrillation ablation. *J Am Coll Cardiol.* 2013;62(6):531-539.

126. Cheng X, Hu Q, Zhou C, et al. The long-term efficacy of cryoballoon vs irrigated radiofrequency ablation for the treatment of atrial fibrillation: A meta-analysis. *Int J Cardiol.* 2015;181:297-302.

127. Luik A, Radzewitz A, Kieser M, et al. Cryoballoon versus open irrigated radiofrequency ablation in patients with paroxysmal atrial fibrillation: the prospective, randomized, controlled, noninferiority FreezeAF study. *Circulation.* 2015;132(14):1311-1319.

128. Mortsell D, Arbelo E, Dagres N, et al. Cryoballoon vs. radiofrequency ablation for atrial fibrillation: a study of outcome and safety based on the ESC-EHRA atrial fibrillation ablation long-term registry and the Swedish catheter ablation registry. *Europace.* 2019;21(4):581-589.

129. Miyazaki S, Tada H. Complications of cryoballoon pulmonary vein isolation. *Arrhythm Electrophysiol Rev.* 2019;8(1):60-64.

130. Stroker E, de Asmundis C, Saitoh Y, et al. Anatomic predictors of phrenic nerve injury in the setting of pulmonary vein isolation using the 28-mm second-generation cryoballoon. *Heart Rhythm.* 2016;13(2):342-351.

131. Verma N, Gillespie CT, Argento AC, et al. Bronchial effects of cryoballoon ablation for atrial fibrillation. *Heart Rhythm.* 2017;14(1):12-16.

14

Atrioventricular Junctional Tachycardias

ATRIOVENTRICULAR NODAL REENTRANT TACHYCARDIA

DEFINITION

Atrioventricular nodal reentrant tachycardia (AVNRT) denotes reentry in the area of the atrioventricular (AV) node. Several models have been proposed to explain the mechanism of the arrhythmia in the context of the complex anatomy of the AV node and its atrial extension, but its exact circuit remains elusive.[1-3]

PATHOPHYSIOLOGY

The concept of dual AV nodal pathways as the substrate for AVNRT dates from 1956 when Moe et al. demonstrated evidence of a dual AV conduction system in dogs. It was postulated that a dual conduction system was present, one having a faster conduction time and longer refractory period (fast pathway), the other having a slower conduction time and shorter refractory period (slow pathway). At a critical coupling interval the premature impulse blocks in the faster pathway and conducts in the still excitable slow pathway, causing a sudden jump in the AV conduction time. After that, the impulse returns to the atria via the fast pathway, and an AV nodal echo beat or sustained tachycardia results (Fig. 14.1).[1] Denes et al. in 1973 ascribed episodes of paroxysmal supraventricular tachycardia to AV node reentry as a result of the presence of dual atrioventricular nodal pathways and, using His bundle recordings and the atrial extrastimulus method, demonstrated sudden prolongation of the AH interval in a patient with dual atrioventricular nodal pathways (so-called atrioventricular conduction jump).[1] In approximately 6% of patients with AV nodal reentry,[4] and at a higher rate in athletes,[5] retrograde conduction is thought to proceed over the slow pathway and may result in an atypical form of AVNRT (Fig. 14.2). In these patients, antegrade conduction curves are not always discontinuous. This pattern of conduction and a potentially incessant nature can also be caused by concealed septal accessory pathways with decremental properties.[6]

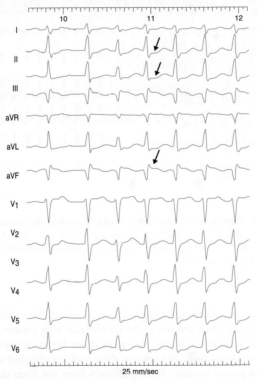

FIG. 14.1. Induction of typical atrioventricular nodal reentrant tachycardia (AVNRT) by atrial ectopy. The first three beats are sinus beats. The next two are atrial ectopic beats conducted with a short PR (apparently over the fast pathway). The next atrial ectopic is conducted with a prolonged PR over the slow pathway because of antegrade block of the fast pathway and initiates AVNRT by returning retrogradely through the fast pathway that has recovered. Retrograde P′ waves are more prominent in lead V₁ and especially the inferior leads *(arrows)*.

I to V6, Electrocardiogram leads. (Katritsis DG, Camm AJ. Atrioventricular nodal re-entrant tachycardia. *Circulation.* 2010;122:831-840.)

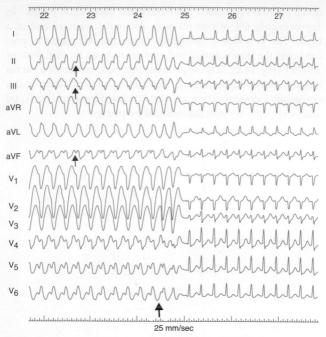

FIG. 14.2. Atypical AVNRT conducted with LBBB aberration (the unusual type). Retrograde P waves are indicated by thin arrows. Following a ventricular extrastimulus (thick arrow), there is ventricular capture followed by a ventricular ectopic and then typical AVNRT.
I to V6: ECG leads.

The concept of longitudinally dissociated dual AV nodal pathways that conduct around a central obstacle with proximal and distal connections can provide explanations for many aspects of the electrophysiologic behavior of these tachycardias, but several obscure points remain. These pathways have not been demonstrated histologically, the exact circuit responsible for the reentrant tachycardia is unknown, and critical questions still remain unanswered. There has been considerable evidence that the right and left inferior extensions of the human AV node may provide the anatomic substrate of the "slow" pathway, whereas inputs to the node especially from the atrial septum may act as the "fast" pathway.[1,7-9] Variable gap junction connectivity due to differential expression of connexin isoforms in the area of the AV nodal extensions,[10] variability in the arrangement of the superficial atrial muscle fibers in the area of the triangle of Koch,[11] and, perhaps, involvement in the circuit of remnants of the primary ring, described as "ring tissues",[12] may also play a role. A probabilistic model of the tachycardia circuit for all forms of atrioventricular nodal reentrant tachycardia based on the concept of atrionodal inputs and connexin expression has been proposed (Fig. 14.3).

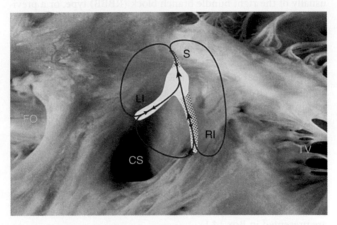

FIG. 14.3. Proposed model of the AVNRT circuit. AVNRT is conceived as one tachycardia with multiple possibilities for atrial retrograde excitation, and typical or atypical forms depending on the conduction properties of the anterogradely and retrogradely conducting input and the resultant AH/HA intervals. Thick arrows indicate the circuits with the higher probability to occur based on the data we have so far (see text for details).

CS, coronary sinus; *FO*, foramen ovale; *LI*, left inferior input; *RI*, right inferior input; *S*, superior ("last") input; *TV*, tricuspid valve. (Katritsis DG. A unified theory for the circuit of atrioventricular nodal reentrant tachycardia. Europace 2020 Sep 26:euaa196).

There is evidence that spontaneous AVNRT can be the first clinical manifestation of concealed Brugada syndrome, and it has been postulated that genetic variants that reduce the sodium current (I_{Na}) may predispose to expression of both phenotypes.[13]

DIAGNOSIS

Typically AVNRT is a narrow-complex tachycardia (i.e., QRS duration < 120 ms) unless there is aberrant conduction, which is usually of the right bundle branch block (RBBB) type, or a previous conduction defect exists. Tachycardia-related ST depression and RR interval variation may be seen. QRS alternans may be seen but is more common in atrioventricular reentrant tachycardia (AVRT).

In the **typical form** of AVNRT (also called slow-fast AVNRT), abnormal (retrograde) P′ waves are constantly related to the QRS and in the majority of cases are indiscernible or very close to the QRS complex. Thus P′ waves are either masked by the QRS complex or seen as a small terminal P′ wave (a pseudo-R′) that is not present during sinus rhythm (see Fig. 14.1).

In the **atypical form** of AVNRT, P′ waves are clearly visible before the QRS (i.e., RP′ > P′R), denoting a "long-RP tachycardia," and are negative or shallow in leads II, III, aVF, and V_6 but positive in V_1 (see Fig. 14.2). Other causes of long-RP tachycardia are presented in Box 14.1.

Although AV dissociation or ventriculoatrial (VA) block is usually not seen, it can occur because neither the atria nor the ventricles are necessary for the reentry circuit. If the tachycardia is initiated by atrial ectopic beats, the initial (ectopic) P′ wave usually differs from the subsequent (retrograde) P′ waves (see Fig. 14.1).

Box 14.1 Long-RP Tachycardias

1. Sinus tachycardia
2. Atrial tachycardia
3. Atypical atrioventricular nodal reentrant tachycardia
4. Atrioventricular reentrant tachycardia caused by slowly conducting concealed accessory pathways
5. Nonparoxysmal junctional tachycardia with 1:1 retrograde conduction

ELECTROPHYSIOLOGIC CLASSIFICATION

The recognition of the fact that AVNRT may present with atypical retrograde atrial activation has made diagnosis of the arrhythmia as well as classification attempts more complicated. Heterogeneity of both fast and slow conduction patterns has been well described, and all forms of AVNRT may display anterior, posterior, and middle or even left atrial retrograde activation patterns.

Typical AVNRT

In the *slow–fast form* of AVNRT the onset of atrial activation appears before, at the onset, or just after the QRS complex, thus maintaining an atrial-His/His-atrial ratio AH/HA greater than 1 (Fig. 14.4).

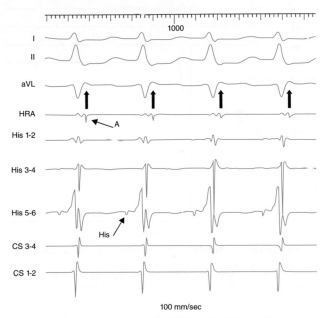

FIG. 14.4. Electrograms during slow–fast AVNRT. The AH interval (as measured from the A on the HRA electrode to the His of the His bundle electrode) is longer than the HA. Small P′ waves at the end of QRS correspond to retrograde atrial conduction *(thick arrows)*.

I, ECG lead; *II*, lead II of the surface ECG; *A*, atrial electrogram; *aVL*, lead aVL of the surface ECG; *CS*, coronary sinus; *ECG*, electrocardiogram; *HRA*, high right atrium; *His*, His bundle electrogram.

The VA interval measured from the onset of ventricular activation on surface electrocardiogram (ECG) to the earliest deflection of the atrial activation in the His bundle electrogram is 60 or less. Although typically the earliest retrograde atrial activation is recorded at the His bundle electrogram, detailed mapping studies have demonstrated that posterior or even left septal fast pathways may occur in up to 7.6% in patients with typical AVNRT (Figs. 14.5–14.7).[14-16]

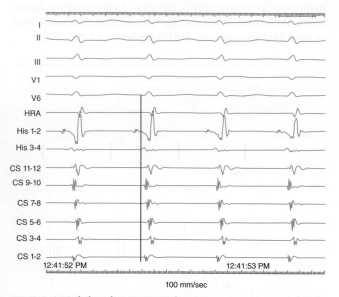

FIG. 14.5. Typical slow–fast AVNRT. Earliest retrograde atrial activation is recorded at proximal His (His 3–4) and distal CS (CS 9–10).

I to V6, 12-Lead electrocardiogram leads; *AVNRT*, atrioventricular nodal reentrant tachycardia; *CS*, coronary sinus; *His*, His bundle electrogram; *HRA*, high right atrium.

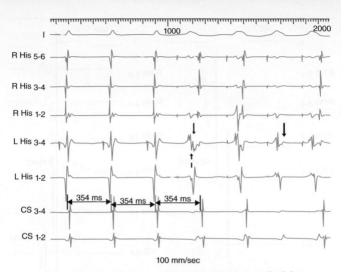

FIG. 14.6. Example of earliest retrograde atrial activation on the left septum during typical AVNRT. Recording was obtained during AVNRT. A right ventricular extrastimulus captures the ventricle without resetting the tachycardia circuit, as judged by constant A-A intervals, results in separation of ventricular and atrial electrograms and allows identification of the beginning of the atrial electrogram on the left His recording electrodes (*thin arrow* pointing down). The third extrastimulus captures the ventricle and produces ventriculoatrial (VA) block *(thick arrow)*, thus verifying identification of the atrial component in previous beats. The sharp electrogram that is adjacent to the first captured ventricular electrogram (*dashed arrow* pointing up) is most probably the His bundle electrogram because it follows the preceding His by exactly 354 ms. The broad electrogram that follows the left atrial one represents either far field from the right atrial electrogram or, most probably, part of the ventricular electrogram because a similar signal is still recorded during VA block. Recordings are at 100 mm/sec.

I, Lead I of the surface electrocardiogram; *AVNRT*, atrioventricular nodal reentrant tachycardia; *CS*, coronary sinus; *L His*, left His bundle recording electrode; *R His*, right His bundle recording electrode. (Katritsis DG, Ellenbogen KA, Becker AE. Atrial activation during atrioventricular nodal reentrant tachycardia: studies on retrograde fast pathway conduction. *Heart Rhythm.* 2006;3:993-1000, with kind permission.)

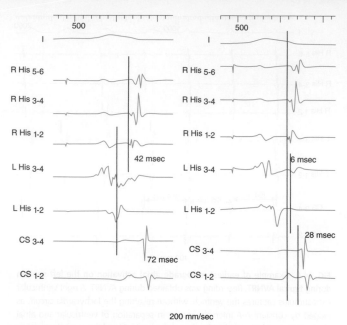

FIG. 14.7. The same recording as in Fig. 14.3 displayed at 200 mm/sec. On the *left panel* the earliest retrograde atrial activation on the left septum during AVNRT precedes atrial activation recorded on the right septum and coronary sinus ostium by 42 and 72 ms, respectively. On the *right panel*, the beat that results in restoration of VA conduction (fourth extrastimulus in Fig. 14.6) after VA block is displayed. The earliest retrograde atrial activation is now recorded by the right His electrode and precedes atrial activation recorded on the left septum and coronary sinus ostium by 6 and 28 ms.

(See Fig. 14.6 for abbreviations.) (Katritsis DG, Ellenbogen KA, Becker AE. Atrial activation during atrioventricular nodal reentrant tachycardia: studies on retrograde fast pathway conduction. *Heart Rhythm.* 2006;3:993-1000.)

Atypical AVNRT

Atypical AVNRT is seen in approximately 6% of all AVNRT cases,[17] and in some patients may coexist with the typical form.[18] A higher incidence of atypical AVNRT has been documented in athletes.[5] In the so-called **fast–slow** form of AVNRT, retrograde atrial electrograms begin well after ventricular activation with an AH/HA ratio less than 1, indicating that retrograde conduction is slower than antegrade conduction. The AH interval is less than 185 to 200 ms. The VA interval measured from the onset of ventricular activation on surface ECG to the earliest deflection of the atrial activation in the His bundle electrogram is more than 60 ms. Earliest retrograde atrial activation generally is at the base of the triangle of Koch, near the coronary sinus ostium, but can be variable, with eccentric atrial activation at the lower septum or even the distal coronary sinus (Figs. 14.8 and 14.9).[19-21]

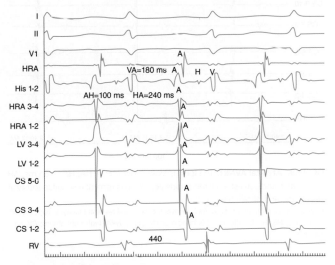

FIG. 14.8. Atypical AVNRT. The form is conventionally fast–slow (AH < HA, HA > 70 ms, AH < 200 ms), and earliest retrograde atrial activation is recorded at the His bundle electrode.
I to V6, 12-Lead electrocardiogram leads; *CS,* coronary sinus; *His,* His bundle electrogram; *HRA,* high right atrium; *LV,* electrode at the left side of the septum; *RV,* right ventricle (Katritsis DG, Josephson ME. Classification of electrophysiological types of atrioventricular nodal re-entrant tachycardia: a reappraisal. *Europace.* 2013;15:1231-1240.)

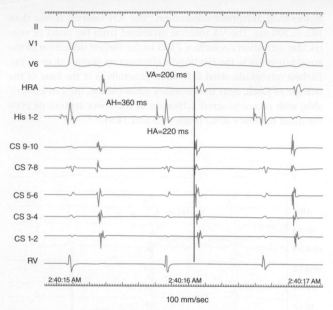

FIG. 14.9. Atypical AVNRT. The form is slow–slow (AH > HA, HA > 60 ms, AH > 200 ms), and earliest atrial retrograde activation is recorded simultaneously at His bundle and distal CS (CS 7–8).

II, V1, Electrocardiogram leads; *AVNRT,* atrioventricular nodal reentrant tachycardia; *CS,* coronary sinus; *His,* His bundle; *His,* His bundle electrogram; *HRA,* high right atrium; *RV,* right ventricle.

In the **slow–slow** form, the AH/HA ratio is greater than 1 and the AH interval greater than 200 ms, but the VA interval is greater than 60 ms, suggesting that two different slow pathways are used for both anterograde and retrograde activation. Earliest retrograde atrial activation is usually at the coronary sinus ostium, but variants of left-sided atrial retrograde activation have also been published.[22,23] The distinction between fast–slow and slow–slow forms is of no practical significance, and certain cases of atypical AVNRT cannot be classified according to described criteria (Fig. 14.10).[24]

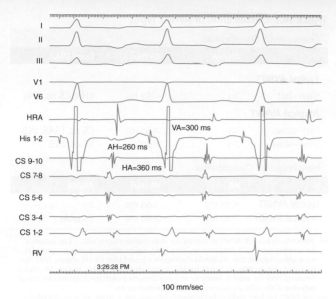

FIG. 14.10. Atypical AVNRT. The form is fast–slow according to the AH < HA definition but slow–slow according to the AH > 200 ms criterion.

II, II, III, V1, V6, Electrocardiogram leads; *AVNRT,* atrioventricular nodal reentrant tachycardia; *CS,* coronary sinus; *His,* His bundle; *His,* His bundle electrogram; *HRA,* high right atrium; *RV,* right ventricle.

There is also evidence that the "fast" pathway during slow–fast AVNRT is not identical to the "fast" component of the so-called fast–slow AVNRT.[18] AVNRT therefore can be classified as typical or atypical according to the HA interval or, when a His bundle electrogram is not reliably recorded, according to the VA interval measured on the His bundle recording electrode (Table 14.1).[24]

TABLE 14.1 Classification of AVNRT types

Conventional Classification			
	AH/HA	VA (His)	Usual ERAA
Typical AVNRT			
Slow–fast	>1	<60 ms	RHis, CS os, LHis
Atypical AVNRT			
Fast–slow	<1	>60 ms	CS os, LRAS, dCS
Slow–slow	>1	>60	CS os, dCS
New Proposed Classification			
	HA	VA (His)	AH/HA
Typical AVNRT	<70 ms	<60 ms	>1
Atypical AVNRT	>70 ms	>60 ms	Variable

AH, Atrium-to-His interval; *AVNRT,* atrioventricular nodal reentrant tachycardia; *CS os,* ostium of the coronary sinus; *dCS,* distal coronary sinus *ERAA,* earliest retrograde atrial activation; *HA,* His-to-atrium interval; *Lhis,* His bundle electrogram recorded from the left septum; *LRAS,* low right atrial septum; *RHis,* His bundle electrogram recorded from the right septum; *VA,* interval measured from the onset of ventricular activation on surface electrocardiogram to the earliest deflection of the atrial activation in the His bundle electrogram.
Atypical AVNRT has been traditionally classified as fast–slow (HA > 70 ms, VA > 60, AH/HA < 1, and AH < 200 ms) or slow–slow (HA > 70 ms, VA > 60 ms, AH/HA > 1, and AH > 200 ms). Not all of these criteria are always met, and atypical AVNRT may not be subclassified accordingly.
Katritsis DG, Camm AJ. Atrioventricular nodal reentrant tachycardia. *Circulation.* 2010;122:831-840, and Katritsis DG, Josephson ME. Classification of electrophysiological types of atrioventricular nodal re-entrant tachycardia: a reappraisal. *Europe.* 2013;Apr 23.

DIFFERENTIAL DIAGNOSIS

In the presence of a **narrow-QRS tachycardia,** AVNRT should be differentiated from the following:

- *Atrial tachycardia*
- *Orthodromic AVRT* caused by a septal accessory pathway
- *Automatic junctional tachycardia*

Atrial tachycardia is usually a narrow-QRS tachycardia. Conduction with aberration or over a bystanding pathway are rare possibilities. Narrow-QRS AVRT in the absence of overt preexcitation is due to a concealed accessory pathway that is responsible for orthodromic tachycardia.

When a **wide-QRS tachycardia** is encountered and ventricular tachycardia is excluded, the possible diagnoses are as follows:

- *AVNRT with aberrant conduction* as a result of bundle branch block

- *Atrial tachycardia with aberrant conduction* as a result of bundle branch block
- *AVNRT with a bystanding accessory pathway*
- *Antidromic AVRT* as a result of an accessory pathway
- *Automatic junctional tachycardia*

Aberrant conduction, although rare, can be seen in AVNRT and is usually, but not invariably, of the RBBB type.

The rare form of verapamil-sensitive atrial tachycardia is due to reentry in the atrial tissue close to the AVN but not the AV nodal conducting system.[25]

Although differential diagnosis is reliably accomplished at electrophysiology study, several electrocardiographic criteria may indicate AVNRT, and they are specific but modestly sensitive (see Chapter 10).[6]

CATHETER ABLATION

A recent randomized clinical trial that compared catheter ablation as first-line treatment with AAD demonstrated significant benefits in arrhythmia-related hospitalizations (Fig. 14.11).[26]

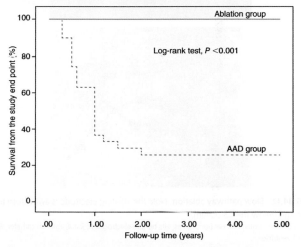

FIG. 14.11. Arrhythmia-free survival after catheter ablation or drugs.
(Katritsis DG, Zografos T, Katritsis GD, et al. Catheter ablation vs. antiarrhythmic drug therapy in patients with symptomatic atrioventricular nodal re-entrant tachycardia: a randomized, controlled trial. *Europace.* 2017;19:602-606.)

Furthermore, catheter ablation for SVT in general, and AVNRT in particular, is the treatment of choice in symptomatic patients because it both substantially improves quality of life,[27-30] and reduces costs.[31-33] Slow pathway modification is effective in both typical and atypical AVNRT.[34] Usually a combined anatomic and mapping approach is employed, with ablation lesions delivered at the inferior part of the triangle of Koch, either from the right or the left septal side (Figs. 14.12–14.14).[34-38]

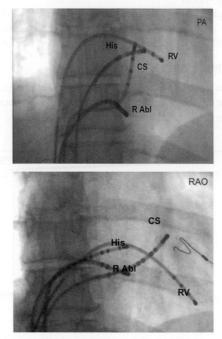

FIG. 14.12. Slow pathway ablation. Note the ablating electrode is away from the His and below the CS ostium.

CS, Coronary sinus; His, His bundle; His, His bundle electrogram; R abl, ablation catheter, RV, right ventricle.

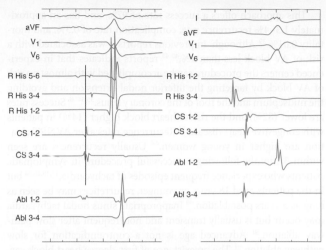

FIG. 14.13. Electrograms at the site of successful outcome. *Left panel:* Right septal ablation of the slow pathway. *Right panel:* Left septal ablation of the slow pathway. Note that the A recorded by the ablation catheter is closer to the CS rather than the His atrial electrogram.

II, aVF, V1, V6, Electrocardiogram leads; *abl,* ablation catheter electrograms; *CS,* coronary sinus; *R His,* His bundle electrogram recorded from the right side of the septum.

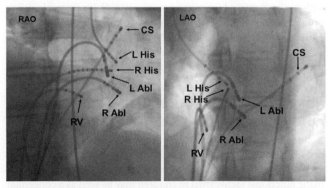

FIG. 14.14. Position of catheters for right- and left-sided slow pathway ablation.
CS, Coronary sinus; *L Abl,* His bundle electrode at the left side of the septum; *L His,* His bundle electrode at the left side of the septum; *R Abl,* His bundle electrode at the right side of the septum; *R His,* His bundle electrode at the right side of the septum; *RV,* right ventricle.

This approach offers a success rate of 97%, and has an approximately 1.3–4% recurrence rate, complication rate of 0.3%, and mortality 0.01%.[39] Although in previous reports it was associated with a risk of AV block less than 1%,[40-43] reports indicates that in experienced centers the procedure can be accomplished with almost no risk of AV block by targeting the inferior nodal extension and avoiding the midseptum and the roof of the coronary sinus.[35,44-46] Success rates are lower (82%) and the risk of heart block higher (14%) in patients with congestive heart disease.[47] Recurrence rates after AVNRT ablation are higher in young women.[48] Usually recurrences are seen within 3 months following a successful procedure in symptomatic patients who experience frequent episodes of tachycardia,[17,18,26,34] but in the patients aged 18 years or younger, recurrences may be seen as long as 5 years postablation.[49] Inappropriate sinus nodal tachycardia may occur but is usually transient and not frequent after slow pathway ablation.[50] Advanced age is not a contraindication for slow pathway ablation.[51] The preexistence of first-degree heart block carries a higher risk for late AV block, and avoidance of extensive slow pathway ablation is preferable under such conditions.[52] There is no procedure-related mortality in most published studies,[40,41,44,53-60] although in the Latin American Catheter Ablation Registry there was one death (corresponding to 0.02% mortality) after tamponade.[56] Cryoablation may carry a lower risk of AV block but is associated with a significantly higher recurrence rate.[61-63] Its favorable safety profile and higher long-term success rate in younger patients make it especially attractive for children.[64] AVNRT is a cause of inappropriate shocks in patients with implantable cardioverter defibrillators, and in the case of frequent episodes, catheter ablation is clearly indicated.[65]

NONREENTRANT JUNCTIONAL TACHYCARDIAS
AUTOMATIC JUNCTIONAL TACHYCARDIA

Automatic junctional tachycardia (or junctional ectopic tachycardia-JET) is an uncommon arrhythmia that arises from abnormal automaticity at the AV node (AVN) or proximal His bundle. Automatic junctional tachycardia in children may be seen as a congenital arrhythmia or, more often, early after infant open heart surgery.[66-68] Junctional tachycardia can also be seen in adult patients with a structurally normal heart[69,70] and can occur during an acute myocardial infarction.[71] The usual ECG finding in JET is a narrow-QRS tachycardia with a short or variable RP interval or VA dissociation. Occasionally the tachycardia is irregular and resembles atrial fibrillation.

Selective catheter ablation at the site of the earliest retrograde atrial activation is feasible but carries a lower success rate and higher AV block risk compared with AVNRT (5% to 10%).[69,72] Cryoablation is safer.[73,74]

OTHER NONREENTRANT VARIANTS

Nonparoxysmal junctional tachycardia was often diagnosed in the past as a junctional rhythm of gradual onset and termination with a rate between 70 and 130 bpm and was considered a typical example of digitalis-induced delayed adterdepoloarizations and triggered activity in the AVN.[75] The RP interval during tachycardia is variable. Myocardial ischemia, hypokalemia, chronic obstructive pulmonary disease, and myocarditis are also associated conditions.

Nonreentrant AV nodal tachycardia caused by *simultaneous multiple nodal pathway conduction* (often called **dual AV nodal tachycardia**) is an uncommon mechanism of AV nodal tachycardia resulting in more QRS than P waves[76-78] and has been associated with *repetitive retrograde concealment or "linking" phenomena*.[79-81] These are expressed in the form of ventricular pauses with consistent AV relationship after the pause and can often be misdiagnosed as atrial fibrillation.[82] These rare tachycardias may cause tachycardiomyopathy that resolves after to slow pathway ablation.

JUNCTIONAL PREMATURE BEATS

Junctional premature beats arise in the AV junction and usually conduct in antegrade fashion to the ventricles and retrogradely to the atria. There are inverted negative P waves in the inferior leads and a positive in aVR, the timing of which relative to the QRS complex depends on the part of the AV junction that is the site of origin and the conduction times to the atria and the ventricles. The retrograde P may occur immediately before, during, or after the QRS complex, which itself may display various degrees of aberration. Concealed His bundle extrasystoles may simulate first- or second-degree AV block and can occur in patients with or without conduction system disease.[83]

References

1. Katritsis DG, Becker A. The atrioventricular nodal reentrant tachycardia circuit: a proposal. *Heart Rhythm.* 2007;4(10):1354-1360.
2. Katritsis DG, Camm AJ. Atrioventricular nodal reentrant tachycardia. *Circulation.* 2010;122(8):831-840.
3. Katritsis DG, Josephson ME. Classification of electrophysiological types of atrioventricular nodal re-entrant tachycardia: a reappraisal. *Europace.* 2013;15(9):1231-1240.
4. Katritsis DG, Sepahpour A, Marine JE, et al. Atypical atrioventricular nodal reentrant tachycardia: prevalence, electrophysiologic characteristics, and tachycardia circuit. *Europace.* 2015;17(7):1099-1106.
5. Miljoen H, Ector J, Garweg C, et al. Differential presentation of atrioventricular nodal re-entrant tachycardia in athletes and non-athletes. *Europace.* 2019;21(6):944-949.
6. Katritsis DG, Josephson ME. Differential diagnosis of regular, narrow-QRS tachycardias. *Heart Rhythm.* 2015;12(7):1667-1676.
7. Katritsis DG, Ellenbogen KA, Becker AE, Camm AJ. Retrograde slow pathway conduction in patients with atrioventricular nodal re-entrant tachycardia. *Europace.* 2007;9(7):458-465.
8. Katritsis DG, Becker AE, Ellenbogen KA, Giazitzoglou E, Korovesis S, Camm AJ. Effect of slow pathway ablation in atrioventricular nodal reentrant tachycardia on the electrophysiologic characteristics of the inferior atrial inputs to the human atrioventricular node. *Am J Cardiol.* 2006;97(6):860-865.
9. Anderson RH, Sanchez-Quintana D, Mori S, Cabrera JA, Back Sternick E. Re-evaluation of the structure of the atrioventricular node and its connections with the atrium. *Europace.* 2020;22(5):821-830.
10. Katritsis DG, Efimov IR. Cardiac connexin genotyping for identification of the circuit of atrioventricular nodal re-entrant tachycardia. *Europace.* 2018.
11. Sanchez-Quintana D, Davies DW, Ho SY, Oslizlok P, Anderson RH. Architecture of the atrial musculature in and around the triangle of Koch: its potential relevance to atrioventricular nodal reentry. *J Cardiovasc Electrophysiol.* 1997;8(12):1396-1407.
12. Yanni J, Boyett MR, Anderson RH, Dobrzynski H. The extent of the specialized atrioventricular ring tissues. *Heart Rhythm.* 2009;6(5):672-680.
13. Hasdemir C, Payzin S, Kocabas U, et al. High prevalence of concealed Brugada syndrome in patients with atrioventricular nodal reentrant tachycardia. *Heart Rhythm.* 2015;12(7):1584-1594.
14. Katritsis DG, Ellenbogen KA, Becker AE. Atrial activation during atrioventricular nodal reentrant tachycardia: studies on retrograde fast pathway conduction. *Heart Rhythm.* 2006;3(9):993-1000.
15. Nam GB, Rhee KS, Kim J, Choi KJ, Kim YH. Left atrionodal connections in typical and atypical atrioventricular nodal reentrant tachycardias: activation sequence in the coronary sinus and results of radiofrequency catheter ablation. *J Cardiovasc Electrophysiol.* 2006;17(2):171-177.
16. Chua K, Upadhyay GA, Lee E, et al. High-resolution mapping of the triangle of Koch: Spatial heterogeneity of fast pathway atrionodal connections. *Heart Rhythm.* 2018;15(3):421-429.

17. Katritsis DG, Sepahpour A, Marine JE, et al. Atypical atrioventricular nodal reentrant tachycardia: prevalence, electrophysiologic characteristics, and tachycardia circuit. *Europace*. 2015;17(7):1099-1106.
18. Katritsis DG, Marine JE, Latchamsetty R, et al. Coexistent types of atrioventricular nodal re-entrant tachycardia. implications for the tachycardia circuit. *Circ Arrhythm Electrophysiol*. 2015;8(5):1189-1193.
19. Nam GB, Rhee KS, Kim JUN, Choi KJ, Kim YH. Left atrionodal connections in typical and atypical atrioventricular nodal reentrant tachycardias: activation sequence in the coronary sinus and results of radiofrequency catheter ablation. *J Cardiovasc Electrophysiol*. 2006;17(2):171-177.
20. Nawata H, Yamamoto N, Hirao K, et al. Heterogeneity of anterograde fast-pathway and retrograde slow-pathway conduction patterns in patients with the fast–slow form of atrioventricular nodal reentrant tachycardia: electrophysiologic and electrocardiographic considerations. *J Am Coll Cardiol*. 1998;32(6):1731-1740.
21. Hwang C, Martin DJ, Goodman JS, et al. Atypical atrioventricular node reciprocating tachycardia masquerading as tachycardia using a left-sided accessory pathway. *J Am Coll Cardiol*. 1997;30(1):218-225.
22. Sakabe K, Wakatsuki T, Fujinaga H, et al. Patient with atrioventricular node reentrant tachycardia with eccentric retrograde left-sided activation treatment with radiofrequency catheter ablation. *Jpn Heart J*. 2000;41(2):227-234.
23. Vijayaraman P, Kok LC, Rhee B, Ellenbogen KA. Unusual variant of atrioventricular nodal reentrant tachycardia. *Heart Rhythm*. 2005;2(1):100-102.
24. Katritsis DG, Josephson ME. Classification, electrophysiological features and therapy of atrioventricular nodal reentrant tachycardia. *Arrhythm Electrophysiol Rev*. 2016;5(2):130-135.
25. Yamabe H, Tanaka Y, Morihisa K, et al. Analysis of the anatomical tachycardia circuit in verapamil-sensitive atrial tachycardia originating from the vicinity of the atrioventricular node. *Circ Arrhythm Electrophysiol*. 2010;3(1):54-62.
26. Katritsis DG, Zografos T, Katritsis GD, et al. Catheter ablation vs. antiarrhythmic drug therapy in patients with symptomatic atrioventricular nodal re-entrant tachycardia: a randomized, controlled trial. *Europace*. 2017;19(4):602-606.
27. Farkowski MM, Pytkowski M, Maciag A, et al. Gender-related differences in outcomes and resource utilization in patients undergoing radiofrequency ablation of supraventricular tachycardia: results from Patients' Perspective on Radiofrequency Catheter Ablation of AVRT and AVNRT Study. *Europace*. 2014;16(12):1821-1827.
28. Goldberg AS, Bathina MN, Mickelsen S, Nawman R, West G, Kusumoto FM. Long-term outcomes on quality-of-life and health care costs in patients with supraventricular tachycardia (radiofrequency catheter ablation versus medical therapy). *Am J Cardiol*. 2002;89(9):1120-1123.
29. Larson MS, McDonald K, Young C, Sung R, Hlatky MA. Quality of life before and after radiofrequency catheter ablation in patients with drug refractory atrioventricular nodal reentrant tachycardia. *Am J Cardiol*. 1999;84(4):471-473.
30. Wood KA, Stewart AL, Drew BJ, Scheinman MM, Froëlicher ES. Patient perception of symptoms and quality of life following ablation in patients with supraventricular tachycardia. *Heart Lung*. 2010;39(1):12-20.

31. Bathina M, Mickelsen S, Brooks C, Jaramillo J, Hepton T, Kusumoto F. Radiofrequency catheter ablation versus medical therapy for initial treatment of supraventricular tachycardia and its impact on quality of life and healthcare costs. *Am J Cardiol.* 1998;82(5):589-593.

32. Cheng CF, Sanders GD, Hlatky MA, et al. Cost-effectiveness of radiofrequency ablation for supraventricular tachycardia. *Ann Intern Med.* 2000;133(11):864-876.

33. Kalbfleisch SJ, Calkins H, Langberg JJ, et al. Comparison of the cost of radiofrequency catheter modification of the atrioventricular node and medical therapy for drug-refractory atrioventricular node reentrant tachycardia. *J Am Coll Cardiol.* 1992;19(7):1583-1587.

34. Katritsis DG, Marine JE, Contreras FM, et al. Catheter ablation of atypical atrioventricular nodal reentrant tachycardia. *Circulation.* 2016;134(21):1655-1663.

35. Kalbfleisch SJ, Strickberger SA, Williamson B, et al. Randomized comparison of anatomic and electrogram mapping approaches to ablation of the slow pathway of atrioventricular node reentrant tachycardia. *J Am Coll Cardiol.* 1994;23(3):716-723.

36. Katritsis DG, Giazitzoglou E, Zografos T, Ellenbogen KA, Camm AJ. An approach to left septal slow pathway ablation. *J Interv Card Electrophysiol.* 2011;30(1):73-79.

37. Katritsis DG, John RM, Latchamsetty R, et al. Left septal slow pathway ablation for atrioventricular nodal reentrant tachycardia. *Circ Arrhythm Electrophysiol.* 2018;11(3):e005907.

38. Stavrakis S, Jackman WM, Lockwood D, et al. Slow/fast atrioventricular nodal reentrant tachycardia using the inferolateral left atrial slow pathway. *Circ Arrhythm Electrophysiol.* 2018;11(9):e006631.

39. Brugada J, Katritsis DG, Arbelo E, et al. 2019 ESC Guidelines for the management of patients with supraventricular tachycardia. *Eur Heart J.* 2020;41(5):655-720.

40. Spector P, Reynolds MR, Calkins H, et al. Meta-analysis of ablation of atrial flutter and supraventricular tachycardia. *The American Journal of Cardiology.* 2009;104(5):671-677.

41. Bohnen M, Stevenson WG, Tedrow UB, et al. Incidence and predictors of major complications from contemporary catheter ablation to treat cardiac arrhythmias. *Heart Rhythm.* 2011;8(11):1661-1666.

42. Morady F. Catheter ablation of supraventricular arrhythmias: State of the art. *Heart Rhythm.* 2004;1(5, Supplement):C67-C84.

43. Van Hare GF, Javitz H, Carmelli D, et al. Prospective assessment after pediatric cardiac ablation: demographics, medical profiles, and initial outcomes. *J Cardiovasc Electrophysiol.* 2004;15(7):759-770.

44. Katritsis SG, Xografos T, Siontis KC, et al. Endpoints for Successful Slow Pathway Catheter Ablation in Typical and Atypical Atrioventricular Nodal Re-Entrant Tachycardia: A Contemporary, Multicenter Study. *JACC Clin Electrophysiol.* 2019 Jan;5(1):113-119.

45. Katritsis DG. Catheter ablation of atrioventricular nodal re-entrant tachycardia: facts and fiction. *Arrhythm Electrophysiol Rev.* 2018;7(4):230-231.

46. Chen H, Shehata M, Ma W, et al. Atrioventricular block during slow pathway ablation: entirely preventable? *Circ Arrhythm Electrophysiol.* 2015;8(3):739-744.

47. Papagiannis J, Beissel DJ, Krause U, et al. Atrioventricular nodal reentrant tachycardia in patients with congenital heart disease. Outcome after catheter ablation. *Circ Arrhythm Electrophysiol.* 2017;10(7):e004869.

48. Feldman A, Voskoboinik A, Kumar S, et al. Predictors of acute and long-term success of slow pathway ablation for atrioventricular nodal reentrant tachycardia: a single center series of 1,419 consecutive patients. *Pacing Clin Electrophysiol.* 2011;34(8):927-933.

49. Backhoff D, Klehs S, Müller MJ, et al. Long-term follow-up after catheter ablation of atrioventricular nodal reentrant tachycardia in children. *Circ Arrhythm Electrophysiol.* 2016;9(11):e004264.

50. Skeberis V, Simonis F, Tsakonas K, Celiker Alp AY, Andries E, Brugada P. Inappropriate sinus tachycardia following radiofrequency ablation of AV nodal tachycardia: incidence and clinical significance. *Pacing Clin Electrophysiol.* 1994;17(5):924-927.

51. Rostock T, Risius T, Ventura R, et al. Efficacy and safety of radiofrequency catheter ablation of atrioventricular nodal reentrant tachycardia in the elderly. *J Cardiovasc Electrophysiol.* 2005;16(6):608-610.

52. Li YG, Gronefeld G, Bender B, Machura C, Hohnloser SH. Risk of development of delayed atrioventricular block after slow pathway modification in patients with atrioventricular nodal reentrant tachycardia and a pre-existing prolonged PR interval. *Eur Heart J.* 2001;22(1):89-95.

53. Spector P, Reynolds MR, Calkins H, et al. Meta-analysis of ablation of atrial flutter and supraventricular tachycardia. *Am J Cardiol.* 2009;104(5):671-677.

54. Bohnen M, Stevenson WG, Tedrow UB, et al. Incidence and predictors of major complications from contemporary catheter ablation to treat cardiac arrhythmias. *Heart Rhythm.* 2011;8(11):1661-1666.

55. Garcia-Fernandez FJ, Ibanez Criado JL, Quesada Dorador A, collaborators of the Spanish Catheter Ablation R, Registry C. Spanish Catheter Ablation Registry. 17th Official Report of the Spanish Society of Cardiology Working Group on Electrophysiology and Arrhythmias (2017). *Rev Esp Cardiol (Engl Ed).* 2018;71(11): 941-951.

56. Keegan R, Aguinaga L, Fenelon G, et al. The first Latin American Catheter Ablation Registry. *Europace.* 2015;17(5):794-800.

57. Steinbeck G, Sinner MF, Lutz M, Muller-Nurasyid M, Kaab S, Reinecke H. Incidence of complications related to catheter ablation of atrial fibrillation and atrial flutter: a nationwide in-hospital analysis of administrative data for Germany in 2014. *Eur Heart J.* 2018;39(45):4020-4029.

58. Konig S, Ueberham L, Schuler E, et al. In-hospital mortality of patients with atrial arrhythmias: insights from the German-wide Helios hospital network of 161 502 patients and 34 025 arrhythmia-related procedures. *Eur Heart J.* 2018;39(44): 3947-3957.

59. Hosseini SM, Rozen G, Saleh A, et al. Catheter ablation for cardiac arrhythmias: utilization and in-hospital complications, 2000 to 2013. *JACC Clin Electrophysiol.* 2017;3(11):1240-1248.

60. Holmqvist F, Kesek M, Englund A, et al. A decade of catheter ablation of cardiac arrhythmias in Sweden: ablation practices and outcomes. *Eur Heart J.* 2018.

61. Deisenhofer I, Zrenner B, Yin Y-h, et al. Cryoablation versus radiofrequency energy for the ablation of atrioventricular nodal reentrant tachycardia (the CYRANO Study): results from a large multicenter prospective randomized trial. *Circulation.* 2010;122(22):2239-2245.

62. Hanninen M, Yeung-Lai-Wah N, Massel D, et al. Cryoablation versus RF ablation for AVNRT: a meta-analysis and systematic review. *J Cardiovasc Electrophysiol.* 2013;24(12):1354-1360.

63. Matta M, Anselmino M, Scaglione M, et al. Cooling dynamics: a new predictor of long-term efficacy of atrioventricular nodal reentrant tachycardia cryoablation. *J Interv Card Electrophysiol.* 2017;48(3):333-341.

64. Pieragnoli P, Paoletti Perini A, Checchi L, et al. Cryoablation of typical AVNRT: younger age and administration of bonus ablation favor long-term success. *Heart Rhythm.* 2015;12(10):2125-2131.

65. Enriquez A, Ellenbogen KA, Boles U, Baranchuk A. Atrioventricular nodal reentrant tachycardia in implantable cardioverter defibrillators: diagnosis and troubleshooting. *J Cardiovasc Electrophysiol.* 2015;26(11):1282-1288.

66. Walsh EP, Saul JP, Sholler GF, et al. Evaluation of a staged treatment protocol for rapid automatic junctional tachycardia after operation for congenital heart disease. *J Am Coll Cardiol.* 1997;29(5):1046-1053.

67. Cools E, Missant C. Junctional ectopic tachycardia after congenital heart surgery. *Acta Anaesthesiol Belg.* 2014;65(1):1-8.

68. Collins KK, Van Hare GF, Kertesz NJ, et al. Pediatric nonpost-operative junctional ectopic tachycardia medical management and interventional therapies. *J Am Coll Cardiol.* 2009;53(8):690-697.

69. Hamdan M, Van Hare GF, Fisher W, et al. Selective catheter ablation of the tachycardia focus in patients with nonreentrant junctional tachycardia. *Am J Cardiol.* 1996;78(11):1292-1297.

70. Ruder MA, Davis JC, Eldar M, et al. Clinical and electrophysiologic characterization of automatic junctional tachycardia in adults. *Circulation.* 1986;73(5):930-937.

71. Fishenfeld J, Desser KB, Benchimol A. Non-paroxysmal A-V junctional tachycardia associated with acute myocardial infarction. *Am Heart J.* 1973;86(6):754-758.

72. Hamdan MH, Badhwar N, Scheinman MM. Role of invasive electrophysiologic testing in the evaluation and management of adult patients with focal junctional tachycardia. *Card Electrophysiol Rev.* 2002;6(4):431-435.

73. Law IH, Von Bergen NH, Gingerich JC, Saarel EV, Fischbach PS, Dick M. Transcatheter cryothermal ablation of junctional ectopic tachycardia in the normal heart. *Heart Rhythm.* 2006;3(8):903-907.

74. Entenmann A, Michel M, Herberg U, et al. Management of postoperative junctional ectopic tachycardia in pediatric patients: a survey of 30 centers in Germany, Austria, and Switzerland. *Eur J Pediatr.* 2017;176(9):1217-1226.

75. Katritsis DG, Boriani G, Cosio FG, et al. European Heart Rhythm Association (EHRA) consensus document on the management of supraventricular arrhythmias, endorsed by Heart Rhythm Society (HRS), Asia-Pacific Heart Rhythm Society (APHRS), and Sociedad Latinoamericana de Estimulación Cardiaca y Electrofisiologia (SOLAECE). *Eur Heart J.* 2018;39(16):1442-1445.

76. Jackowska-Zduniak B, Forys U. Mathematical model of the atrioventricular nodal double response tachycardia and double-fire pathology. *Math Biosci Eng.* 2016;13(6):1143-1158.

77. Peiker C, Pott C, Eckardt L, et al. Dual atrioventricular nodal non-re-entrant tachycardia. *Europace.* 2016;18(3):332-339.

78. Fadahunsi OO, Elsokkari I, AbdelWahab A. Irregular narrow complex tachycardia. *Circulation.* 2019;139(15):1848-1850.
79. Yokoshiki H, Sasaki K, Shimokawa J, Sakurai M, Tsutsui H. Nonreentrant atrioventricular nodal tachycardia due to triple nodal pathways manifested by radiofrequency ablation at coronary sinus ostium. *J Electrocardiol.* 2006;39(4):395-399.
80. Itagaki T, Ohnishi Y, Inoue T, Yokoyama M. Linking phenomenon in dual atrioventricular nodal pathways. *Jpn Circ J.* 2001;65(11):937-940.
81. Arena G, Bongiorni MG, Soldati E, Gherarducci G, Mariani M. Incessant nonreentrant atrioventricular nodal tachycardia due to multiple nodal pathways treated by radiofrequency ablation of the slow pathways. *J Cardiovasc Electrophysiol.* 1999;10(12):1636-1642.
82. Wang NC. Dual atrioventricular nodal nonreentrant tachycardia: a systematic review. *Pacing Clin Electrophysiol.* 2011;34(12):1671-1681.
83. Ameen A, Dharawat A, Khan A, Turitto G, El-Sherif N. His bundle extrasystoles revisited: the great electrocardiographic masquerader. *Pacing Clin Electrophysiol.* 2011;34(6):e56-e59.

15

Wolff-Parkinson-White Syndrome and Atrioventricular Reentrant Tachycardias

DEFINITIONS

The anatomic basis of atrioventricular reentrant tachycardia (AVRT) is an abnormal connection (**accessory pathway [AP]**) between the atrial and ventricular myocardium. One limb of the reentrant circuit is the atrioventricular (AV) node and the other is the AP. On rare occasions the circuit includes two or more APs.

The term **preexcitation** refers to earlier activation of the ventricle by a wave front arising in the atrium than would be expected if conduction occurred via the normal atrioventricular conduction pathway.

Wolff-Parkinson-White (WPW) syndrome refers to the combination of preexcitation on an electrocardiogram and episodic tachycardias using the AP (Fig. 15.1).[1]

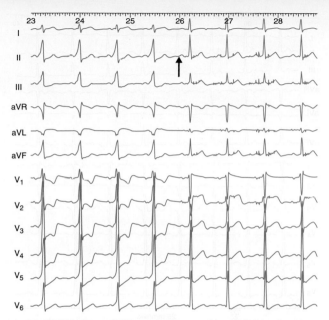

FIG. 15.1. Wolff-Parkinson-White syndrome caused by a left lateral accessory pathway. Application of radiofrequency energy during catheter ablation *(arrow)* results in loss of preexcitation and restoration of normal conduction.

The AP is located along the mitral or tricuspid annulus, and during sinus rhythm a typical pattern with the following characteristics is present on the electrocardiogram (ECG): (1) short PR interval (≤120 ms), (2) slurred upstroke or downstroke of the QRS complex ("delta wave"), and (3) a widened QRS complex during sinus rhythm. However, WPW patients with a *fasciculoventricular* pathway have a QRS width 120 ms or less.[2,3] Occasionally, preexcitation may not be fully apparent because of fusion of wave fronts progressing through the AP and the normal conduction system (Figs. 15.2 and 15.3). In most cases accessory pathways giving rise to the WPW pattern are seen in structurally normal hearts.

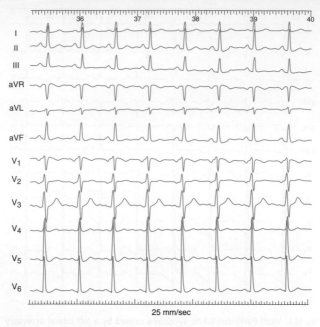

FIG. 15.2. A 12-lead electrocardiogram (ECG) of a patient with frequent episodes of narrow-QRS tachycardia. The ECG superficially looks normal, but there is a short PR interval and a hint of delta waves.

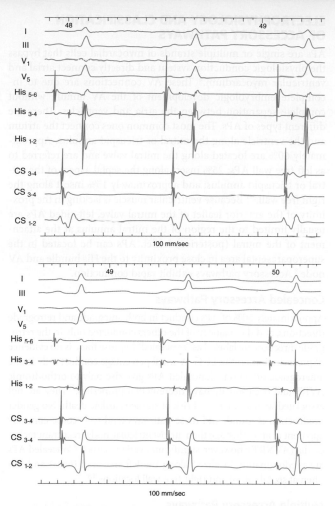

FIG. 15.3. Same patient as in Fig. 15.2. *Upper panel:* A relatively slowly antegrade conducting left-sided pathway that allows fusion of conduction with that through the His bundle. Note the close A and V electrograms at the CS catheter electrodes. Mapping identified its location in the posterior aspect of the mitral annulus, close to the septum. *Lower panel:* After successful ablation, A and V electrograms are clearly separated in the CS catheter electrodes.

I, III, V1, V5, Electrocardiogram leads; *CS,* coronary sinus; *His,* His bundle.

ELECTROPHYSIOLOGY AND CLASSIFICATION OF ACCESSORY PATHWAYS

APs are single or multiple strands of myocardial cells that bypass the physiologic conduction system and directly connect atrial and ventricular myocardium.[4] These AV connections are due to incomplete embryologic development of the AV annuli, without complete separation between the atria and ventricles. There are different types of APs. The most common ones connect the atrium and the ventricle along the mitral or tricuspid annulus. Approximately 60% are located along the mitral valve and are referred to as left free wall APs; 25% insert along the septal aspect of the mitral or tricuspid annulus; and approximately 15% insert along the right free wall.[5-7] Because ventricular muscle is lacking in the proximity of the anterior leaflet of the mitral valve, left-sided APs are usually limited to the region of the mitral annulus at the attachment of the mural (posterior) leaflet. APs can be located in the superoparaseptal area in close proximity to the His bundle and AV node.[8] Accessory pathways exhibit rapid conduction.

Concealed Accessory Pathways

Approximately 50% of APs conduct in both antegrade and retrograde directions, and the majority of the others conducted only in the retrograde direction are labeled as "concealed" because there is no evidence of preexcitation on the ECG. A small percentage conduct only in the anterograde direction. Concealed APs give rise only to orthodromic AVRT and occasionally have decremental properties.[9] They are not associated with an increased risk of sudden cardiac death. No gender predilection is found, and these pathways tend to become clinically apparent at an earlier age than atrioventricular nodal reentrant tachycardia (AVNRT); however, significant overlap exists.[10] Concealed APs are predominantly localized along the left free wall (65%) and less often at septal (30%) and right free wall locations.[4,9]

Multiple Accessory Pathways

Multiple APs occur in up to 12% of patients with preexcitation and in up to 50% in patients with Ebstein anomaly.[11] Characteristics suggestive of two or more APs are as follows:
1. Delta wave pattern not typical of any single location.
2. Changes in delta wave during atrial fibrillation or during right atrial versus coronary sinus (CS) pacing.

3. Retrograde fusion during orthodromic AVRT.
4. Changes in retrograde atrial activation sequence during ortho-dromic AVRT, either spontaneous or during radiofrequency (RF) ablation

Atypical Accessory Pathways

Atypical APs (previously called Mahaim fibers) are connections between the right atrium or the AV node (AVN) and the right ventricle into or close to the right bundle branch.[12-18] Pathways with atypical characteristics can be *atriofascicular, nodofascicular,* or *nodoventricular,* depending on their proximal and distal inser-tions.[16,17] Left-sided atypical pathways have also been described but are extremely rare.[19-21] They usually contain accessory nodal tissue, which results in decremental properties, and connect the atrium to the fascicles by crossing the lateral aspect of the tricuspid annulus, but posteroseptal locations can also be found in rare cases. Conduction is usually anterograde only, but concealed nodoventricular and nodofascicular fibers have also been de-scribed and may give rise to incessant tachycardias.[15,22] The base-line QRS of patients with atypical APs is normal or displays differ-ent degrees of manifest preexcitation with left bundle branch block morphology. Programmed or incremental atrial pacing results in manifest preexcitation when there has been sufficient delay in the AH interval. An increase in AV interval plus shortening of the HV interval and QRS widening is observed at shorter pacing cycle lengths. Atypical pathways can participate in antidromic AVRT (Fig. 15.4).

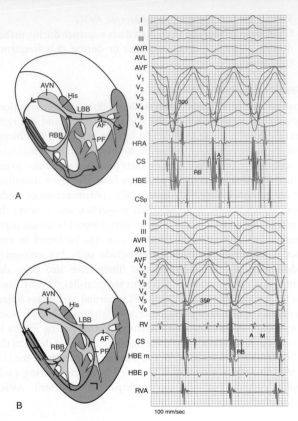

FIG. 15.4. Atypical AP physiology. Change in QRS morphology from short to long V-A AVRT. (A) During short V-A AVRT (tachycardia cycle length 300 ms), there is also antegrade activation over the left anterior fascicle to produce a fused QRS complex with a normal axis. (B) With retrograde right bundle branch block, antegrade conduction over the left anterior fascicle is no longer possible and conduction to the left ventricle proceeds only via the right free wall. Therefore the long V-A AVRT (tachycardia cycle length 350 ms) has a leftward axis. During the change from short V-A AVRT to long V-A AVRT, the QRS width also increases from 120 to 150 ms.

A, Atrial electrogram; *AF,* anterior fascicle; *AVN,* atrioventricular node; *AVRT,* atrioventricular reentrant tachycardia; *LBB,* left bundle branch catheter; *M,* Mahaim potential; *PF,* posterior fascicle; *RB,* right bundle potential; *RBB,* right bundle-branch catheter. (Gandhavadi M, Sternick EB, Jackman WM, et al. Characterization of the distal insertion of atriofascicular accessory pathways and mechanisms of QRS patterns in atriofascicular antidromic tachycardia. *Heart Rhythm.* 2013;10:1385-1392.)

DIAGNOSIS

Patients present with symptoms of paroxysmal tachycardia or with preexcited AF. AVRT is the most common tachycardia associated with the WPW syndrome. WPW predisposes to development of AF, which may or may not be eliminated after ablation of the pathway.[23,24] It is more common in patients with WPW syndrome than in the general population and may be the presenting arrhythmia in affected patients.[25]

Antegrade-conducting APs may produce a typical WPW pattern on the ECG or may be latent. Latent pathways, when conducting antegrade, may be revealed by infusion of adenosine, which not only that blocks the AV node but also facilitates AP conduction. A small percentage of APs are dependent on sympathetic activation and become manifest only during infusion of isoprenaline. In the presence of a WPW pattern, localization of the AP may be accomplished from the 12-lead ECG (Figs. 15.5 and 15.6).

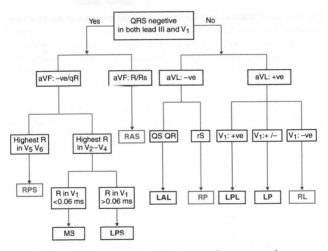

FIG. 15.5. The St. George algorithm for localization of accessory pathways.
+, Positive QRS complex; −, negative QRS complex; ±, equiphasic QRS complex; *LAL*, left anterolateral; *LP*, left posterior; *LPL*, left posterolateral; *LPS*, left posteroseptal; *MS*, midseptal; *RAS*, right anteroseptal; *RP*, right posterior; *RPS*, right posteroseptal; *RL*, right lateral; *RW*, R wave width in V1; *RWH*, the highest R wave recorded in precordial leads; *YES*, QRS complex negative in both lead III and lead V1. (Xie B, Heald SC, Bashir Y, et al. Localization of accessory pathways from the 12-lead electrocardiogram using a new algorithm. *Am J Cardiol.* 1994;74:161-165.)

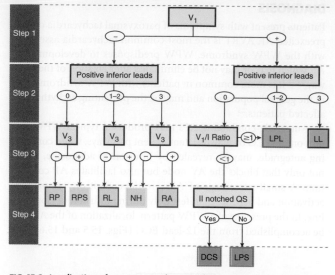

FIG. 15.6. Localization of accessory pathway in the presence of maximum pre-excitation. Accessory pathway (AP) locations are green when right sided and red when left sided. LPL APs can have 0, 1, or 2 inferior leads with positive polarity, whereas NH APs can have 1, 2, or 3 inferior leads with positive polarity. Right-sided APs are framed orange or yellow when the V3 lead is negative or positive, respectively. Left posterior APs are framed blue when V1/I ratio is less than 1 or purple when V1/I ratio is 1 or more.

DCS, Deep coronary sinus; LPL, left posterolateral; LL, left lateral; LPS, left paraseptal; NH, nodo-Hisian; RA, right anterior; RL, right lateral; RP, right posterior; RPS, right paraseptal. (Pambrun T, El Bouazzaoui R, Combes N, et al. Maximal pre-excitation based algorithm for localization of manifest accessory pathways in adults. JACC Clin Electrophysiol. 2018;4: 1052-1061.)

Orthodromic AVRT

Orthodromic AVRT refers to a reentrant tachycardia that uses the AV node–His bundle axis as the antegrade limb and the AP as the retrograde limp (Figs. 15.7 and 15.8).

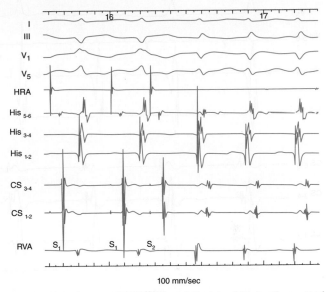

100 mm/sec

FIG. 15.7. Orthodromic AVRT caused by a left posterolateral pathway. Atrial pacing results in a preexcited electrocardiogram (ECG) with close A and V electrograms in the CS. After the last atrial extrastimulus, the AH interval gets prolonged because of refractoriness of the accessory pathway, as indicated by the absence of a V component in the CS electrograms and decremental conduction through the AVN. This allows retrograde conduction through the pathway and induction of an orthodromic tachycardia with antegrade conduction through the AVN-His axis.

I, III, Vt, V5, ECG leads; *AVN*, atrioventricular node; *CS*, coronary sinus *His*, his bundle; *HRA*, high right atrium; *RVA*, right ventricular apex.

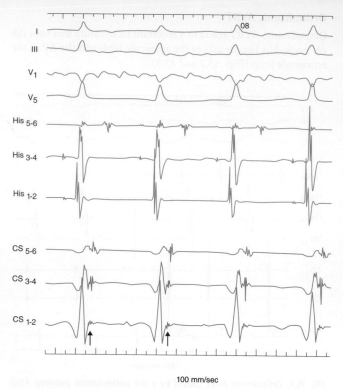

FIG. 15.8. Orthodromic AVRT with earliest atrial activation at the distal CS, consistent with a left-lateral AP. The sharp component recorded by the distal CS electrodes *(arrows)* may represent an early atrial electrogram or a pathway potential. *I, III, V1, V5,* Electrocardiogram leads; *AP,* accessory pathway; *AVRT,* atrioventricular reentrant tachycardia; *CS,* coronary sinus; *His,* His bundle.

Orthodromic AVRT accounts for more than 90% of AVRTs and 20% to 30% of all sustained SVTs.[26,27] The rate usually is 170 to 220 beats per minute. During tachycardia, the QRS is narrow unless there is a functional or underlying bundle branch block. ST segment depression often is present and has been shown to usually not be due to myocardial ischemia.[28] Ipsilateral bundle branch block during AVRT results in an increase in VA time, which can also increase the cycle length of the tachycardia, although no change in rate may also be seen because of a compensatory reduction in AH interval. A contralateral bundle branch block has no effect on the tachycardia, as it is not a part of the tachycardia circuit.

The differential diagnosis of narrow-QRS complex tachycardias is discussed in Chapter 10. In certain cases of tachycardias with atypical characteristics, multiple pacing techniques are required to reach a diagnosis. Figs. 15.9 to 15.11 present a case of a narrow-QRS tachycardia with prolonged RP intervals that was easily induced by both atrial and ventricular pacing.

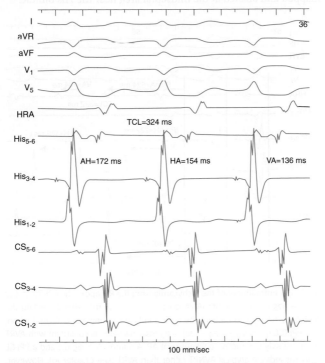

FIG. 15.9. Electrograms during narrow-QRS tachycardia with prolonged RP intervals.
I, aVR, aVF, V1, V5, Electrocardiogram leads; *AH,* atrial-to-His interval; *CS,* coronary sinus; *HA,* His-to-atrium interval; *His,* His bundle; *HRA,* high right atrium; *TCL,* tachycardia cycle length; *VA,* ventriculoatrial interval measured at the His bundle electrode.

The tachycardia was interrupted by ventricular extrastimulation and an A-V response or with single ventricular extrastimuli that were not conducted to the atria, while His-synchronous ventricular extrastimuli failed to reset the tachycardia. Thus the differential diagnosis is between atypical AVNRT and AVRT because of a concealed midseptal accessory pathway. For differential diagnosis, entrainment by ventricular pacing attempted both from the RV apex and RV base was necessary. After entrainment maneuvers as indicated in Figs. 15.10 and 15.11, an accessory pathway was mapped and ablated at the midseptal area near the His bundle.[29]

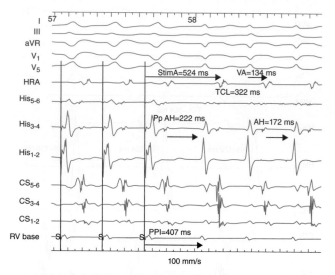

FIG. 15.10. Entrainment of the tachycardia from the RV apex. The PPI-TCL is 447 − 322 = 125 ms and the StimA-VA is 592 − 134 = 458 ms. After correcting the PPI-TCL by taking into account the pacing induced AV incremental conduction, the cPPI-TCL ms is 125 − (224 − 172) = 73 ms. This value is consistent with AVRT using a slowly conducting posteroseptal AP. A StimA-VA > 85 ms and a PPI-CL > 115 ms indicate atypical AVNRT rather than AVRT (see Chapter 10). However, correcting the PPI-TCL by taking into account the pacing induced incremental AV nodal conduction results in a cPPI-TCL = 125 − (224 − 172) ms = 73 ms. This suggests AVRT rather than AVNRT because the cutoff value is 110 ms.

AVNRT, atrioventricular nodal reentrant tachycardia; *AVRT,* atrioventricular reentrant tachycardia; *Pp AH,* postpacing AH interval; *PPI,* postpacing interval; *RV,* right ventricle; *Stim-AQ,* stimulus-atrial interval measured on the HRA electrograms; *TCL,* tachycardia cycle length; *VA,* ventriculoatrial interval measured on the HRA electrograms; other abbreviations as in Fig. 15.9. (Katritsis DG. A tachycardia with narrow-QRS morphology and prolonged RP intervals. Europace. 2013;15:969.)

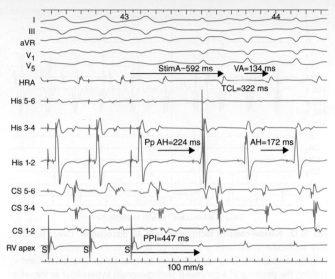

FIG. 15.11. Entrainment of the tachycardia from the RV base. The PPI-TCL is 407 − 322 = 85 ms, the StimA-VA is 524 − 134 = 390 ms, and the cPPI-TCL = 85 − (222 − 172) = 35 ms. The RV apex is closer to the AVNRT circuit in the vicinity of the AV node than the RV base because the impulse is conducted retrogradely through the His-Purkinje network. Thus basal entrainment produces longer cPPI-TCL and StimA-VA intervals in atypical AVNRT.

Pp AH, postpacing AH interval; *PPI,* postpacing interval; *RV,* right ventricle; *Stim-A,* stimulus-atrial interval measured on the HRA electrograms; *TCL,* tachycardia cycle length; *VA,* ventriculoatrial interval measured on the HRA electrograms; other abbreviations as in Fig. 15.9. (Katritsis DG. A tachycardia with narrow-QRS morphology and prolonged RP intervals. Europace. 2013;15:969.)

Fig. 15.12 presents a rare case of an orthodromic AVRT caused by a concealed nodoventricular pathway and AV dissociation.[30]

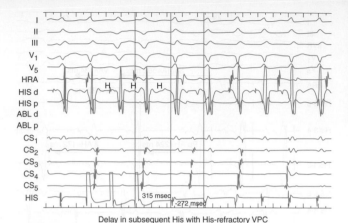

Delay in subsequent His with His-refractory VPC

FIG. 15.12. Narrow-complex tachycardia with AV dissociation. Three His-refractory ventricular extrastimuli are delivered during supraventricular tachycardia with AV dissociation. The third ventricular stimulus delays the next His and V, proving the presence of a concealed ventriculonodal bypass tract as the retrograde limits.

I, II, III, V1, V6, Electrocardiogram leads; *ABL,* ablation catheter; *CS,* coronary sinus; *His,* His bundle; *HRA,* high right atrium; *RVa,* right ventricular apex. (Josephson ME. Electrophysiology at a crossroads. *Heart Rhythm.* 2007;4:658-661.)

Permanent Junctional Reciprocating Tachycardia (PJRT)

PJRT represents a rare form of a long RP tachycardia using a concealed AP. Usually these APs are located in the posteroseptal region and are associated with retrograde decremental conduction properties.[31] The incessant nature of PJRT may result in tachycardiomyopathy that usually resolves after successful treatment by RF catheter ablation, particularly in younger patients.[32]

Antidromic AVRT

Antidromic AVRT refers to a reentrant circuit that uses the AP as the antegrade limb, and the AV node–His bundle axis (or, rarely, another AP) as the retrograde limp. Antidromic AVRT occurs in 3% to 8% of patients with WPW syndrome.[33-35] In patients with spontaneous antidromic AVRT, multiple APs (manifest or concealed), which may or may not serve as the retrograde limb of the AVRT, may be present. Antidromic AVRT is a wide QRS complex (fully preexcited) tachycardia. In the presence of atrial tachycardia, atrial flutter, AF, or AVNRT, the QRS complexes can also be preexcited when the AP acts as a **bystander** and is not a critical part of the reentry circuit.

The differential diagnosis of wide complex tachycardias is discussed in Chapter 11.

RISK STRATIFICATION OF PATIENTS WITH ASYMPTOMATIC PREEXCITATION

More than 20% of patients with an asymptomatic WPW pattern develop an arrhythmia related to their AP during follow-up.[36-45] The most common arrhythmia in patients with WPW syndrome is AVRT (80%), followed by a 20% to 30% incidence of AF. Sudden cardiac death (SCD) secondary to preexcited AF that conducts rapidly to the ventricle over the AP resulting in ventricular fibrillation (VF) is the most feared manifestation of the WPW syndrome.[46-49] The risk of cardiac arrest/VF was recently estimated at 2.4 per 1000 person-years, but no deaths were reported in this registry of 2169 patients over an 8-year follow-up.[46] However, in a Danish registry of 310 individuals with preexcitation (age range 8 to 85 years), there was a higher hazard of AF and heart failure in the presence of a right anteroseptal AP and in patients older than 65 years.[44] Recent data support the notion of left ventricular dysfunction related to *electrical asynchrony* in patients, especially children, with asymptomatic preexcitation.[50-53]

Electrophysiology Testing

Electrophysiologic data that identify patients with a high-risk AP include a shortest preexcited RR interval during AF (SPERRI) 250 ms or less, AP ERP 250 ms or less, multiple APs and an inducible AP-mediated tachycardia in the baseline state or during isoproterenol infusion, especially in children.[37-40,46-48,54-57] However, even the absence of these factors does not rule out the possibility of a potentially high-risk AP. In a retrospective study of 912 patients 21 years and younger with WPW syndrome, 96 patients experienced life-threatening events. Of those, 49% had rapidly conducted preexcited AF. In patients with events subjected to EPS risk stratification, 22 of 60 (37%) did not have EPS-determined high-risk characteristics, and 15 of 60 (25%) had neither high-risk AP characteristics nor inducible AVRT.[45]

Noninvasive Testing

With noninvasive testing, identification of an abrupt and complete normalization of the PR interval with loss of delta wave during exercise testing or after procainamide, propafenone, or disopyramide administration have been considered to be markers of low risk.[47,58-60] Autonomic tone can be a major confounding factor in all tests, both invasive[54,55] and noninvasive.[47,58,59] Intermittent loss of preexcitation on a resting ECG or ambulatory monitoring has also been associated with APs with longer ERPs and previously was considered to be a credible risk stratification tool.[61,62] However, a number of studies in both symptomatic and asymptomatic individuals have indicated that more than 20% of patients with intermittent preexcitation have an AP ERP less than 250 ms. Thus intermittent preexcitation is no longer considered to be a reliable indicator of a low-risk AP.[59,63-67]

CATHETER ABLATION

Recurrent AVRT or Pre-Excited AF

The treatment of choice for patients with recurrent AVRT or pre-excited AF is catheter ablation. In patients with overt preexcitation this can be accomplished during sinus rhythm, with the target being an AP potential or V electrogram preceding the delta wave as much as possible. At the successful ablation site the AV interval is minimum and a pathway potential may be found (Fig. 15.13).[68]

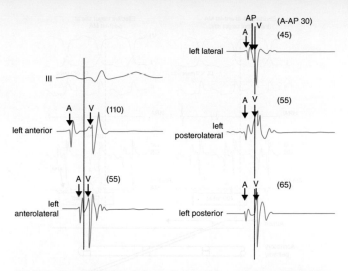

FIG. 15.13. Map of left free wall along mitral annulus recorded from left ventricular catheter in a patient with a left lateral accessory pathway. Shown are bipolar endocardial electrograms from five annular sites and surface electrocardiographic lead III. Vertical line denotes onset of the delta wave; numbers in parentheses represent, except where noted, local atrioventricular (AV) conduction times in milliseconds. Note the recording in the left lateral electrogram of the shortest AV interval (45 ms), which coincides with the appearance of an accessory pathway (AP) potential between the atrial (A) and ventricular (V) potential. The A-AP interval measures 30 ms.
(Kuck KH, Schluter M. Single-catheter approach to radiofrequency current ablation of left-sided accessory pathways in patients with Wolff-Parkinson-White syndrome. *Circulation.* 1991;84:2366-2375.)

For **left-sided APs,** two approaches are available: an antegrade transseptal and a retrograde aortic approach. There is evidence that the transseptal approach in experienced hands results in reduced radiation and procedure time.[69,70] Left-sided APs often have an oblique fiber orientation, and the site of earliest ventricular activation is not necessarily the effective target site. Successful ablation may be accomplished at a site where V activation is not the earliest but where an AP potential is recorded (Fig. 15.14).[71]

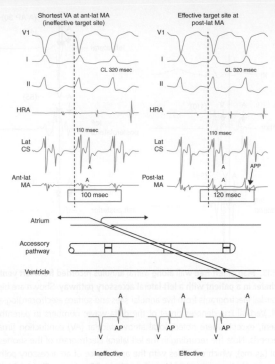

FIG. 15.14. Ablation of an oblique left-sided AP. The shortest VA interval is at the anterolateral mitral annulus, but at this site the AP potential is relatively late. An RF application at the ventricular aspect of the mitral annulus at this site was ineffective because the site was not close enough to the ventricular insertion site of the AP and the ablation lesion was not deep enough to cross the annulus and reach the atrial insertion site. The effective target site was at the posterolateral mitral annulus where the VA interval was longer but where an earlier AP potential was recorded. Identification of the site of the earliest AP potential allows the catheter to be positioned closer to the ventricular insertion site where RF ablation is likely to be successful. The *right panel* depicts this is graphic fashion.

I, II, V1, Electrocardiogram leads; *AP,* accessory pathway; *HRA,* high right atrium; *CS,* coronary sinus; *MA,* mitral annulus; *RF,* radiofrequency; *VA,* ventriculoatrial. (Jackman WM, Friday KJ, Yeung-Lai-Wah JA, et al. New catheter technique for recording left free-wall accessory atrioventricular pathway activation. Identification of pathway fiber orientation. *Circulation.* 1988;78:598-611.)

With **septal APs** close to the AV node, the electrocardiogram typically displays a positive delta wave in leads avF and avL and a narrow positive delta wave in lead V1 that has a prominently negative QRS complex.[8] RF ablation of para-Hisian AP without creating AV block is possible,[72] but with cryoenergy the incidence of AV block is lower.[73] However, the recurrence rate of AP conduction is significantly higher after cryoablation.[74] In some patients with anteroseptal pathways, the successful ablation site can be in the right coronary cusp and noncoronary cusp noncoronary cusp of the aortic valve, which lie in close anatomical proximity to the anterior septum (Fig. 15.15).[75]

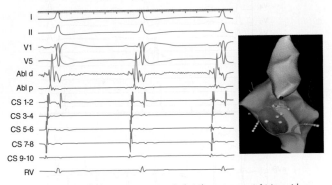

FIG. 15.15. *Left panel:* Electrograms recorded at the anteroseptal tricuspid annulus, where both a His bundle depolarization and an AP potential were recorded. An attempt at RF ablation was quickly aborted because of junctional ectopy indicating impending AV block. An effective ablation site was found in the noncoronary cusp. At this site, AP conduction block was created within a few seconds and there was no junctional ectopy or prolongation of the PR interval during a 60-second application at 25 watts. *Right panel:* Electroanatomic map in a left anterior oblique (LAO) view showing the ineffective ablation site at the anteroseptal TV annulus *(blue tag)* and the effective target site in the noncoronary cusp *(red tag).*

I, II, V1, V5, Electrocardiogram leads; *Abl,* ablation catheter; *AV,* atrioventricular; *AP* accessory pathway; *CS,* coronary sinus; *RF,* radiofrequency; *RV,* right ventricle.

Epicardial APs occur in less than 10% of all cases and can be approached from the coronary sinus or the pericardial space (<1%) (Fig. 15.16).

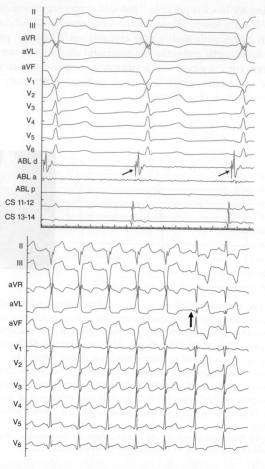

FIG. 15.16. *Left panel:* Electrograms recorded in the pericardial space near the posterior septum. The electrogram recorded by the distal electrodes of the ablation catheter *(Abl d)* show a large AP potential *(arrow)* and early ventricular activation. *Right panel:* AP conduction block *(arrow)* occurred within the first few seconds of an application of RF energy at this site in the pericardial space (4-mm tip, 40 watts, 55°–60°C).

II, III, aVR, aVL, aVF, V1–V6, Electrocardiogram leads; *ABL,* ablation catheter; *AP,* accessory pathway; *CS,* coronary sinus; *RF,* radiofrequency.

In patients with **concealed** or latent pathways, ablation is usually performed during ventricular pacing or AVRT by targeting the site of the earliest retrograde atrial activation (Fig. 15.17) or earliest retrograde AP potential. Bracketing of the pathway by the CS electrodes may be useful in identifying its approximate position.

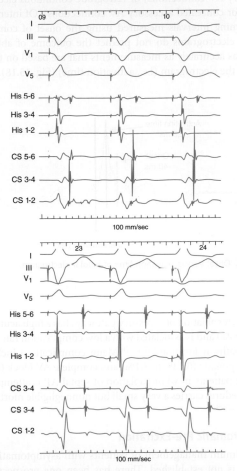

FIG. 15.17. *Upper panel:* V pacing reveals earliest retrograde atrial activation at distal CS. The first, sharp component of the atrial electrogram (CS 1-2) may represent a pathway potential. *Lower panel:* After successful ablation at this site through a transseptal approach, concentric retrograde atrial activation (through the His bundle) is revealed. *I, III, V1, V5,* Electrocardiogram leads; *CS,* coronary sinus; *His,* his bundle.

In general, the local electrogram parameters of greatest importance in predicting the success or failure of radiofrequency catheter ablation of accessory AV connections are electrogram stability, the presence of an accessory AV connection potential, and the timing of ventricular activation relative to the QRS complex (for manifest accessory AV connections) or retrograde continuous electrical activity (for concealed accessory AV connections). Of interest, however, timing intervals measured using the onset of conventional bipolar electrograms do not predict the outcome of ablation attempts as accurately as measurements that are based on the tallest peak of the electrogram (i.e., activation time) (Fig. 15.18).[76]

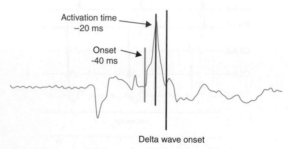

Activation time
−20 ms

Onset
-40 ms

Delta wave onset

FIG. 15.18. Onset versus activation time of bipolar electrogram.

Catheter ablation of accessory pathways has a high acute success rate (≥95%) and is associated with a low complication rate depending on pathway location.[37,74,77,78] Major complications include cardiac tamponade (0.13% to 1.1%) and complete AV block (0.17% to 2.7%) in patients in whom ablation of septal AP is attempted, and the procedures carries a very small but nonnegligible mortality risk (0.1%).[26,27,79-86]

Asymptomatic Pre-Excitation

The optimum management of patients with asymptomatic preexcitation is not established. There has been one prospective randomized clinical trial of patients with asymptomatic preexcitation pattern.[87] Catheter ablation was associated with a 92% risk reduction of developing an arrhythmia during follow-up, but no fatalities were reported in the untreated group. If a patient undergoes screening with an EPS and is found to have an AP with "high-risk" characteristics, catheter ablation should be considered given that catheter ablation of an AP, when performed by an experienced operator, is associated with a high success rate (>95%) and low risk (<0.5%) of major complications.[37,74,77,87] In the CASPED registry of 182 children and adolescents with asymptomatic preexcitation, catheter ablation achieved a 91% success rate without significant complications.[88] It also seems reasonable to consider ablation if a link between preexcitation and left ventricular dysfunction can be made.[50-53] In patients with atypical pathways, preventive ablation for prognostic reasons is not routinely recommended, not even in patients with preexcitation or bundle branch block in the surface ECG, because fast conduction via the AP is unlikely as a result of decremental conduction properties.

The approach to patients with asymptomatic preexcitation that does not exhibit high-risk characteristics at EPS depends on the experience and expertise of the electrophysiologist performing the procedure as well as patient preference. The location of the pathway is important. The risk of heart block associated with ablation of anteroseptal or midseptal AP may preclude attempts at ablation of such a pathway in an asymptomatic patient.

References

1. Bhatia A, Sra J, Akhtar M. Preexcitation syndromes. *Curr Probl Cardiol.* 2016;41(3):99-137.
2. Suzuki T, Nakamura Y, Yoshida S, Yoshida Y, Shintaku H. Differentiating fasciculoventricular pathway from Wolff-Parkinson-White syndrome by electrocardiography. *Heart Rhythm.* 2014;11(4):686-690.
3. Anderson RH, Smerup M, Sanchez-Quintana D, Loukas M, Lunkenheimer PP. The three-dimensional arrangement of the myocytes in the ventricular walls. *Clin Anat.* 2009;22(1):64-76.
4. Ho SY. Accessory Atrioventricular pathways: getting to the origins. *Circulation.* 2008;117(12):1502-1504.
5. Jackman WM, Wang XZ, Friday KJ, et al. Catheter ablation of accessory atrioventricular pathways (Wolff-Parkinson-White syndrome) by radiofrequency current. *N Engl J Med.* 1991;324(23):1605-1611.
6. Katritsis D, Bashir Y, Heald S, Poloniecki J, Ward DE. Radiofrequency ablation of accessory pathways: implications of accumulated experience and time dedicated to procedures. *Eur Heart J.* 1994;15(3):339-344.

7. Schluter M, Geiger M, Siebels J, Duckeck W, Kuck KH. Catheter ablation using radiofrequency current to cure symptomatic patients with tachyarrhythmias related to an accessory atrioventricular pathway. *Circulation*. 1991;84(4):1644-1661.

8. Liu Q, Shehata M, Lan DZ, et al. Accurate localization and catheter ablation of superoparaseptal accessory pathways. *Heart Rhythm*. 2018;15(5):688-695.

9. Kuck KH, Friday KJ, Kunze KP, Schluter M, Lazzara R, Jackman WM. Sites of conduction block in accessory atrioventricular pathways. Basis for concealed accessory pathways. *Circulation*. 1990;82(2):407-417.

10. Katritsis DG, Boriani G, Cosio FG, et al. European Heart Rhythm Association (EHRA) consensus document on the management of supraventricular arrhythmias, endorsed by Heart Rhythm Society (HRS), Asia-Pacific Heart Rhythm Society (APHRS), and Sociedad Latinoamericana de Estimulación Cardiaca y Electrofisiologia (SOLAECE). *Eur Heart J*. 2018;39(16):1442-1445.

11. Cappato R, Schluter M, Weiss C, et al. Radiofrequency current catheter ablation of accessory atrioventricular pathways in Ebstein's anomaly. *Circulation*. 1996;94(3):376-383.

12. Kottkamp H, Hindricks G, Shenasa H, et al. Variants of preexcitation—specialized atriofascicular pathways, nodofascicular pathways, and fasciculoventricular pathways: electrophysiologic findings and target sites for radiofrequency catheter ablation. *J Cardiovasc Electrophysiol*. 1996;7(10):916-930.

13. Gandhavadi M, Sternick EB, Jackman WM, Wellens HJJ, Josephson ME. Characterization of the distal insertion of atriofascicular accessory pathways and mechanisms of QRS patterns in atriofascicular antidromic tachycardia. *Heart Rhythm*. 2013;10(9):1385-1392.

14. Haissaguerre M, Cauchemez B, Marcus F, et al. Characteristics of the ventricular insertion sites of accessory pathways with anterograde decremental conduction properties. *Circulation*. 1995;91(4):1077-1085.

15. Hluchy JAN, Schlegelmilch P, Schickel S, Jörger URS, Jurkovicova O, Sabin GV. Radiofrequency ablation of a concealed nodoventricular mahaim fiber guided by a discrete potential. *J Cardiovasc Electrophysiol*. 1999;10(4):603-610.

16. Katritsis DG, Wellens HJ, Josephson ME. Mahaim accessory pathways. *Arrhythm Electrophysiol Rev*. 2017;6(1):29-32.

17. de Alencar Neto JN, Ramalho de Moraes SR, Back Sternick E, Wellens HJJ. Atypical bypass tracts: can they be recognized during sinus rhythm? *Europace*. 2019;21(2):208-218.

18. Anderson RH, Sanchez-Quintana D, Mori S, et al. Unusual variants of preexcitation: from anatomy to ablation: part i—understanding the anatomy of the variants of ventricular pre-excitation. *J Cardiovasc Electrophysiol*. 2019;30(10):2170-2180.

19. Francia P, Pittalis MC, Ali H, Cappato R. Electrophysiological study and catheter ablation of a Mahaim fibre located at the mitral annulus-aorta junction. *J Interv Card Electrophysiol*. 2008;23(2):153-157.

20. Johnson CT, Brooks C, Jaramillo J, Mickelsen S, Kusumoto FM. A left free-wall, decrementally conducting, atrioventricular (Mahaim) fiber: diagnosis at electrophysiological study and radiofrequency catheter ablation guided by direct recording of a Mahaim potential. *Pacing Clin Electrophysiol*. 1997;20(10 Pt 1):2486-2488.

21. Yamabe H, Okumura K, Minoda K, Yasue H. Nodoventricular Mahaim fiber connecting to the left ventricle. *Am Heart J.* 1991;122(1 Pt 1):232-234.

22. Han FT, Riles EM, Badhwar N, Scheinman MM. Clinical features and sites of ablation for patients with incessant supraventricular tachycardia from concealed nodofascicular and nodoventricular tachycardias. *JACC Clin Electrophysiol.* 2017;3(13):1547-1556.

23. Centurion OA, Shimizu A, Isomoto S, Konoe A. Mechanisms for the genesis of paroxysmal atrial fibrillation in the Wolff Parkinson-White syndrome: intrinsic atrial muscle vulnerability vs. electrophysiological properties of the accessory pathway. *Europace.* 2008;10(3):294-302.

24. Haissaguerre M, Fischer B, Labbe T, et al. Frequency of recurrent atrial fibrillation after catheter ablation of overt accessory pathways. *Am J Cardiol.* 1992;69(5):493-497.

25. Etheridge SP, Escudero CA, Blaufox AD, et al. Life-threatening event risk in children with Wolff-Parkinson-White Syndrome: a multicenter international study. *JACC Clin Electrophysiol.* 2018;4(4):433-444.

26. Garcia-Fernandez FJ, Ibanez Criado JL, Quesada Dorador A, collaborators of the Spanish Catheter Ablation R, Registry C. Spanish Catheter Ablation Registry. 17th Official Report of the Spanish Society of Cardiology Working Group on Electrophysiology and Arrhythmias (2017). *Rev Esp Cardiol (Engl Ed).* 2018;71(11):941-951.

27. Holmqvist F, Kesek M, Englund A, et al. A decade of catheter ablation of cardiac arrhythmias in Sweden: ablation practices and outcomes. *Eur Heart J.* 2019; 40(10):820-830.

28. Nelson SD, Kou WH, Annesley T, de Buitleir M, Morady F. Significance of ST segment depression during paroxysmal supraventricular tachycardia. *J Am Coll Cardiol.* 1988;12(2):383-387.

29. Katritsis DG. A tachycardia with narrow-QRS morphology and prolonged RP intervals. *Europace.* 2013;15(7):969.

30. Josephson ME. Electrophysiology at a crossroads. *Heart Rhythm.* 2007;4(5): 658-661.

31. Kang KT, Potts JE, Radbill AE, et al. Permanent junctional reciprocating tachycardia in children: a multicenter experience. *Heart Rhythm.* 2014;11(8):1426-1432.

32. Moore JP, Patel PA, Shannon KM, et al. Predictors of myocardial recovery in pediatric tachycardia-induced cardiomyopathy. *Heart Rhythm.* 2014;11(7): 1163-1169.

33. Packer DL, Gallagher JJ, Prystowsky EN. Physiological substrate for antidromic reciprocating tachycardia. Prerequisite characteristics of the accessory pathway and atrioventricular conduction system. *Circulation.* 1992;85(2):574-588.

34. Brembilla-Perrot B, Pauriah M, Sellal JM, et al. Incidence and prognostic significance of spontaneous and inducible antidromic tachycardia. *Europace.* 2013;15(6): 871-876.

35. Ceresnak SR, Tanel RE, Pass RH, et al. Clinical and electrophysiologic characteristics of antidromic tachycardia in children with Wolff-Parkinson-White syndrome. *Pacing Clin Electrophysiol.* 2012;35(4):480-488.

36. Obeyesekere MN, Leong-Sit P, Massel D, et al. Risk of arrhythmia and sudden death in patients with asymptomatic preexcitation. A meta-analysis. *Circulation.* 2012;125(19):2308-2315.

37. Pappone C, Vicedomini G, Manguso F, et al. Wolff-Parkinson-White Syndrome in the era of catheter ablation: insights from a registry study of 2169 patients. *Circulation*. 2014;130(10):811-819.
38. Santinelli V, Radinovic A, Manguso F, et al. The natural history of asymptomatic ventricular pre-excitation: a long-term prospective follow-up study of 184 asymptomatic children. *J Am Coll Cardiol*. 2009;53(3):275-280.
39. Pappone C, Vicedomini G, Manguso F, et al. Risk of malignant arrhythmias in initially symptomatic patients with Wolff-Parkinson-White Syndrome: results of a prospective long-term electrophysiological follow-up study. *Circulation*. 2012;125(5):661-668.
40. Santinelli V, Radinovic A, Manguso F, et al. Asymptomatic ventricular preexcitation: a long-term prospective follow-up study of 293 adult patients. *Circ Arrhythm Electrophysiol*. 2009;2(2):102-107.
41. Beckman KJ, Gallastegui JL, Bauman JL, Hariman RJ. The predictive value of electrophysiologic studies in untreated patients with Wolff-Parkinson-White syndrome. *J Am Coll Cardiol*. 1990;15(3):640-647.
42. Bunch TJ, May HT, Bair TL, et al. Long-term natural history of adult Wolff–Parkinson–White Syndrome patients treated with and without catheter ablation. *Circ Arrhythm Electrophysiol*. 2015;8(6):1465-1471.
43. Cain N, Irving C, Webber S, Beerman L, Arora G. Natural history of Wolff-Parkinson-White Syndrome diagnosed in childhood. *Am J Cardiol*. 2013;112(7):961-965.
44. Skov MW, Rasmussen PV, Ghouse J, et al. Electrocardiographic preexcitation and risk of cardiovascular morbidity and mortality: results from the Copenhagen ECG Study. *Circ Arrhythm Electrophysiol*. 2017;10(6):e004778.
45. Etheridge SP, Escudero CA, Blaufox AD, et al. Life-threatening event risk in children with Wolff-Parkinson-White syndrome. A multicenter international study. *JACC Clin Electrophysiol*. 2018;4:433-444.
46. Klein GJ, Bashore TM, Sellers TD, Pritchett ELC, Smith WM, Gallagher JJ. Ventricular fibrillation in the Wolff-Parkinson-White syndrome. *N Engl J Med*. 1979;301(20):1080-1085.
47. Sharma AD, Yee R, Guiraudon G, Klein GJ. Sensitivity and specificity of invasive and noninvasive testing for risk of sudden death in Wolff-Parkinson-White syndrome. *J Am Coll Cardiol*. 1987;10(2):373-381.
48. Montoya PT, Brugada P, Smeets J, et al. Ventricular fibrillation in the Wolff-Parkinson-White syndrome. *Eur Heart J*. 1991;12(2):144-150.
49. Pappone C, Vicedomini G, Manguso F, et al. Wolff-Parkinson-White syndrome in the era of catheter ablation: insights from a registry study of 2169 patients. *Circulation*. 2014;130(10):811-819.
50. Dai C, Guo B, Li W, et al. The effect of ventricular pre-excitation on ventricular wall motion and left ventricular systolic function. *Europace*. 2018;20(7):1175-1181.
51. Kohli U, Pumphrey KL, Ahmed A, Das S. Pre-excitation induced ventricular dysfunction and successful berlin heart explantation after accessory pathway ablation. *J Electrocardiol*. 2018;51(6):1067-1070.
52. Nagai T, Hamabe A, Arakawa J, Tabata H, Nishioka T. The impact of left ventricular deformation and dyssynchrony on improvement of left ventricular ejection fraction following radiofrequency catheter ablation in Wolff-Parkinson-White

syndrome: a comprehensive study by speckle tracking echocardiography. *Echocardiography.* 2017;34(11):1610-1616.

53. Kwon EN, Carter KA, Kanter RJ. Radiofrequency catheter ablation for dyssynchrony-induced dilated cardiomyopathy in an infant. *Congenit Heart Dis.* 2014;9(6):E179-E184.

54. Moore IP, Kannankeril PJ, Fish FA. Isoproterenol administration during general anesthesia for the evaluation of children with ventricular preexcitation. *Circ Arrhythm Electrophysiol.* 2011;4(1):73-78.

55. Kubuš P, Vít P, Gebauer RA, Materna O, Janoušek J. Electrophysiologic profile and results of invasive risk stratification in asymptomatic children and adolescents with the Wolff–Parkinson–White electrocardiographic pattern. *Circ Arrhythm Electrophysiol.* 2014;7(2):218-223.

56. Leitch JW, Klein GJ, Yee R, Murdock C. Prognostic value of electrophysiology testing in asymptomatic patients with Wolff-Parkinson-White pattern [published erratum appears in Circulation 1991 Mar;83(3):1124]. *Circulation.* 1990;82(5):1718-1723.

57. Rinne C, Klein GJ, Sharma AD, Yee R, Milstein S, Rattes MF. Relation Between clinical presentation and induced arrhythmias in the Wolff-Parkinson-White syndrome. *Am J Cardiol.* 1987;60(7):576-579.

58. Daubert C, Ollitrault J, Descaves C, Mabo P, Ritter P, Gouffault J. Failure of the exercise test to predict the anterograde refractory period of the accessory pathway in Wolff Parkinson White syndrome. *Pacing Clin Electrophysiol.* 1988;11(8):1130-1138.

59. Wackel P, Irving C, Webber S, Beerman L, Arora G. Risk stratification in Wolff-Parkinson-White syndrome: the correlation between noninvasive and invasive testing in pediatric patients. *Pacing Clin Electrophysiol.* 2012;35(12):1451-1457.

60. Gaita F, Giustetto C, Riccardi R, Mangiardi L, Brusca A. Stress and pharmacologic tests as methods to identify patients with Wolff-Parkinson-White syndrome at risk of sudden death. *Am J Cardiol.* 1989;64(8):487-490.

61. Page RL, Joglar JA, Caldwell MA, et al. 2015 ACC/AHA/HRS Guideline for the management of adult patients with supraventricular tachycardia: executive summary: a report of the American College of Cardiology/American Heart Association Task Force on Clinical Practice Guidelines and the Heart Rhythm Society. *J Am Coll Cardiol.* 2016;67(13):1575-1623.

62. Pediatric and Congenital Electrophysiology Society, Heart Rhythm Society, American College of Cardiology Foundation, et al. PACES/HRS expert consensus statement on the management of the asymptomatic young patient with a Wolff-Parkinson-White (WPW, ventricular preexcitation) electrocardiographic pattern: developed in partnership between the Pediatric and Congenital Electrophysiology Society (PACES) and the Heart Rhythm Society (HRS). Endorsed by the governing bodies of PACES, HRS, the American College of Cardiology Foundation (ACCF), the American Heart Association (AHA), the American Academy of Pediatrics (AAP), and the Canadian Heart Rhythm Society (CHRS). *Heart Rhythm.* 2012;9(6):1006-1024.

63. Jastrzebski M, Kukla P, Pitak M, Rudzinski A, Baranchuk A, Czarnecka D. Intermittent preexcitation indicates "a low-risk" accessory pathway: time for a paradigm shift? *Ann Noninvasive Electrocardiol.* 2017;22(6).

64. Kiger ME, McCanta AC, Tong S, Schaffer M, Runciman M, Collins KK. Intermittent versus persistent wolff-parkinson-white syndrome in children: electrophysiologic properties and clinical outcomes. *Pacing Clin Electrophysiol.* 2016;39(1): 14-20.

65. Cohen M. Intermittent preexcitation: should we rethink the current guidelines? *Pacing Clin Electrophysiol.* 2016;39(1):9-11.

66. Mah DY, Sherwin ED, Alexander ME, et al. The electrophysiological characteristics of accessory pathways in pediatric patients with intermittent preexcitation. *Pacing Clin Electrophysiol.* 2013;36(9):1117-1122.

67. Spar DS, Silver ES, Hordof AJ, Liberman L. Relation of the utility of exercise testing for risk assessment in pediatric patients with ventricular preexcitation to pathway location. *Am J Cardiol.* 2012;109(7):1011-1014.

68. Kuck KH, Schluter M. Single-catheter approach to radiofrequency current ablation of left-sided accessory pathways in patients with Wolff-Parkinson-White syndrome. *Circulation.* 1991;84(6):2366-2375.

69. Katritsis D, Giazitzoglou E, Korovesis S, Zambartas C. Comparison of the transseptal approach to the transaortic approach for ablation of Left-Sided accessory pathways in patients with Wolff-Parkinson-White syndrome. *Am J Cardiol.* 2003;91(5):610-613.

70. Manolis AS, Wang PJ, Estes NA, 3rd. Radiofrequency ablation of left-sided accessory pathways: transaortic versus transseptal approach. *Am Heart J.* 1994;128(5): 896-902.

71. Jackman WM, Friday KJ, Yeung-Lai-Wah JA, et al. New catheter technique for recording left free-wall accessory atrioventricular pathway activation. Identification of pathway fiber orientation. *Circulation.* 1988;78(3):598-611.

72. Liang M, Wang Z, Liang Y, et al. Different approaches for catheter ablation of para-hisian accessory pathways: implications for mapping and ablation. *Circ Arrhythm Electrophysiol.* 2017;10(6):e004882.

73. Marazzato J, Fonte G, Marazzi R, et al. Efficacy and safety of cryoablation of para-Hisian and mid-septal accessory pathways using a specific protocol: single-center experience in consecutive patients. *J Interv Card Electrophysiol.* 2019;55(1):47-54.

74. Bravo L, Atienza F, Eidelman G, et al. Safety and efficacy of cryoablation vs. radiofrequency ablation of septal accessory pathways: systematic review of the literature and meta-analyses. *Europace.* 2018;20(8):1334-1342.

75. Kovach JR, Mah DY, Abrams DJ, et al. Outcomes of catheter ablation of anteroseptal and midseptal accessory pathways in pediatric patients. *Heart Rhythm.* 2020;17(5 Pt A):759-767.

76. Calkins H, Kim YN, Schmaltz S, et al. Electrogram criteria for identification of appropriate target sites for radiofrequency catheter ablation of accessory atrioventricular connections. *Circulation.* 1992;85(2):565-573.

77. Xue Y, Zhan X, Wu S, et al. Experimental, pathologic, and clinical findings of radiofrequency catheter ablation of para-hisian region from the right ventricle in dogs and humans. *Circ Arrhythm Electrophysiol.* 2017;10(6):e005207.

78. Brado J, Hochadel M, Senges J, et al. Outcomes of ablation in Wolff-Parkinson-White-syndrome: Data from the German Ablation Registry. *Int J Cardiol.* 2020.

79. Spector P, Reynolds MR, Calkins H, et al. Meta-analysis of ablation of atrial flutter and supraventricular tachycardia. *Am J Cardiol.* 2009;104(5):671-677.
80. Keegan R, Aguinaga L, Fenelon G, et al. The first Latin American Catheter Ablation Registry. *Europace.* 2015;17(5):794-800.
81. Spector P, Reynolds MR, Calkins H, et al. Meta-analysis of ablation of atrial flutter and supraventricular tachycardia. *Am J Cardiol.* 2009;104(5):671-677.
82. Bohnen M, Stevenson WG, Tedrow UB, et al. Incidence and predictors of major complications from contemporary catheter ablation to treat cardiac arrhythmias. *Heart Rhythm.* 2011;8(11):1661-1666.
83. Steinbeck G, Sinner MF, Lutz M, Muller-Nurasyid M, Kaab S, Reinecke H. Incidence of complications related to catheter ablation of atrial fibrillation and atrial flutter: a nationwide in-hospital analysis of administrative data for Germany in 2014. *Eur Heart J.* 2018;39(45):4020-4029.
84. Konig S, Ueberham L, Schuler E, et al. In-hospital mortality of patients with atrial arrhythmias: insights from the German-wide Helios hospital network of 161 502 patients and 34 025 arrhythmia-related procedures. *Eur Heart J.* 2018;39(44):"3947-3957.
85. Katritsis DG, Zografos T, Siontis KC, et al. Endpoints for successful slow pathway catheter ablation in typical and atypical atrioventricular nodal re-entrant tachycardia: a contemporary, multicenter study. *JACC Clin Electrophysiol.* 2019;5(1):113-119.
86. Hosseini SM, Rozen G, Saleh A, et al. Catheter ablation for cardiac arrhythmias: utilization and in-hospital complications, 2000 to 2013. *JACC Clin Electrophysiol.* 2017;3(11):1240-1248.
87. Pappone C, Santinelli V, Manguso F, et al. A randomized study of prophylactic catheter ablation in asymptomatic patients with the Wolff-Parkinson-White Syndrome. *N Engl J Med.* 2003;349(19):1803-1811.
88. Telishevska M, Hebe J, Paul T, et al. Catheter ablation in ASymptomatic PEDiatric patients with ventricular preexcitation: results from the multicenter "CASPED" study. *Clin Res Cardiol.* 2019;108(8):683-690.

16

Ventricular Arrhythmias

DEFINITIONS

Ventricular tachycardia (VT) is defined as a tachycardia (rate > 100 beats per minute [bpm]) with three or more consecutive beats that originates in the ventricles.[1,2]

Accelerated idioventricular rhythm denotes a ventricular rhythm less than 100 bpm.

Sustained ventricular tachycardia lasts more than 30 seconds (unless requiring termination because of hemodynamic collapse), whereas **nonsustained tachycardia** terminates spontaneously within 30 seconds.

Monomorphic ventricular tachycardia has only one morphology during each episode (Fig. 16.1).

Pleomorphic ventricular tachycardia has more than one morphology of monomorphic VT during the same or different episodes of VT, but the QRS is not continuously changing. In patients with implantable cardioverter defibrillators (ICDs), pleomorphic VT is associated with increased risk.[3]

In **polymorphic** ventricular tachycardia there is a constant change in QRS configuration indicating a changing ventricular activation sequence, usually at a heart rate less than 333 bpm (cycle length > 180 ms). Rapid polymorphic ventricular tachycardia cannot easily be distinguished from ventricular fibrillation.

Bidirectional ventricular tachycardia is a rare form of tachycardia with two alternating morphologies, usually right bundle branch block with alternating left and right axis deviation. This typically occurs in digitalis intoxication, catecholaminergic polymorphic ventricular tachycardia, or other conditions that predispose cardiac myocytes to delayed afterdepolarizations (DADs) and triggered activity.[4]

Incessant VT denotes hemodynamically stable VT lasting hours.

VT storm indicates very frequent episodes of VT (more than three episodes in 24 hours), monomorphic or polymorphic, requiring cardioversion.[5]

Torsades de pointes is a form of polymorphic ventricular tachycardia with characteristic beat-by-beat changes (twisting around the baseline) in the QRS complex associated with prolongation of the QT interval.

Ventricular flutter indicates a monomorphic, regular ventricular arrhythmia with a rate of approximately 300 bpm (cycle length 200 ms) with no isoelectric interval between QRS complexes.

Ventricular fibrillation (VF) usually has a rate greater than 300 bpm (cycle length ≤ 200 ms) and is a grossly irregular ventricular rhythm with marked variability in QRS morphology and amplitude. Fine VF is low-amplitude VF that superficially could mimic asystole.

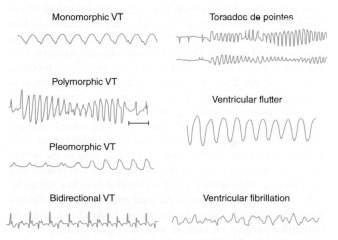

FIG. 16.1. Types of ventricular tachycardia.

ELECTROPHYSIOLOGIC MECHANISMS

Ventricular Tachycardia

Monomorphic VT may be focal or macroreentrant. Focal VT has a point source of earliest ventricular activation with a spread of activation away in all directions from that site. The mechanism can be triggered activity, automaticity, or microreentry. The site of origin can be endocardial or epicardial with focal endocardial breakthrough (see Chapter 2). Macroreentry is due to myocardial scars secondary to prior myocardial infarction or other disease process.

Triggered activity as a result of delayed afterdepolarizations is the usual mechanism of idiopathic outflow tract tachycardias.[6] Termination of idiopathic ventricular outflow tract tachycardias by an intravenous bolus of adenosine or infusion of a calcium channel blocker or by vagotonic maneuvers is consistent with triggered activity as the likely mechanism for some of these tachycardias. These tachycardias can be difficult to induce at electrophysiology testing; rapid-burst pacing and/or isoproterenol infusion is often required.

Automaticity that is provoked by adrenergic stimulation (not triggered) or disease processes that diminish cell-to-cell coupling may less commonly cause focal VT. This type of VT may become incessant under stress or during isoproterenol administration but cannot be initiated or terminated by programmed electrical stimulation; it can sometimes be suppressed by calcium channel blockers or beta blockers. Automaticity from damaged Purkinje fibers has been suggested as a mechanism for catecholamine-sensitive, focal origin VT. Automaticity can also occur in partially depolarized myocytes, as has been shown for VTs during the early phase of myocardial infarction and in some patients with ventricular scars. Automatic premature beats may, in addition, initiate reentrant VTs.

Reentry around a myocardial scar (scar-related reentry) characterized by regions of slow conduction and anatomic or functional unidirectional conduction block at some point in the reentry path is the cause of the majority of monomorphic VT in patients with heart disease.[7] Myocardial scarring is identified from low-voltage regions on ventricular voltage maps, areas with fractionated electrograms, unexcitability during pace mapping, evidence of scarring on myocardial imaging, or from an area of surgical incision. Normal myocardium is typically characterized by bipolar voltage greater than

1.5 mV, dense scarring by bipolar voltage less than 0.5 mV, and border zone tissue by bipolar voltage of 0.5 to 1.5 mV. It should be noted, however, that voltage mapping has several limitations, include variation of bipolar and unipolar amplitudes as a result of wave front direction, electrode size and spacing, and annotation of multiple component signals to the largest peak.[8] Prior myocardial infarction is the most common cause, but scar-related VT also occurs in cardiomyopathies and after cardiac surgery for congenital heart disease or valve replacement. Evidence supporting reentry includes initiation and termination by programmed stimulation (although this does not exclude triggered activity), demonstrable entrainment or resetting with fusion, continuous diastolic electrical activity, and isolated diastolic potentials that cannot be dissociated from VT by perturbations introduced by pacing.

After myocardial infarction, ion channel remodeling and regional reductions in I_{Na} and I_{Ca} are present within the scar, as well as reduced coupling between myocytes by increased collagen, alterations in gap junction distribution and function, and intervening patchy fibrosis resulting in a zigzag pattern of transverse conduction. Thus scar remodeling contributes to the formation of channels and regions where conduction time is prolonged, facilitating reentry. Many reentry circuits contain a protected isthmus or channel of variable length, isolated by arcs of conduction block (Fig. 16.2).[9] Typical isthmus sites are located in areas with low voltages, with dimensions ranging from 21 to 59 mm length by 15 to 47 mm width.[10] Circuit exit sites, defined by local activation coincident with the onset of the QRS, are observed in the infarct border zone as described by voltage mapping. Multiple VT morphologies caused by multiple reentry circuits are often inducible in the same patient. The majority of reentrant circuits are located in the subendocardium, but subepicardial or intramyocardial reentry may also occur.[11]

Macroreentry through the bundle branches occurs in patients with slowed conduction through the His-Purkinje system and is usually associated with severe left ventricular dysfunction as a result of dilated cardiomyopathy, valvular heart disease, and, less often, ischemic heart disease.[12,13] Although these tachycardias are usually unstable, the 12-lead electrocardiogram (ECG), when obtainable, may show either a left bundle branch block (LBBB) or right bundle branch block (RBBB) pattern. The necessary condition for bundle branch reentry is prolonged conduction in the

His-Purkinje system, and this is reflected in the HV interval, which is prolonged during sinus rhythm and prolonged or equal to the baseline sinus rhythm during VT. The circuit involves the right and left brunch bundles with antegrade conduction occurring most of the time through the right bundle, and the HV interval during tachycardia is usually, but not invariably, equal to or greater than the HV interval measured during sinus rhythm.[14] The HH interval variation usually precedes any VV interval variation, in contrast to what happens in microreentrant ventricular tachycardia with retrograde activation of the His bundle.

Left ventricular, fascicular, verapamil-sensitive VT occurs in patients without structural heart disease. The mechanism is reentry that appears to involve a portion of the Purkinje fibers, most often in the region of the left posterior fascicle, giving rise to a characteristic RBBB superior axis QRS configuration and a QRS duration that is only slightly prolonged.[15,16]

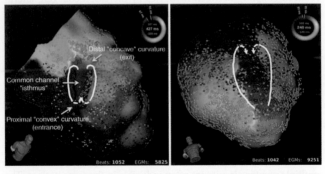

FIG. 16.2. Activation map of reentrant ventricular tachycardias. Activation maps of ventricular tachycardias (VT) in the anterior-septum of the left ventricle. The left panel shows a reentrant figure-eight circuit with a separate entrance, common channel, and exit. The entrance is characterized by convergence of the two activation wavefronts, forming a convex-shaped curvature with a wavefront propagating toward the common channel. The common channel "isthmus" is bounded by two lateral lines of block (or pseudoblock, allowing very slow conduction). The exit is characterized by concave-shaped curvature with divergence of wavefronts in front and lateral to the common-channel. The right panel is another example of figure-eight reentrant VT with an opposite axis. The arrowheads mark the proximal curvature (entrance) into the common channel.

(Anter E, Tschabrunn CM, Buxton AE, Josephson ME. High-resolution mapping of postinfarction reentrant ventricular tachycardia: electrophysiological characterization of the circuit. Circulation. 2016;134(4):314-327.

Ventricular Fibrillation

The mechanism of VF remains elusive, and both reentrant mechanisms (caused by multiple wavelets, mother rotor, or a combination of both) and focal mechanisms (rapidly firing focus initiated by triggered activity or automaticity) have been implicated.[17] Rapid pacing–induced VF generally is attributed to reentrant mechanisms. Ischemia, drugs, and genetic defects that prolong repolarization and alter intracellular calcium promote polymorphic ventricular arrhythmias degenerating to VF. In certain cases focal mechanisms may be involved in VF initiation and maintenance.

DIAGNOSIS

With **monomorphic VT** the ECG displays a wide-QRS (>120 ms) tachycardia. A relatively narrow QRS (100 to 120 ms) may be seen in fascicular VT or in septal VT arising close to the His-Purkinje network. Prior MI, idiopathic VT, and arrhythmogenic cardiomyopathies (most often arrhythmogenic right ventricular cardiomyopathy/dysplasia [ARVC/D][18]) are the most common causes.

Polymorphic VT is usually seen in the context of QT prolongation (in the form of torsades de pointes), in patients with other genetic channelopathies (Brugada syndrome, short QT, or early repolarization syndrome) and nonischemic cardiomyopathies, and in patients with acute ST-elevation myocardial infarction (STEMI) or myocardial ischemia. In STEMI, polymorphic VT may be seen during the acute phase or up to 8 days after the MI,[19] and these patients are at high risk of developing arrhythmic storm.

Torsades de pointes occurs in most commonly in congenital long-QT syndrome (LQTS), drug-related QT prolongation, and metabolic abnormalities such as hypokalemia and during marked bradycardia in patients with third-degree atrioventricular (AV) block with premature ventricular contractions (PVCs).

Polymorphic VT/VF storm in a patient with coronary disease is strongly suggestive of acute myocardial ischemia; pauses may occur before polymorphic VT even in the absence of QT prolongation. Usually, severe underlying heart disease is present. More rarely, VT storm can occur in patients who have a structurally normal heart, such as in Brugada syndrome, LQTS, or catecholaminergic VT, or in drug overdoses.

The **differential diagnosis** of wide-QRS tachycardias is discussed in Chapter 11.

ELECTROPHYSIOLOGY TESTING

Electrophysiology study may be required for establishment of the **diagnosis** in patients presenting with nonsustained ventricular rhythms. Indications include the need for differentiation from supraventricular tachycardia (SVT) with aberration, AF in the context of an accessory pathway, or other forms of aberration; risk stratification in patients with repaired tetralogy of Fallot or sarcoidosis; and programmed electrical stimulation for induction of VT.

Programmed electrical stimulation (PES) may also be used for **risk stratification** purposes.[20] In postinfarction patients with nonsustained ventricular tachycardia (NSVT), the induction of sustained ventricular tachycardia is associated with a two- to threefold increased risk of arrhythmia-related death.[21] In patients with reduced left ventricular ejection fraction (LVEF; <40%) and NSVT, inducibility of sustained monomorphic ventricular tachycardia at baseline PES is associated with a 2-year actuarial risk of sudden death or cardiac arrest of 50% compared with a 6% risk in patients without inducible ventricular tachycardia.[22] Analysis of patients enrolled in the MUSTT (Multicenter UnSustained Tachycardia Trial) and of those in the registry revealed that noninducible patients have a significantly lower risk of cardiac arrest or sudden death compared with inducible patients at 2 and 5 years (12% vs 24% and 18% vs 32%, respectively).[23] Noninducibility after VT ablation in patients with postinfarction VT is also independently associated with lower mortality during long-term follow-up.[24] Still, as these results indicate, patients with noninducible sustained VT are not free of risk of sudden death, although in a recent trial, revascularized patents with noninducible arrhythmias 4 days after the infarction and an LVEF less than 30% had a similar long-term survival free of death or arrhythmia as patients with LVEF greater than 40%.[25]

The MUSTT investigators have further analyzed the relationship of ejection fraction and inducible ventricular tachyarrhythmias to mode of death in 1791 patients who did not receive antiarrhythmic therapy. Total and arrhythmic mortality were higher in patients with an ejection fraction less than 30% compared with those whose ejection fractions were 30% to 40%. The relative contribution of arrhythmic events to total mortality was significantly higher in patients with inducible VT and among patients with an ejection fraction of 30% or greater. This study therefore suggested that the major utility of electrophysiologic testing may be restricted to patients having an ejection fraction between 30% and 40%.[26] There has been some evidence that programmed stimulation performed as early as 3 days after myocardial infarction (MI) in patients with LVEF 40% or less induces VT in up to one-third of patients and may identify patients at high risk for spontaneous VT and sudden cardiac death.[27] Noninducibility after VT ablation in patients with postinfarction VT is independently associated with lower mortality during long-term follow-up.[24]

The ventricular stimulation protocol and the type of VT induced are important. Inducible monomorphic VT identifies patients at high risk of arrhythmia even when it is very fast (cycle length 200 to 250 ms, rate 240 to 300 bpm)[27,28] or is induced by three or four extrastimuli or by burst pacing.[29,30] Inducibility of ventricular fibrillation or flutter (usually with a cycle length less than 200 to 250 ms) has been considered a nonspecific finding,[27,31,32] especially when induced with three extrastimuli at very short coupling intervals.[33] In the MUSTT, VF with one to two extrastimuli did confer an adverse prognostic significance.[23]

These results should be considered in the context of evidence from analysis of stored ICD data that have shown little association between spontaneous and induced ventricular arrhythmias.[34] The remodeling process after MI is ongoing, with a resultant low correlation between induced and clinically occurring VT in the long term.[35]

In patients with coronary artery disease and relatively preserved left ventricular function (LVEF > 40%), the role of PES is not established, but there has been observational evidence that it may be of value for risk stratification.[36] Inducible monomorphic VT might prompt catheter ablation and, if needed, an ICD, whereas inducibility of VF may be a nonspecific sign, especially if three extrastimuli are used.[33] However, further investigations for ischemia, cardiomyopathies, or inherited channelopathies may be appropriate. The prognostic usefulness of programmed stimulation in patients with nonischemic dilated cardiomyopathy, including those with NSVT, remains controversial.[37,38] There has been some evidence that inducibility of ventricular arrhythmias,[39] and especially polymorphic VT or VF,[40] indicates increased likelihood of subsequent ICD therapies and might be considered a useful risk stratifier.

Inducible sustained monomorphic or polymorphic VT is an independent risk factor for subsequent events in patients with repaired tetralogy of Fallot[41] and sarcoidosis.[42]

CATHETER ABLATION

RATIONALE

Catheter ablation is currently indicated for VT in various clinical settings either for eradication of the arrhythmia, as occurs in idiopathic VT, or for reducing the arrhythmia burden and consequent ICD shocks in patients with ischemic or structural heart disease.[43,44] ICD shocks are associated with diminished quality of life and increased mortality.[45,46] Antiarrhythmic drugs have an important role in shock reduction; however, these agents often have limited efficacy and significant side effects.[47,48] Amiodarone reduces VT recurrence and ICD shocks[49] but may be associated with increased mortality in this respect.[50] Thus, in cases of frequent monomorphic VT or VT storm in patients with ischemic cardiomyopathy who already have an ICD, ablation can reduce the number of ICD shocks and is preferable to drug therapy escalation (according to the VANISH, SMASH-VT, and VTACH randomized trials).[51-56] Preventive VT ablation before ICD implantation does not reduce mortality or hospitalization for arrhythmia or worsening heart failure during 1 year of follow-up, but patients subjected to ablation have fewer ventricular arrhythmias and ICD interventions (per the BERLIN VT randomized trial).[57]

In-hospital **mortality rates** for VT catheter ablation depend on the clinical condition of the patient.[58] On average, they are 2.5% for ischemic heart disease, 1.5% for nonischemic structural heart disease, and 0.1% for patients without apparent heart disease, although no mortality has been reported for idiopathic VT ablation in experienced centers (see also specific VT entities, and Table 16.1).[59,60]

Although catheter ablation has not been proven to improve mortality in any randomized trial, retrospective cohort studies have provided evidence that successful ablation may be associated with both a higher rate of freedom from VT and also improved survival. A retrospective analysis of outcomes of VT ablation demonstrated that freedom from recurrent VT is associated with a significant reduction in all-cause mortality, independent of ejection fraction and heart failure status.[61] A meta-analysis of 8 cohort studies with 928 postinfarction VT patients demonstrated that patients who have VT rendered noninducible by an ablation procedure have a lower VT recurrence rate compared with those who still have inducible arrhythmias after the ablation. Noninducibility translated to a significant reduction in all-cause mortality compared with partial success.[62] In a multicenter observational study of postinfarction patients, noninducibility was associated with a 35% reduction in mortality.[24] A similar finding has been reported in dilated cardiomyopathy patients.[63]

PROCEDURAL CONSIDERATIONS

Anticoagulation with intravenous heparin is necessary for all left ventricular (LV) procedures, as well as for right ventricular (RV) procedures in patients at high risk for thromboembolism.[64] Endocardial mapping often is also done in epicardial procedures. In fully anticoagulated patients, pericardial access for epicardial mapping/ablation can be performed without interruption of anti-coagulation[65,66] or after protamine reversal.[64]

Most laboratories use **general anesthesia** (GA) for scar-related VTs and **conscious sedation** for idiopathic PVC/VT. Conscious sedation and GA can potentially suppress spontaneous or inducible arrhythmia by reducing sympathetic tone and is preferred for complex ablation procedures that can last for several hours, during which the patients are required to remain still to facilitate stability of the electroanatomic map. The frequency and depth of breathing play an important role in determining good catheter contact and stability. Epicardial access is often easier when respiratory motion can be controlled as under GA. However, patients with severe LV dysfunction can experience hemodynamic deterioration during prolonged procedures under GA.

Acute hemodynamic decompensation, defined as persistent hypotension despite vasopressors requiring mechanical support or discontinuation of the procedure, is reported to occur in 11% of patients and portends increased mortality.[67] To identify patients at highest risk for hemodynamic decompensation, the PAAINESD (Pulmonary disease, Age older than 60 years, general Anesthesia, Ischemic cardiomyopathy, New York Heart Association class III or IV, LVEF < 25%, VT Storm, Diabetes mellitus),[67] and the I-VT (LVEF, age, electrical storm, type of cardiomyopathy and diabetes mellitus [www.vtscore.org])[58] risk scores have been developed.

An inotropic agent, intraaortic balloon pump, or percutaneous LV assist device (LVAD) or extracorporeal membrane oxygenation (ECMO) have been used to maintain hemodynamic stability during VT ablation.[56,68] Although more complicated to use, ECMO provides maximal hemodynamic support (>4.5 L/min) and is of most benefit when placed preemptively in high-risk patients undergoing VT ablation or as a bailout measure when intraprocedural hemodynamic deterioration occurs. These devices maintain end-organ perfusion during prolonged periods of VT and may allow a longer time for detailed entrainment/activation mapping.[56]

Electroanatomic mapping and multielectrode catheters (see Chapters 5 and 7) are now used for VT substrate mapping in most laboratories. They allow rapid acquisition of multiple sites at high spatial resolution,[9] and the increased current density during pacing from smaller electrodes can achieve capture at relatively low pacing stimulus strength.[69] However, various shapes of multielectrode configurations may induce ectopy, spatial sampling is not uniform, and none of them is well suited for mapping of papillary muscles or the epicardium.

Coronary angiography or imaging of the coronary ostia with **intracardiac echocardiography** in relevant cases is necessary for epicardial ablation and for ablation in the sinuses of Valsalva. A distance of more than 5 mm from the ablation catheter tip to an epicardial coronary artery and more than 10 mm of the catheter tip to the coronary ostium are considered safe for ablation.[64]

MAPPING TECHNIQUES

Mapping During VT

12-Lead ECG Mapping. A 12-lead ECG obtained during tachycardia may provide certain clues about the origin of the arrhythmia, as discussed in the Clinical Forms section.

Body Surface Mapping. Electrocardiographic imaging (ECGI) integrates unipolar electrograms obtained during the arrhythmia while the patient is wearing a 256-electrode vest, with ventricular anatomy derived from a computed tomography (CT) or cardiac magnetic resonance (CMR) scan with the vest in place. An activation map during the arrhythmia is then mathematically derived using the inverse solution and is plotted on the epicardial surface as designated by the CT or CMR scan. ECGI maps have shown good correlations with endo- and epicardial mapping results in patients with and without ischemic cardiomyopathy, and outflow arrhythmias.[64,70] Their efficacy is diminished in reentrant VTs over myocardial scarring or over slowly conducting tissue.[71] Clinical experience with this modality is limited.

Activation Mapping. During hemodynamically tolerated scar-related VT, the onset of the surface QRS corresponds temporally to the emergence of the diastolic VT circuit from the scar. Recordings from the exit site of a VT circuit with conventional catheters demonstrate electrograms that precede the onset of the surface QRS complexes. Electroanatomic activation mapping using multielectrode catheters (see Chapter 5) is now usually employed for identifying the VT exit site. Electroanatomic activation mapping involves the identification of the earliest site of electrical activation in a cardiac chamber compared with an arbitrary reference electrogram during VT. This information can be color coded and recorded on a three-dimensional (3D) electroanatomic map so that the earliest site of local electrical activation can be identified. This is particularly useful for focal VT that has a single earliest site with centrifugal activation away from that location. Because electrical activity is continuous, activation mapping in reentrant VT is not useful to delineate early and late activation, but it can be used to identify VT exit sites along the scar border and identification of diastolic corridors (isthmuses) during VT. The VT reentry circuit isthmus is a critical component of the VT circuit and may not necessarily correspond to channels identified by electroanatomic voltage mapping.[72,73]

Electrograms at isthmus sites occur earlier during diastole, typically have very low voltage amplitude (<0.5 mV), and can have multiple components, but the mere presence of **diastolic potentials** during VT cannot discriminate between isthmus and bystander sites (Fig. 16.3).[8] The inability to dissociate a diastolic potential from the next ventricular electrogram by pacing maneuvers makes it more likely that the diastolic potential does originate in a critical isthmus. Diastolic potentials, together with the recording of bipolar myocardial signal amplitude less than 1.5 mV, allow orientation toward the areas where pace or entrainment mapping should be performed.[51]

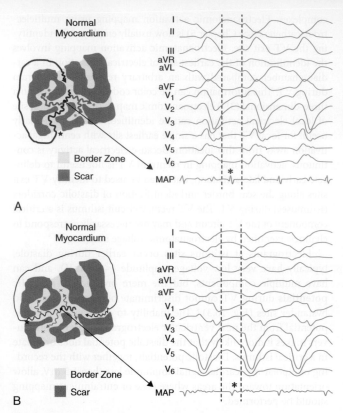

FIG. 16.3. Myocardial scar and mechanism of reentrant VT. (A) A VT circuit *(red arrow)* is dependent on slow and circuitous electrical activity through border zone tissue during the diastolic period *(orange dashed lines)*, which is recorded as diastolic electrograms *(black asterisk)* on the MAP. Locations distal to the VT circuit *(orange asterisks)* may also demonstrate diastolic electrograms as a result of passive activation *(orange arrows)*. Critical locations are identified only with entrainment and termination of VT with ablation. The QRS morphology of the VT is dependent on the exit site from border zone tissue to the normal myocardium *(red star)*. (B) Another VT circuit with a different exit site would demonstrate a different QRS morphology on electrocardiography.

MAP, Mapping catheter; *VT,* ventricular tachycardia. (Dukkipati SR, Koruth JS, Choudry S, et al. Catheter ablation of ventricular tachycardia in structural heart disease: indications, strategies, and outcomes—Part II. *J Am Coll Cardiol.* 2017;70(23):2924-2941.)

Electrograms can also be fractionated and immediately precede the onset of the QRS complex at the exit site from a VT reentry circuit. Ablation at exit sites can terminate the tachycardia, but it may also result in a change of the tachycardia circuit and/or cycle length (CL) in which the diastolic pathway exits at different locations from the scar.[8] Both central and exit sites have been the preferred ablation targets,[51] but zones of slow conduction are more functionally relevant than the latest activated regions.[74]

A limitation of endocardial activation mapping is that scar-related circuits, particularly in patients with a nonischemic substrate, can have intramural or epicardial components that might not be recorded on the surface.

VT Entrainment. As discussed, electrogram timing alone is not entirely reliable as a guide to successful ablation sites due to the frequent presence of multiple conduction channels, some of which are bystanders, and entrainment techniques are used to determine relevance to the VT circuit. Entrainment principles are the same as discussed for any reentrant tachycardia (see Chapter 10) provided that we are dealing with one VT circuit.[75] Responses to pacing from various sites in and around the circuit are indicated in Fig. 16.4. *Critical isthmus sites are defined by concealed entrainment—that is, no change of QRS morphology, S-QRS interval less than 70% of the VT cycle length (ideally equal to the electrogram to QRS during VT), and a postpacing interval–VT cycle length difference 30 ms or less (ideally equal to the VT cycle length).*

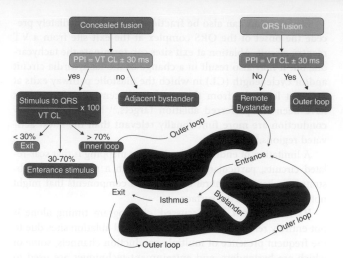

FIG. 16.4. Entrainment responses from components of reentrant VT circuit.
CL, Cycle length; *PPI,* postpacing interval; *VT,* ventricular tachycardia. (Cronin EM, Bogun FM, Maury P, et al. 2019 HRS/EHRA/APHRS/LAHRS expert consensus statement on catheter ablation of ventricular arrhythmias: Executive summary. *Heart Rhythm.* 2020;17(1):e155-e205.)

With pacing site outside the reentry circuit during VT, the stimulated wave front that propagates out from the pacing site collides with the orthodromically propagating wave front of the reentry circuit and produces a fused QRS complex (classic entrainment). During pacing from within a protected region or in a bystander site communicating with the critical isthmus near the reentry circuit, pacing entrains the VT without changing the QRS configuration (concealed entrainment or entrainment with concealed fusion).[76]

The S-QRS interval is indicative of the conduction time from the pacing site to the point of the VT exit from the scar. A short S-QRS suggests a stimulus closer to the exit, whereas a long S-QRS indicates an entrance to the channel. If pacing is performed from a site in the circuit, the stimulus-QRS interval should be equal to the electrogram-QRS interval during VT. If pacing is performed from a bystander site, the stimulus-QRS interval is longer than the electrogram-QRS interval during tachycardia.[7,77] The stimulus-QRS/VTCL ratio is therefore a reflection of the pacing site location within the critical zone of the reentry circuit.

The postpacing interval (PPI) measures the interval from the pacing stimulus to the following nonstimulated depolarization recorded at the pacing site and is also used to verify whether the pacing site is within the circuit or is in a bystander area (Fig. 16.5).[68] To prove that a specific site is an integral part of the reentrant circuit (i.e., entrance, isthmus, or exit site), the PPI should approximate the tachycardia CL (<30 ms).[75] Care is needed not to pace at a very fast rate that may result in slower conduction and erroneous prolongation of the PPI and to distinguish tachycardia depolarizations from far-field electrograms generated by remote tissue.[78]

Successful entrainment mapping satisfying all criteria identifies critical isthmus sites where a few radiofrequency lesions can reliably eliminate VT.[77,79]

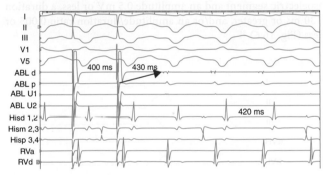

FIG. 16.5. Entrainment of VT. Pacing in the scar at a cycle length (CL) 20 ms shorter than the tachycardia CL accelerates all electrograms and QRS complexes to the paced CL. QRS complexes during pacing match those during ventricular tachycardia. The postpacing interval *(blue arrow)* approximates the tachycardia CL.
(Nof E, Stevenson WG, John RM. Catheter ablation for ventricular arrhythmias. *Arrhythm Electrophysiol Rev.* 2013;2(1):45-52.)

Mapping During Sinus Rhythm

Although entrainment mapping is the preferred method for characterizing the VT circuit, hemodynamic instability during tachycardia and the need to induce clinical VT may make this approach challenging. The presence of multiple VT morphologies also makes entrainment mapping cumbersome. In the Thermocool VT ablation trial, 54% of induced VT morphologies were unmappable, most commonly because of hemodynamic instability.[80] Even in patients with well-tolerated clinical VT, approximately 70% will have at least one unmappable VT induced at electrophysiology (EP) study.[10]

Late Potentials and Fractionated Electrograms. Diastolic activity is detected in the form of **late or isolated potentials** after the QRS complex and separated from the ventricular electrogram by an isoelectric interval of more than 20 ms or as fractionated electrograms with multiple components without an isoelectric segment and an amplitude 0.5 mV or less, a duration 130 ms or greater, and/or an amplitude/duration ratio 0.005 or less (Fig. 16.6).[81]

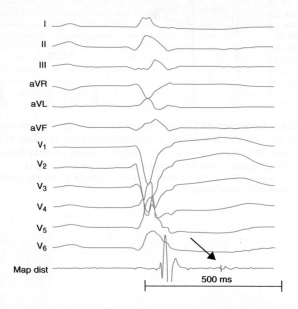

FIG. 16.6. Example of an isolated potential recorded within a posterior left ventricular scar. The isolated potential *(arrow)* is separated from the ventricular electrogram by an isoelectric segment of 120 ms. The amplitude of the isolated potential is 0.035 mV. The electrogram width is 260 ms. In this patient there were 11 different inducible ventricular tachycardias (VTs); after the ablation procedure and the displayed lesions, these VTs were no longer inducible. *Map dist,* distal electrode pair of the mapping catheter.

(Bogun F, Good E, Reich S, et al. Isolated potentials during sinus rhythm and pace-mapping within scars as guides for ablation of post-infarction ventricular tachycardia. *J Am Coll Cardiol.* 2006;47(10):2013-2019.)

Potentials within the QRS may also be identified with high-density mapping during sinus rhythm. These potentials are defined as local abnormal ventricular activations (**LAVAs**) and have been described as credible targets for VT ablation (Figs. 16.7 and 16.8), although the absence of inducible VT at the end of the procedure was not predictive of VT-free survival in this study.[82] Mapping of abnormal electrograms during RV pacing may be more sensitive than during normal sinus rhythm because of a change in the direction of the activation wave front (Fig. 16.9).[83] A limitation of fractionated electrograms and late potentials is that they are markedly influenced by factors such as the direction of wave front activation, catheter orientation, and electrode confiduration.[8,84]

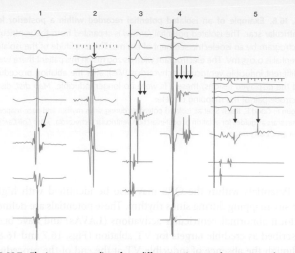

FIG. 16.7. Electrogram recordings from different patients to show various characteristics of local abnormal ventricular electrograms (LAVAs; *arrows*). 1. The potential representing LAVA is fused with the terminal portion of the far-field ventricular signal, making it difficult to identify the LAVA as a separate signal. 2. LAVA potential occurs just after and with a slightly higher frequency than the far-field ventricular potential. LAVAs in 1 and 2 occur within the QRS complex. 3. LAVA is a double-component potential that closely follows the farfield ventricular signal. The early component is a high-frequency potential that is almost fused with the preceding far-field ventricular potential. It occurs within the terminal portion of the QRS complex. Another low-amplitude signal follows an isoelectric interval and represents the late component of LAVA, which occurs after the QRS complex. 4. LAVAs are represented by multicomponent signals without isoelectric intervals. These signals can be visualized distinctly from the preceding far-field ventricular signal. 5. Double-component LAVA signal. Although the early component is recorded just after the QRS complex, the late component is recorded after the inscription of the T wave on the surface ECG.

(Jais P, Maury P, Khairy P, et al. Elimination of local abnormal ventricular activities: a new end point for substrate modification in patients with scar-related ventricular tachycardia. *Circulation.* 2012;125(18):2184-2196.)

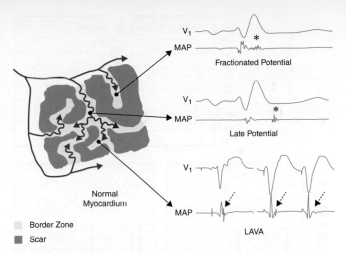

FIG. 16.8. Myocardial scar and substrate for reentrant VT. *(Left)* Electrical activation from the normal myocardium through border zone tissue is slow and delayed *(red arrows)*. Multiple myocardial channels are present and can be identified by characteristic electrograms that can be classified as fractionated electrograms *(top, asterisk)*, late potentials *(middle, asterisk)*, or local abnormal ventricular activity *(bottom)*. In this case, LAVA is best appreciated with ventricular pacing, which separates the local abnormal electrogram *(dashed arrow)* from the far-field electrogram with demonstration of local entrance block to the site with the third complex. These myocardial channels may all serve as potential pathways for different VTs.

LAVA, Local abnormal ventricular activity; *MAP,* mapping catheter; *VT,* ventricular tachycardia. (Dukkipati SR, Koruth JS, Choudry S, et al. Catheter ablation of ventricular tachycardia in structural heart disease: indications, strategies, and outcomes—part II. *J Am Coll Cardiol.* 2017;70(23): 2924-2941.)

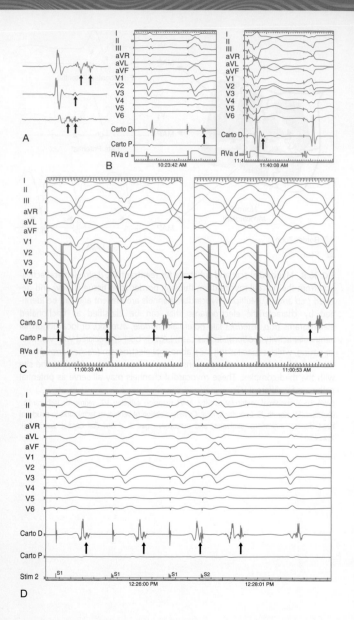

FIG. 16.9. (A) Sinus rhythm electrograms (EGMs) demonstrating late potentials and multicomponent EGMs *(arrows)*. (B) Right ventricular (RV) pacing used to expose late potentials *(arrows)* hidden within the QRS during sinus rhythm *(left panel)* and biventricular pacing *(right panel)*. (C) Entrainment mapping with capture of the far field EGM *(left panel)*. A reduction in pacing output *(right panel)* results in successful capture of the local EGM *(arrow)* and evidence of concealed entrainment. (D) EGMs recorded from abnormal substrate are poorly coupled to the rest of the myocardium. RV pacing results in separation of the late potential (hidden within the sinus QRS beat), and extrastimulus results in further delay.

(Sadek MM, Schaller RD, Supple GE, et al. Ventricular tachycardia ablation: the right approach for the right patient. *Arrhythm Electrophysiol Rev.* 2014;3(3):161-167.)

Scar Identification. Scar tissue identification is based on bipolar electrogram amplitude using a 4-mm-tip mapping catheter and 1-mm ring interelectrode spacing with a 2-mm ring filtered at 10 to 400 Hz. Normal ventricular tissue has a bipolar voltage more than 1.5 mV, dense scar is defined by voltages less than 0.5 mV, and a border zone is defined by voltages between 0.5 and 1.5 mV.[85] However, unipolar pacing in the area of the so-called dense scar shows local capture, suggesting presence of viable myocardium, and a bipolar voltage of less than 0.1 mV has also been used to define electrical inexcitability.[8] Changing the bipolar viability voltage range to 0.1 to 0.5 mV increases the heterogeneity within the area of previously defined "dense scar." In patients with nonischemic cardiomyopathy in particular, heart biopsies have demonstrated that the amount of viable myocardium shows a linear association with both bipolar and unipolar voltage, in a way that any cutoff to delineate fibrosis is unreliable.[86] In addition, bipolar voltage amplitude depends on several factors,[8] as discussed in Chapter 5 (see Figs. 5.2 and 5.3). The addition of filtered unipolar to bipolar voltage mapping may be useful in this respect.[8,64]

Cardiac magnetic resonance is considered the gold standard for identification of scarring in the human myocardium, although its current resolution is limited for the purpose of reliable tissue characterization.[8]

Pace Mapping. Pace mapping involves pacing at a rate close to the tachycardia CL from the site presumed to be close to the VT origin as judged on the 12-lead SCG during VT, in an attempt to match exactly the clinical VT morphology. Computer programs are now available that use template-matching algorithms to generate a correlation coefficient between VT morphology and pace maps.[87]

Pace mapping can identify the site of origin of focal VTs[88] and the tachycardia exit site in reentrant VTs.[89,90] Usually, pacing mapping within the scar reveals a paced QRS morphology similar to that during VT and a prolonged S-QRS interval (>40 ms).[89] In particular, pace mapping at sites of isolated potentials detected during sinus rhythm (SR) in areas of scarring is helpful in identifying critical VT isthmuses.[81] An abrupt transition between a paced QRS that matches the clinical VT (exit site) and a nonmatched paced QRS (entrance site) can also identify an isthmus.[87] VT exit site pacing will yield a matched QRS with a short S-QRS, and entrance site pacing will often yield a nonmatched QRS because the stimulus wave front can exit antidromically in the opposite direction as the VT.[73] Inherent limitations of pace mapping are that pacing in noncritical areas adjacent to the exit may also generate an adequate pace match that is similar in morphology to a pace map from the VT exit, whereas a perfect pace map can be observed at sites up to 2 cm away from the VT origin.[91,92] In addition, varying the pacing rate may alter the paced-QRS morphology. To minimize this, pacing should be conducted at the VT cycle length,[93] and at the lowest possible pacing output to reduce the possibility of far field capture. For practical purposes, pacing is started at an output of 10 mA at 2 ms pulse width.[64]

ABLATION TECHNIQUES

Patients without Structural Heart Disease

Catheter ablation is based on **activation mapping** either with conventional catheters or electroanatomic mapping. **Pace mapping** may also be useful in this respect.[43,44]

Patients with Structural Heart Disease

Conventional and substrate ablation may be used. Initial results with VT catheter ablation have been obtained with traditional VT mapping techniques, such as **entrainment/activation mapping** of hemodynamically stable VT and pace mapping, and limited substrate ablation for poorly tolerated VT.[43,44]

In predominantly substrate ablation strategies, abnormal electrograms including **late potentials** and **fractionated/late potentials** and LAVA in and around the scar are targeted in an attempt to ablate all potential channels that can support VT reentry.[81,82] However, as discussed, the presence of abnormal electrograms does not necessarily predict involvement in the VT circuit, it can be difficult to eliminate abnormal potentials even with long ablation lesions, and standard mapping may fail to detect all abnormal electrograms. Diastolic potentials that cannot be dissociated from the following ventricular activation during pacing maneuvers are much more likely to indicate a potentially effective target site for ablation.

The creation of **empiric ablation lines** during sinus rhythm has also been proposed. Such lines, composed of multiple sequential lesions placed approximately 5 mm apart, can be either single or multiple and transect from the middle of the scar or area identified as an isthmus to the border zones (≤ 1.0 mV).[55,85]

Techniques involving electrical **isolation of the scar** have been developed. In patients with ischemic heart disease, electrical isolation of the entire low-voltage area with a circumferential line along the border zone was associated with a reduction in VT recurrence.[94] This approach is particularly attractive in the case of smaller identifiable infarcts with poor pace map sites and no late potentials.

Because of the probabilistic nature of substrate modification, a more extensive endocardial and epicardial scar ablation strategy (**scar homogenization**) has also been proposed.[95] However, there is concern about the hemodynamic consequence of extensively ablating in proximity to normal myocardium at the edge of scar, and ablation of the **core** portion of the scar has also been advocated.[10] Other approaches also under study.[96]

Substrate ablation may offer similar or even higher success rates to conventional ablation.[82,97-103] In the VISTA trial,[104] ischemic cardiomyopathy patients with hemodynamically tolerated VT were randomly assigned to target clinical VTs using entrainment, activation, and pace mapping versus an extensive substrate-based ablation strategy targeting all abnormal electrograms within the scar. Substrate ablation was associated with a 67% lower risk of VT recurrence compared with clinical VT ablation.

Substrate-guided ablation is less cumbersome than mapping during VT but does not distinguish bystander regions from reentry circuit sites, and therefore broad areas of ablation are often necessary. Thus when only the clinical monomorphic VT is inducible in the EP laboratory and the patient remains hemodynamically stable, entrainment/activation mapping is preferable. A combination of approaches, such as entrainment mapping, pace mapping, and substrate modification, often is justified when there are multiple VT morphologies or recurrences after conventional ablation. In hemodynamically unstable and thus unmappable VTs, substrate modification is the only option.

EPICARDIAL ABLATION

Indications for epicardial mapping include an unsuccessful prior endocardial ablation procedure and VT unrelated to coronary artery disease (e.g., dilated cardiomyopathy [DCM], ARVC/D, hypertrophic cardiomyopathy [HCM], and Chagas cardiomyopathy) (Fig. 16.10). The presence of midmyocardial or subepicardial scarring on CMR may be useful in identifying patients who are likely to require epicardial mapping for successful abolition of VT.[105]

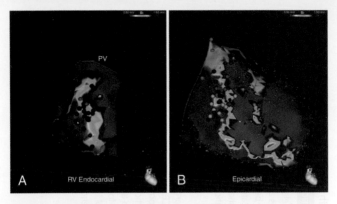

FIG. 16.10. Bipolar voltage maps of the RV endocardium and epicardium in a patient with ARVC/D and recurrent VT. (A) The bipolar voltage map of the RV endocardium (anterior posterior view) shows a large area of scar *(red area)* on the inferior and free walls. (B) There is also a large area of scar seen on the RV epicardial surface. Radiofrequency ablation *(red points)* was required on the endocardial and epicardial surfaces of the RV to successfully abolish the multiple VTs that were induced. All late potentials *(black points)* and fractionated potentials *(pink points)* were also targeted.

ARVC/D, Arrhythmogenic right ventricular cardiomyopathy/dysplasia; *PV,* pulmonary valve; *RV,* right ventricular; *VT,* ventricular tachycardia. (Dukkipati SR, Koruth JS, Choudry S, et al. Catheter ablation of ventricular tachycardia in structural heart disease: indications, strategies, and outcomes—part II. *J Am Coll Cardiol.* 2017,70(23):2924-2941.)

VT circuits in post-MI patients are usually subendocardial, but up to 30% of patients may require epicardial ablation for midmyocardial or subepicardial circuits.[95] A number of ECG criteria suggest an epicardial VT exit.[106] The most helpful criterion is delayed onset of ventricular activation with a pseudodelta greater than 34 ms and an RS greater than 121 ms.[107] It should be noted, however, that proposed 12-lead ECG features for differentiation of epicardial versus endocardial sites for nonischemic LV-VTs do not reliably identify VTs that require ablation from the epicardium.[108,109] Especially in patients with ischemic cardiomyopathy, endocardial mapping should be the first approach to catheter ablation for VT.[108]

Table 16.1 Major Complications of Ventricular Arrhythmia Ablation in Patients With Structural Heart Disease

COMPLICATION	INCIDENCE	MECHANISMS	PRESENTATION	PREVENTION	TREATMENT
In-hospital mortality	0%–3%	VT recurrence, heart failure, complications of catheter ablation	Not applicable	Correct electrolyte disturbances and optimize medical status before ablation	—
Long-term mortality	3%–35% (12–39) months of follow-up)	VT recurrence and progression of heart failure	Cardiac nonarrhythmic death (heart failure) and VT recurrence	Identification of patients with indication for heart transplantation	—
Neurologic complication (stroke, TIA, cerebral hemorrhage)	0%–%2.7%	Emboli from left ventricle, aortic valve, or aorta; cerebral bleeding	Focal or global neurologic deficits	Careful anticoagulation control; ICE can help detection of thrombus formation, and of aortic valve calcification; TEE to assess aortic arch	Thrombolytic therapy
Pericardial complications: cardiac famponade, hemopericardium, pericarditis	0%–2.7%	Catheter manipulation, RF delivery, epicardial perforation	Abrupt or gradual fall in blood pressure; arterial line is recommended in ablation of complex VT	Contact force can be useful, careful in RF delivery in perivenous foci and RVOT	Pericardiocentesis; if necessary, surgical drainage, reversal heparin, steroids and colchicine in pericarditis

AV block	0%–1.4%	Energy delivery near the conduction system	Fall in blood pressure and ECG changes	Careful monitoring when ablation is performed near the conduction system; consider cryoablation	Pacemaker; upgrade to a biventricular pacing device might be necessary
Coronary artery damage/MI	0.4%–1.9%	Ablation near coronary artery, unintended coronary damage during catheter manipulation in the aortic root or crossing the aortic valve	Acute coronary syndrome; confirmation with coronary catheterization	Limit power near coronary arteries and avoid energy delivery <5 mm from coronary vessel; ICE is useful to visualize the coronary ostium	Percutaneous coronary intervention
Heart failure/pulmonary edema	0%–3%	External irrigation, sympathetic response due to ablation, and VT induction	Heart failure symptoms	Urinary catheter and careful attention to fluid balance and diuresis, optimize clinical status before ablation, reduce irrigation volume if possible (decrease flow rates or use closed irrigation catheters)	New/increased diuretics

Continued

Table 16.1 Major Complications of Ventricular Arrhythmia Ablation in Patients With Structural Heart Disease—cont'd

COMPLICATION	INCIDENCE	MECHANISMS	PRESENTATION	PREVENTION	TREATMENT
Valvular injury	0%–0.7%	Catheter manipulation, especially retrograde crossing the aortic valve and entrapment in the mitral valve; energy delivery to subvalvular structures, including papillary muscle	Acute cardiovascular collapse, new murmurs, progressive heart failure symptoms	Careful catheter manipulation; ICE can be useful for identification of precise location of energy delivery	Echocardiography is essential in the diagnosis; medical therapy, including vasodilators and dobutamine before surgery; IABP is useful in acute mitral regurgitation and is contraindicated in aortic regurgitation
Acute periprocedural hemodynamic decompensation, cardiogenic shock	0%–11%	Fluid overloading, general anesthesia, sustained VT	Sustained hypotension despite optimized therapy	Close monitoring of fluid infusion and hemodynamic status —Optimize medical status before ablation —pLVAD —Substrate mapping preferred, avoid VT induction in higher-risk patients	Mechanical HS

Vascular injury: hematomas, pseudoaneurysm, AV fistulae	0%–6.9%	Access to femoral arterial and catheter manipulation	Groin hematomas, groin pain, fall in hemoglobin	Ultrasound-guided access	Ultrasound-guided compression, thrombin injection, and surgical closure
Overall major complications with SHD	3.8%–11.24%				
Overall all complications	7%–14.7%				

AV, Atrioventricular; ECG, electrocardiogram; HS, hemodynamic support; IABP, intra-aortic balloon pump; ICE, intracardiac echocardiography; MI, myocardial infarction; pLVAD, percutaneous left ventricular assist device; RF, radiofrequency; RVOT, right ventricular outflow tract; SHD, structural heart disease; TEE, transesophageal echocardiography; TIA, transient ischemic attack; VT, ventricular tachycardia.
Cronin EM, Bogun FM, Maury P, et al. 2019 HRS/EHRA/APHRS/LAHRS expert consensus statement on catheter ablation of ventricular arrhythmias: executive summary. Heart Rhythm. 2020;17(1):e155-e205.

CLINICAL FORMS OF VENTRICULAR ARRHYTHMIAS
IDIOPATHIC VT

Approximately two-thirds of idiopathic VTs originate in the RV, and the rest in the LV (Fig. 16.11). NSVT originating from the right ventricular outflow tract (RVOT) may occasionally cause syncope, but the risk of death is very low. However, malignant ventricular arrhythmias and sudden death have been reported in patients with RVOT ectopic activity (see PVC-induced VF).[110-112] Thus catheter ablation may be indicated in certain cases.[64]

The prevalence of NSVT in apparently healthy persons has been reported to be in the range of 0.5% to 1%.[113] A distinction between monomorphic and polymorphic NSVT is essential for prognostic and diagnostic purposes, and patients should be thoroughly evaluated for underlying cardiac disease.[114]

Ventricular Outflow Tract Tachycardias

Idiopathic ventricular outflow arrhythmias mainly arise in the RVOT (80%) and rarely below it, and 20% from the left ventricular outflow tract (LVOT), and most probably are due to triggered activity secondary to cyclic adenosine monophosphate (cAMP)–mediated delayed after-depolarizations.[6] Defects of connexins (proteins involved in cell-to-cell connections) may also be responsible.[115] Inducibility of sustained monomorphic VT (adenosine sensitive) is possible with concomitant administration of isoprenaline in less than 50% of the cases of outflow tract tachycardias. RVOT tachycardias produce an LBBB pattern with inferior axis and R/S transition at or beyond V_3. R/S transmission beyond V_4 and notching in the inferior leads indicates a free wall rather than septal site of origin and a positive R wave in lead I posterior rather than anterior septal and free-wall sites.[116] LVOT tachycardias may produce an RBBB morphology with inferior axis and R/S transition at V_1 or V_2 because of the more posterior location of LVOT compared with RVOT.[117] If the R/S transition is in V_3, the tachycardia may originate from either the RVOT (usually) or the LVOT. A V_2 transition ratio 0.60 or greater predicts LVOT origin.[118] The transition ratio represents percentage R wave during VT divided by percentage R wave during SR, $[R / (R + S)_{VT}$ divided by $[R / (R + S)]_{SR}$, and is calculated by measuring R wave amplitude (highest point to isoelectric line) and S wave (lowest point to isoelectric line) durations in millivolts during VT and SR.

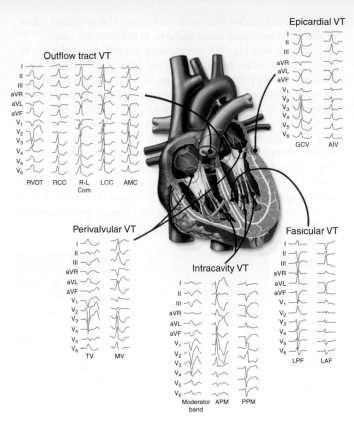

FIG. 16.11. Twelve-lead electrocardiogram morphology of different sites of origin in idiopathic ventricular tachycardia.

AIV, Anterior interventricular vein; *AMC,* aortomitral continuity; *APM,* anterior PAP; *GCV,* greater cardiac vein; *LAF,* left anterior fascicle; *LCC,* left coronary cusp; *LPF,* left posterior fascicle; *MV,* mitral annulus; *APM,* anterior papillary muscle; *PPM,* posterior papillary muscle; *RCC,* right coronary cusp; *R–L com,* right–left coronary cusp commissure; *RVOT,* right ventricular outflow tract; *TV,* tricuspid annulus. (Tanawuttiwat T, Nazarian S, Calkins H. The role of catheter ablation in the management of ventricular tachycardia. *Eur Heart J.* 2016;37(7):594-609.)

Ventricular outflow tract tachycardias may also originater below or above the semilunar valves and arise at the coronary cusps.[119-121] They have a variable QRS morphology depending on the site of origin: Tachycardias originating in the *left coronary cusp* have a QRS morphology consistent with an M or W pattern in lead V_1, tachycardias originating in the *right coronary cusp* or the *left ventricular side of the septum* may have an LBBB pattern, and tachycardias arising from the commissure between the left and right cusps display a QS morphology in lead V_1 with notching on the downward deflection and precordial transition in V_3 (Fig. 16.12). LBBB morphology with an R wave in V_1 and large R waves in the inferior leads suggests the *pulmonary artery cusps* as site of origin.[120] Catheter ablation is the treatment of choice.[121] Rarely (<10%) there can also be an *epicardial* site of origin (prominent r in V_1, delayed QRS onset to maximal deflection interval).[122]

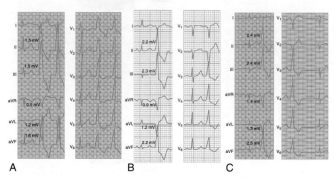

FIG. 16.12. Typical electrocardiograms (ECGs) from three patients with ventricular arrhythmias (VAs) originating from the left ventricular outflow tract (LVOT) below the left coronary cusp (LCC), LCC/right coronary cusp (RCC) junction, and the RCC. **A,** ECG recording from a 15-year-old woman in whom the VA origin was located below the LCC, with two previous failed ablation attempts in the great cardiac vein, LVOT, and LCC; **B,** ECG recording from a 60-year-old woman with VAs originating from below the RCC/LCC junction; **C,** ECG recording from a 47-year-old woman with VAs originating below the RCC. Note that (1) II, III, and aVF have high amplitudes and there is QS morphology in aVR and aVL during clinical arrhythmias; (2) absolute values of the R-wave amplitudes in II, III, and aVF and the Q-wave amplitude in aVR and aVL are marked on the surface ECG; and (3) there is no S wave in V_5 and V_6, with early transition in the precordial leads before V_3.
(Ouyang F, Mathew S, Wu S, et al. Ventricular arrhythmias arising from the left ventricular outflow tract below the aortic sinus cusps: mapping and catheter ablation via transseptal approach and electrocardiographic characteristics. *Circ Arrhythm Electrophysiol.* 2014;7(3):445-455.)

Fascicular Tachycardias

Idiopathic left ventricular tachycardias typically are due to reentry within the Purkinje network, are verapamil sensitive, and originate within one of the fascicles of the left bundle branch. Usually the posterior fascicle is involved, resulting in a tachycardia with RBBB and left axis deviation (90%), but cases with inferior axis from an anterior or high septal fascicular origin may also occur. Tachycardias or premature ventricular beats originating from the proximal left anterior fascicle have a morphology close to that during sinus rhythm and can be safely ablated from the right coronary cusp.[123] Upper septal VT is the least common variant.[121] Catheter mapping during VT demonstrates characteristic potentials thought to represent activation of abnormal Purkinje fibers (Fig. 16.13).[15,124]

AV Annuli

Tachycardias may also originate in the AV annuli either in the tricuspid (LBBB pattern) or the mitral annulus (RBBB pattern or RS in V_1 and monophasic R or RS in V_2–V_6).[125]

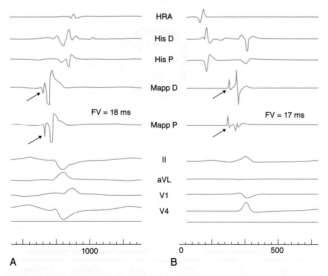

FIG. 16.13. Mapping during (A) left posterior fascicular tachycardia and (B) sinus rhythm. A discrete potential consistent with a fascicular potential) precedes the earliest ventricular electrogram, as indicated.

(Katritsis D, Heald S, Ahsan A, et al. Catheter ablation for successful management of left posterior fascicular tachycardia: an approach guided by recording of fascicular potentials. *Heart.* 1996;75(4):384-388.)

Papillary Muscles

Idiopathic VTs originating in the **left ventricular papillary muscles** present with an RBBB morphology and arise in the posterior papillary muscle much more often than in the anterolateral papillary muscle.[121,126] Papillary muscle ventricular arrhythmias are distinguished electrocardiographically from fascicular VAs by longer QRS durations and lower prevalence of r<R' V1 QRS morphology and from mitral annular VAs by lower prevalence of positive precordial lead concordance.[126] Distinct morphologies of pappilary (anterolateral or posteromedial) VAs are Rr', R with slurred downstroke, and RR (double-peak R), as well as shorter intrinsicoid deflection compared to other idiopathic forms (Fig. 16.14).[127]

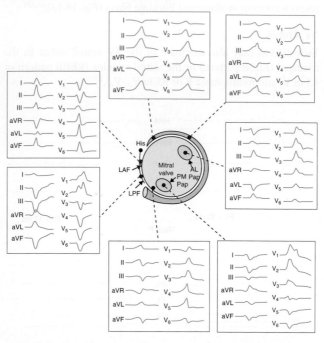

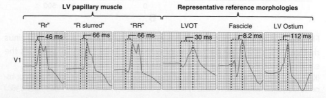

FIG. 16.14. Upper panel. Representative 12-lead ECGs of papillary muscle, fascicular, and mitral annular ventricular arrhythmias with corresponding locations on schematic diagram. AL indicates anterolateral; LAF, left anterior fascicle; LPF, left posterior fascicle; Pap, papillary muscle; and PM, posteromedial. **Lower panel.** QRS intrinsicoid measurements of lead V1 for PVCs from the papillary muscles (left) and other sites in the LV (right). LV 5 left ventricular; LVOT 5 left ventricular outflow tract; PVC 5 premature ventricular complex.

(Upper panel): Al'Aref SJ, Ip JE, Markowitz SM, Liu CF, et al. Differentiation of papillary muscle from fascicular and mitral annular ventricular arrhythmias in patients with and without structural heart disease. *Circ Arrhythm Electrophysiol.* 2015;8:616-24. *(Lower pannel):* Briceno DF, Santangeli P, Frankel DS, et al. QRS morphology in lead V1 for the rapid localization of idiopathic ventricular arrhythmias originating from the left ventricular papillary muscles: A novel electrocardiographic criterion. *Heart Rhythm.* 2020;17(10):1711-1718.

Intraventricular Septum

Tachycardias may also originate around the His bundle or in the intraventricular septum (LBBB with inferior axis).[128]

Differential Diagnosis

Differentiation of idiopathic VT from **ARVC** is crucial.[129] The diagnosis of ARVC should be ruled out in patients with exercise-related palpitations and/or syncope; survivors of sudden cardiac arrest (particularly during exercise); and individuals with frequent ventricular premature beats (>500 in 24 hours) and/or VT of LBBB morphology in the absence of other heart disease.[18] A normal baseline ECG, normal cardiac magnetic resonance imaging, the presence of a single VT morphology both clinically and by programmed stimulation, and a normal endocardial voltage map are evidence of the VT being idiopathic.[130]

Prolonged terminal activation duration (TAD) is measured from the nadir of the S wave to the end of all depolarization deflections. A TAD 55 ms or greater in any of the V_1-V_3 leads in the absence of complete RBBB differentiates ARVC from idiopathic RVOT-VT (Fig. 16.15).[18]

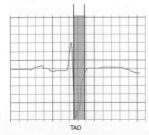

TAD

FIG. 16.15. Terminal activation duration (TAD) is measured from the nadir of the S wave to the end of all depolarization deflections and is prolonged if 55 ms or greater in any of the V_1-V_3 leads in the absence of complete right bundle branch block.

(Towbin JA, McKenna WJ, Abrams DJ, et al. 2019 HRS expert consensus statement on evaluation, risk stratification, and management of arrhythmogenic cardiomyopathy. *Heart Rhythm.* 2019.)

QRS duration in lead I of more than 120 ms, earliest onset QRS in lead V1, QRS notching, and a transition of V_5 or later predict the presence of ARVC (Fig. 16.16).[131]

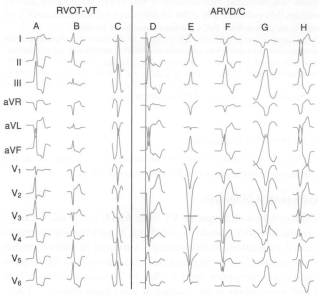

FIG. 16.16. Differentiation between RVOT VT and ARVC. Twelve-lead electrocardiograms from patients with right ventricular outflow tract ventricular tachycardia (RVOT-VT) (A–C) and arrhythmogenic right ventricular dysplasia/cardiomyopathy (ARVC/C) (D–H) showing characteristic features. (A) RVOT-VT from an anterior-septal location showing precordial transition at V2 and narrow QRS duration in lead I (78 ms). (B) RVOT-VT originating superior to His bundle region showing precordial transition at V4, positive R-wave in aVL, and narrow QRS in lead I (86 ms). (C) RVOT-VT from a posterior-septal location showing precordial transition at V3 and narrow QRS duration in lead I (118 ms). (D) ARVC/C ventricular tachycardia (VT) showing late precordial transition V5, wide QRS duration in lead I (124 ms), and earliest onset QRS in V1 *(vertical line)*. (E) ARVC/C-VT shows very late precordial transition V6 and wide QRS duration in lead I (126 ms). (F) ARVC/C-VT shows very late precordial transition V6 and wide QRS duration in lead I (150 ms). (G) ARVC/C-VT shows late precordial transition V5, wide QRS duration in lead I (160 ms), and notching of the QRS (II, III, aVF, V4–V6). (H) ARVC/C-VT shows wide QRS duration in lead I (128 ms) and notching of the QRS (II, III, aVF, V4–V6). (Hoffmayer KS, Machado ON, Marcus GM, et al. Electrocardiographic comparison of ventricular arrhythmias in patients with arrhythmogenic right ventricular cardiomyopathy and right ventricular outflow tract tachycardia. *J Am Coll Cardiol.* 2011;58(8):831-838.)

QRS notching in multiple leads is defined as a QRS complex deflection on the upstroke or downstroke of less than 0.05/mV that does not cross the baseline and is present in at least two leads (Fig. 16.17).

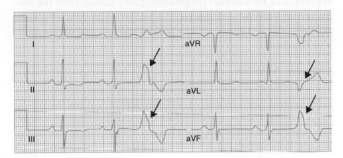

FIG. 16.17. Example of QRS notching. *Arrows* show QRS notching in ectopic beats lead II, III, aVF, and aVL.

(Hoffmayer KS, Machado ON, Marcus GM, et al. Electrocardiographic comparison of ventricular arrhythmias in patients with arrhythmogenic right ventricular cardiomyopathy and right ventricular outflow tract tachycardia. *J Am Coll Cardiol.* 2011;58(8):831-838.)

Table 16.2 presents the criteria for distinguishing idiopathic VT from ARVC-related VT.[131] A score of 5 or greater suggests ARVC. A QRS duration of more than 180 ms in PVCs makes ARVC more likely than idiopathic PVCs.[132]

Table 16.2 Electrocardiographic Scoring System for Distinguishing RVOT Arrhythmias in Patients With ARVC/D From Idiopathic VT

ECG CHARACTERISTIC	POINTS
Anterior T wave inversions (V$_1$–V$_3$) in sinus rhythm	3
VT/PVC:	
Lead I QRS duration ≥ 120 ms	2
QRS notching (multiple leads)	2
V$_3$ transition or later	1

Anterior T wave inversion is defined as T wave negativity in, at least, leads V$_1$, V$_2$, V$_3$.
Lead I QRS duration ≥ 120 ms is defined as the duration from the initial deflection of the QRS complex to the end of the QRS complex in lead I.
QRS notching in multiple leads is defined as a QRS complex deflection on the upstroke or downstroke of >0.5 mV that did not cross the baseline occurring in, at least, two leads.
The precordial transition point is designated as the earliest precordial lead where the R wave amplitude exceeded the S wave amplitude.
Hoffmayer KS, et al. An electrocardiographic scoring system for distinguishing right ventricular outflow tract arrhythmias. *Heart Rhythm.* 2013;10:477-82.

Older age at symptom onset, presence of cardiovascular co-morbidities, nonfamilial pattern of disease, PR interval prolongation, high-grade atrioventricular block, significant left ventricular dysfunction, myocardial delayed enhancement of the septum, and mediastinal lymphadenopathy should raise the suspicion for **cardiac sarcoidosis**.[133] Usually VT is either Purkinje related (QRS < 170 ms) or scar related and may respond to catheter ablation.[134]

Catheter Ablation

Catheter ablation is the treatment of choice for idiopathic VT with success rates exceeding 80% for RVOT VT and fascicular tachycardias. Catheter ablation of tachycardias from the papillary muscles may be difficult because of the contraction of the muscle. Success rates also are lower with epicardial or intraseptal sites of origin. The most common major complication is tamponade or pericardial effusion, reported to occur in 1% to 2% of cases, whereas no mortality is usually reported.[135,136]

ISCHEMIC HEART DISEASE

Compared with the pre-reperfusion era, late VT now is less common but still occurs in approximately 20% of patients between 1 week and 2 years postinfarction when the ejection fraction is less than 0.40.[137]

NSVT is detected 2 to 9 days after admission in 18% to 25% of patients with an acute coronary syndrome, and even short episodes of VT lasting 4 to 7 beats are independently associated with the risk of sudden cardiac death (SCD) over the subsequent year, especially when associated with myocardial ischemia.[138] Earlier episodes within 48 hours after admission do not carry the same risk. In patients with a STEMI, NSVT occurs in up to 75% of reperfused patients and during the first 13[139] to 24 hours[140] does not carry a prognostic significance. In-hospital NSVT after this period indicates increased in-hospital mortality. However, in patients who had a prior myocardial infarction treated with reperfusion and beta blockers, NSVT is not an independent predictor of long-term mortality when other covariates such as LVEF are taken into account.[114] It may carry an adverse prognostic significance in patients with LVEF greater than 35%.[141]

Monomorphic VT usually is due to scar-related reentry, and its incidence has been reduced from 3% to 1% to 2% in the reperfusion era. An LBBB configuration in lead V_1 (dominant S wave) suggests an exit site in the right ventricle or the interventricular septum. A dominant R wave or RBBB pattern in V_1 indicates a LV exit site. The QRS axis defines VT origins in the vertical plane; an inferiorly directed QRS axis suggests a superior or anterior wall exit, whereas a superiorly directed axis indicated an inferior wall exit. The precordial leads are more indicative of directionality in the horizontal plane. Deep S waves in the apical leads (V_3–V_6) indicate exit sites at the apex, whereas prominent R waves in these leads point to a basal origin of activation. Subepicardial origin of VT is suggested by wider QRS complexes and delayed initial upstrokes in the precordial leads. Several algorithms have been published for identification of the exit site if postinfarction VT from the 12-lead ECG (Fig. 16.18).[142-144]

Polymorphic VT or VF may be due to acute ischemia (acute coronary syndrome or spasm) or in the context of scar-related VT that degenerates into VF.[145,146]

Ventricular storm is mainly scar related and often triggered by a PVC, although His-Purkinje related reentry may also be responsible.[147]

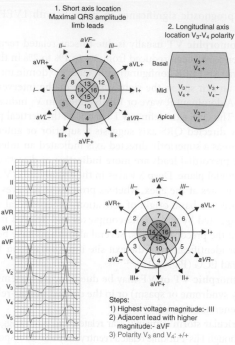

FIG. 16.18. Localization of the origin of scar-related VT. *Left panel:* The QRS axis–based algorithm. The figure shows the 17-segment model from the American Heart Association superimposed on a representation of the QRS axis and all the limb leads. Steps to identify the segment of origin of a ventricular arrhythmia: (1) Identify the limb lead with the highest voltage magnitude (positive or negative). If this magnitude is in lead I, II, or III, analyze the adjacent leads. The adjacent limb lead with higher magnitude will determine the group of segments suggested as a possible site of origin. (2) Identify the positivity or negativity of the precordial leads V_3 and V_4; concordance indicates a basal or apical origin, respectively. Other combinations indicate a medial origin. *Right panel:* Example of the application of the QRS axis–based algorithm. (A) An ECG of VT. (B) The application of the QRS axis–based graphical algorithm. In the ECG of panel (A), the lead with the highest voltage magnitude is III2. Applying the first step of the algorithm, the segment of origin of VT is one of the groups selected by the *red circle*. By analyzing the voltage magnitude of the adjacent leads of III2 (aVF2 and aVL1), it is possible to determine that aVF2 has more voltage magnitude than aVL1. As a result, the group of segments selected by the algorithm is the one marked with the *blue circle*. The last step of the algorithm (positivity or negativity in leads V_3 and V_4) indicates a basal origin of VT (leads V_3 and V_4 are both more positive than negative). The final selected segment by the algorithm is 4, marked with the green circle.

ECG, Electrocardiogram; *VT,* ventricular tachycardia. (Andreu D, Fernandez-Armenta J, Acosta J, et al. A QRS axis-based algorithm to identify the origin of scar-related ventricular tachycardia in the 17-segment American Heart Association model. *Heart Rhythm.* 2018;15(10):1491.1497.)

Catheter Ablation

Catheter ablation is useful for reducing ICD discharges and can be accomplished even for unmappable VTs. In postinfarction patients, several studies have reported that all inducible VTs were eliminated by ablation in 56% to 77% of patients. The procedure-related mortality rate was 0.5% to 5%, the VT recurrence rate within the next year was 12% to 50%.[54,55,61,80,148-150] Early referral of patients for catheter ablation results in improved freedom from VT compared with later referral.[151] Catheter ablation may also be effective in the treatment of VT storm.[147]

Procedure-related complications have been reported to occur in approximately 7% of patients.[56,61,,64,80,149,152] Ablation-related early (<30 days) mortality ranges up to 3% in experienced centers, with more than one-half of patients dying before hospital discharge, most often because of refractory VT or heart failure (Table 16.2). Predictors of early mortality include LVEF, chronic kidney disease, presentation with VT storm, and presence of unmappable VTs.[149]

The reported 1-year mortality rate after VT ablation is 18%, with the primary causes of death being recurrent VT (37.5%) and heart failure (35%).[80] Other complications consist of cardiac perforation in 1.5%, major vascular injury in 2.3%, uncontrollable VT in up to 2.6%, high-degree AV block in 0.9%, coronary artery injury in 0.2%, and stroke or transient ischemic attack in 0.5% (Table 16.1).

HEART FAILURE

In patients with heart failure and LVEF less than 30% to 40%, the reported prevalence of NSVT is 30% to 80%.[114,153] Although the GE-SICA-GEMA investigators identified NSVT as an independent predictor of total mortality in patients with heart failure (35% to 40% with ischemic heart disease) and LVEF 35% or less,[154] in the CHF STAT cohort (70% to 75% with ischemic heart disease), after adjusting other variables and especially for LVEF, NSVT was not an independent predictor of sudden death or total mortality in patients with heart failure and LVEF less than 35% to 50%.[155] Similar results were published by the PROMISE investigators.[156] Only during the recovery period after exercise has frequent ventricular ectopy been found to carry an adverse prognostic significance in patients with heart failure.[157] However, in an analysis of ICD interrogation data in the SCD-HeFT population, long runs of rapid rate NSVT were associated with subsequent appropriate ICD shocks and an increase in mortality.[158]

Sustained VT in patients with heart failure is discussed in relevant sections according to its cause.

CARDIOMYOPATHIES

Dilated Cardiomyopathy

NSVT may be detected in 40% to 50% of patients with DCM, but results on its independent prognostic significance have been conflicting. LVEF and NSVT have been found to be significant predictors of arrhythmic events,[159] but after medical stabilization with angiotensin-converting enzyme inhibitor and beta blocker, the number and length of NSVT runs did not increase the risk of ventricular arrhythmias in patients with LVEF of 0.35 or less, as opposed to those with LVEF greater than 0.35.[160] In the Marburg Cardiomyopathy Study,[161] on univariate analysis nonsustained VT and frequent ventricular premature beats showed a significant association with a higher arrhythmia risk, but on multivariate analysis only LVEF was found to be a significant predictor of major arrhythmic events. The combination of LVEF 30% or less and NSVT denoted an eightfold higher risk for subsequent arrhythmic events compared with LVEF 30% or less and no NSVT.

The mechanism of VT in patients with dilated cardiomyopathy is usually scar-related reentry, but Purkinje reentry (bundle branch reentry VT) and focal automaticity or triggered activity may also occur.[162] Scarring in DCM may be midmyocardial or epicardial and most often occurs in the basal anteroseptal and inferolateral LV regions.[105,163] The use of contrast-enhanced CMR helps identify an endocardial versus epicardial origin.[164,165] An EP study may be useful in inducing a monomorphic VT that could be amenable to catheter ablation[166] and as a risk stratifier because inducibility of ventricular arrhythmias,[39] and especially polymorphic VT or VF,[40] indicates increased likelihood of subsequent ICD therapies in patients with such a device.

In a small percentage of the cases of idiopathic dilated cardiomyopathy, VT is due to **bundle branch reentry**. Bundle branch reentrant tachycardia may also occur in patients with ischemic cardiomyopathy, intraventricular conduction defects, and, rarely, in the absence of structural heart disease.[13] Genetic causes have been identified.[12]

Patients with **myotonic muscular dystrophy type 1,** certain **lamin A/C** (LMNA, a cause of limb-girdle dystrophy) mutations, and **desmin mutations** are especially at risk for VT and nonischemic dilated cardiomyopathy.[18,167-169]

When there is no established cause for DCM and there has been an arrhythmia with rates consistently greater than 100 bpm, **tachycardia-induced cardiomyopathy** should be considered.[170-173] Usually, LV end-diastolic diameter is less than 65 and LV end-systolic dimension is less than 50 mm in patients with LVEF less than 30% as a result of tachycardiomyopathy.[174] Larger volumes suggest another cause of dilated cardiomyopathy, although there may be overlap. The diagnosis is established by demonstrating recovery of LV function within 3 months after elimination of the arrhythmia or control of the ventricular rate.

Catheter Ablation. The overall success rate with catheter ablation for patients with nonischemic cardiomyopathy (38% to 67%) is lower than that for patients with postinfarction ischemic cardiomyopathy (56% to 77%),[61,175-178] and an epicardial approach may be necessary. Complication rates are shown in Table 16.1. Catheter ablation is more efficacious for bundle branch reentry with up to 100% success rates having been reported, but at a risk of up to 40% for inadvertent complete heart block.[64]

Arrhythmogenic Right Ventricular Cardiomyopathy/Dysplasia

Compared with patients with nonischemic dilated cardiomyopathy, patients with arrhythmogenic ARVC/D have better outcomes of ablation.[178] With the addition of epicardial mapping to the ablation strategy for ARVC/D patients, the success rates of catheter ablation have markedly improved.[179-182] A large, single-center study reported a 71% rate of freedom from recurrent VT after multiple procedures during a mean follow-up of nearly 5 years.[182]

Hypertrophic Cardiomyopathy

In HCM 20% to 30% of patients may have NSVT,[114] which is a risk factor for VT/VF.[183] There are little published data on the results of VT ablation in patients with hypertrophic cardiomyopathy. Catheter ablation, often using a combined endocardial/epicardial approach, appears to be reasonably efficacious and safe in the treatment of drug-refractory VT in these patients.[178,184-187]

Cardiac Sarcoidosis

Catheter ablation in patients with cardiac sarcoidosis is challenging because of the complex underlying substrate. However, it is feasible in selected patients and results in reduced arrhythmia burden.[187-189] Reported success rates approach 50% with a 5% risk of complications.[64]

MITRAL VALVE PROLAPSE

In approximately 2.4% of the general population mitral valve prolapse (MVP) can be detected.[190] Sudden cardiac death may occur in the context of prominent prolapse, especially in young athletes and women with arrhythmias and particular charcateristics.[191] Patients with MVP who may experience sudden cardiac death are mostly females with bileaflet prolapse, ventricular arrhythmias of LV origin (outflow tract alternating with papillary muscle/fascicular origin), and frequent ECG repolarization abnormalities on inferior leads.[192,193] Contrast-enhanced CMR can identify fibrosis of the papillary muscles and inferobasal LV free wall, which correlates well with arrhythmia morphology.[193] **Mitral annulus disjunction (MAD),** an abnormal atrial displacement of the mitral valve leaflet hinge point, has also been associated with mitral valve prolapse and sudden cardiac death.[194] Ventricular arrhythmias detected are frequent but mostly in the form of ventricular ectopy but the presence of arrhythmia, particularly severe, is associated with long-term excess mortality and lower event-free survival, independent of other characteristics, including MR severity and MAD.[195]

GENETIC CHANNELOPATHIES

Epicardial ablation of the RVOT arrhythmogenic substrate in patients with **Brugada syndrome** is feasible, and good results have been reported (Fig. 16.19).[196-199] However, the procedure should not be considered curative or adequate to avoid the need for an ICD in high-risk patients.

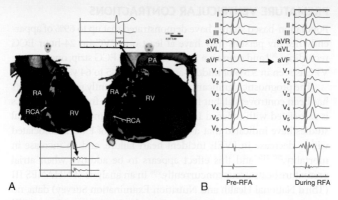

FIG. 16.19. Epicardial substrate ablation in a patient with Brugada syndrome and appropriate ICD shocks for VF. Image integration of a preacquired CT with the electroanatomic epicardial substrate map is shown in (A). Purple represents bipolar voltage greater than 1.5 mV. Fractionated potentials *(arrows)* are tagged with black dots, and a representative example is displayed. Widespread fractionated potentials were recorded from the epicardial aspect of the RVOT extending down into the basal RV body. Ablation lesions are tagged with red dots. Some fractionated potentials could not be ablated because of the proximity of the acute marginal branches of the right coronary artery. Panel (B) shows the significant transient accentuation of the Brugada ECG pattern during the application of radiofrequency energy at one of these sites.

CT, Computed tomography; *ECG,* electrocardiogram; *ICD,* implantable cardioverter defibrillator; *PA,* pulmonary artery; *RA,* right atrium; *RCA,* right coronary artery; *RFA,* radiofrequency ablation; *RV,* right ventricle; *RVOT,* right ventricular outflow tract; *VF,* ventricular fibrillation. (Cronin EM, Bogun FM, Maury P, et al. 2019 HRS/EHRA/APHRS/LAHRS expert consensus statement on catheter ablation of ventricular arrhythmias: executive summary. *Heart Rhythm.* 2020;17(1):e155-e205.)

Catheter ablation has also been proposed for patients with the **early repolarization syndrome** by targeting the RV inferolateral epicardium or VF triggers at Purkinje sites.[200] Clinical experience with this approach is limited.

ADULT CONGENITAL HEART DISEASE

Most data on patients with adult congenital heart disease are derived from patients with operated **tetralogy of Fallot.** Anatomic isthmuses critical to the VT reentrant circuit often are identified between the septal defect patch or ventriculotomy and the pulmonary valve and between the tricuspid annulus and the outflow patch or septal defect patch. Part of the circuit may also be mapped at the left side of the ventricular septum, and left-sided ablation may be successful.[201] Ablation offers an approximately 80% freedom from VT within the next 10 years.[202,203]

PREMATURE VENTRICULAR CONTRACTIONS

Population-based studies have demonstrated that up to 69% of apparently healthy persons may have at least one PVC on 24-hour ECG recordings,[204] and even on a 2-minute rhythm ECG strip, one or more VPC is seen in 5.5% of middle-aged patients (45 to 64 years old).[205]

The prognostic significance of PVC in apparently normal subjects has been controversial, but it seems that a higher frequency of PVCs is associated with reduced LVEF and increased mortality.[206] Several studies have indicated that a higher frequency of PVC is associated with a decrease in LVEF, incident heart failure, and an increase in mortality,[207-210] and this effect appears to be additive when atrial premature beats occur concurrently.[208] In an analysis of NHANES III (Third National Health and Nutrition Examination Survey) data, no significant association of PVC with total mortality was detected,[211] but atrial premature beats were associated with total and cardiovascular mortality.[211] Rarely, right and left ventricular Purkinje-related or even RVOT PVCs may trigger polymorphic VT/VF.

Frequent ventricular ectopy and NSVT, when detected during exercise in apparently healthy persons, and especially during recovery, indicates increased cardiovascular mortality within the next decades.[212,213] However, exercise-induced NSVT in older persons (>60 years) has not been found to carry an adverse prognosis.[214] In trained athletes, frequent PVC and NSVT may occur at ambulatory monitoring or during exercise and are benign.[215-217] NSVT in athletes without structural heart disease or evidence of genetic channelopathy appears to be part of "athlete's heart syndrome" and carries no adverse prognostic significance. Electroanatomic substrate mapping may help diagnose subclinical myocardial diseases in competitive athletes presenting with recent-onset ventricular arrhythmias and an apparently normal heart.[218]

In patients with heart disease, PVCs have adverse prognostic significance. They are an important risk factor after the acute phase of myocardial infarction and in patients with heart failure.[206]

PVC-Triggered VT/VF

Certain cases of idiopathic VF and/or polymorphic ventricular tachycardia can be triggered by isolated spontaneous PVC that can be mapped and ablated.[219,220] PVC are localized to the right or left Purkinje system[221] and rarely may be present in patients with idiopathic ventricular arrhythmias arising from the RVOT.[222,223] These RVOT extrasystoles may have a very short coupling interval, especially a second cycle length of NSVT less than 317 ms,[111,222] as opposed to the long coupling interval seen in the truly benign RVOT-VT, but intermediate coupling intervals may also be seen with VF-inducing PVC.[111,112]

Focal PVC triggers arising in Purkinje fibers may also trigger VT/VF in patients with idiopathic VF, in post–myocardial infarction patients,[224] and in those with early repolarization syndrome,[200] and PVCs arising from the RVOT may trigger VF in patients with the Brugada syndrome,[225] and torsades de pointes in patients with the long-QT syndrome.[225,226] PVC triggers from the papillary muscles of the right and left ventricle and the right ventricular moderator band have also been implicated in polymorphic VT and VF.[227,228] VF storm in post-MI patients often is triggered by PVCs originating in the Purkinje fibers at the borders of scar and also may respond to catheter ablation.[53,224] Published data on the long-term results of catheter ablation in all of these settings are limited.

PVC-Induced Cardiomyopathy

Frequent PVCs are an established cause of cardiomyopathy that is an entity phenotypically distinct from a tachycardia-induced cardiomyopathy.[170-172,229,230] The mechanism is not established, but dyssynchrony appears to play a major role.[229,230] In a swine model, cardiomyopathy severity was strongly associated with severity of the hemodynamic derangement associated with the paced ectopic beats, particularly the extent of LV dyssynchrony.[231]

A precise threshold number of daily PVCs associated with PVC-induced cardiomyopathy does not exist. In addition to PVC frequency, factors such as the PVC coupling interval, site of PVC origin, and QRS duration may play a role. Nevertheless, the PVC burden in patients with a PVC-induced cardiomyopathy generally is more than 15,000 to 20,000 per day, or alternatively a 24-hour burden of more than 15% to 20% on continuous ambulatory monitoring.[232,233] However, PVC-induced cardiomyopathy has been reported in a patient with only 5502 beats per day,[234] and deterioration of the LV function has been reported with more than 1000 PVCs per day.[235] The presence of interpolated PVCs may play an important role in the generation of PVC-induced cardiomyopathy.[236] A PVC QRS duration 150 ms or greater and a non-RVOT origin are also predictive of impaired LV function.[237]

Cardiomyopathy induced by monomorphic PVC is a reversible condition and is an appropriate indication for catheter ablation. Success rates are approximately 85% with no reported mortality.[230,238,239]

References

1. Priori SG, Blomstrom-Lundqvist C, Mazzanti A, et al. 2015 ESC Guidelines for the management of patients with ventricular arrhythmias and the prevention of sudden cardiac death: The Task Force for the Management of Patients with Ventricular Arrhythmias and the Prevention of Sudden Cardiac Death of the European Society of Cardiology (ESC). Endorsed by: Association for European Paediatric and Congenital Cardiology (AEPC). *Eur Heart J.* 2015;36(41):2793-2867.

2. Al-Khatib SM, Stevenson WG, Ackerman MJ, et al. 2017 AHA/ACC/HRS Guideline for management of patients with ventricular arrhythmias and the prevention of sudden cardiac death: executive summary: a report of the American College of Cardiology/American Heart Association Task Force on Clinical Practice Guidelines and the Heart Rhythm Society. *Heart Rhythm.* 2018;15(10):e190-e252.

3. Hadid C, Almendral J, Ortiz M, et al. Incidence, determinants, and prognostic implications of true pleomorphism of ventricular tachycardia in patients with implantable cardioverter-defibrillators: a substudy of the DATAS Trial. *Circ Arrhythm Electrophysiol.* 2011;4(1):33-42.

4. Baher AA, Uy M, Xie F, Garfinkel A, Qu Z, Weiss JN. Bidirectional ventricular tachycardia: ping pong in the His-Purkinje system. *Heart Rhythm.* 2011;8(4):599-605.

5. Credner SC, Klingenheben T, Mauss O, Sticherling C, Hohnloser SH. Electrical storm in patients with transvenous implantable cardioverter-defibrillators: incidence, management and prognostic implications. *J Am Coll Cardiol.* 1998;32(7):1909-1915.

6. Kim RJ, Iwai S, Markowitz SM, Shah BK, Stein KM, Lerman BB. Clinical and electrophysiological spectrum of idiopathic ventricular outflow tract arrhythmias. *J Am Coll Cardiol.* 2007;49(20):2035-2043.

7. Stevenson WG, Khan H, Sager P, et al. Identification of reentry circuit sites during catheter mapping and radiofrequency ablation of ventricular tachycardia late after myocardial infarction. *Circulation.* 1993;88(4 Pt 1):1647-1670.

8. Josephson ME, Anter E. Substrate mapping for ventricular tachycardia: assumptions and misconceptions. *JACC Clin Electrophysiol.* 2015;1(5):341-352.

9. Anter E, Tschabrunn CM, Buxton AE, Josephson ME. High-resolution mapping of postinfarction reentrant ventricular tachycardia: electrophysiological characterization of the circuit. *Circulation.* 2016;134(4):314-327.

10. Sadek MM, Schaller RD, Supple GE, et al. Ventricular tachycardia ablation—the right approach for the right patient. *Arrhythm Electrophysiol Rev.* 2014;3(3):161-167.

11. Tung R, Raiman M, Liao H, et al Simultaneous endocardial and epicardial delineation of 3D reentrant ventricular tachycardia. *J Am Coll Cardiol.* 2020;75(8):884-897.

12. Roberts R. Bundle branch reentrant ventricular tachycardia: novel genetic mechanisms in a life-threatening arrhythmia. *JACC Clin Electrophysiol.* 2017;3(3):276-288.

13. Blanck Z, Jazayeri M, Dhala A, Deshpande S, Sra J, Akhtar M. Bundle branch reentry: a mechanism of ventricular tachycardia in the absence of myocardial or valvular dysfunction. *J Am Coll Cardiol.* 1993;22(6):1718-1722.

14. Asirvatham SJ, Stevenson WG. Bundles branch reentry. *Circ Arrhythm Electrophysiol.* 2013;6(6):e92-e94.

15. Katritsis D, Heald S, Ahsan A, et al. Catheter ablation for successful management of left posterior fascicular tachycardia: an approach guided by recording of fascicular potentials. *Heart.* 1996;75(4):384-388.

16. Lopera G, Stevenson WG, Soejima K, et al. Identification and ablation of three types of ventricular tachycardia involving the His-Purkinje system in patients with heart disease. *J Cardiovasc Electrophysiol.* 2004;15(1):52-58.

17. Nash MP, Mourad A, Clayton RH, et al. Evidence for multiple mechanisms in human ventricular fibrillation. *Circulation.* 2006;114(6):536-542.

18. Towbin JA, McKenna WJ, Abrams DJ, et al. 2019 HRS expert consensus statement on evaluation, risk stratification, and management of arrhythmogenic cardiomyopathy. *Heart Rhythm.* 2019;16(11):e301-e372.

19. Viskin S, Chorin E, Viskin D, et al. Quinidine-responsive polymorphic ventricular tachycardia in patients with coronary heart disease. *Circulation.* 2019;139(20): 2304-2314.

20. Katritsis DG, Zografos T, Hindricks G. Electrophysiology testing for risk stratification of patients with ischaemic cardiomyopathy: a call for action. *Europace.* 2018;20(FI2):fI48-fI52.

21. Kowey PR, Taylor JE, Marinchak RA, Rials SJ. Does programmed stimulation really help in the evaluation of patients with nonsustained ventricular tachycardia? Results of a meta-analysis. *Am Heart J.* 1992;123(2):481-485.

22. Wilber DJ, Olshansky B, Moran JF, Scanlon PJ. Electrophysiological testing and nonsustained ventricular tachycardia. Use and limitations in patients with coronary artery disease and impaired ventricular function. *Circulation.* 1990;82(2): 350-358.

23. Buxton AE, Lee KL, DiCarlo L, et al. Electrophysiologic testing to identify patients with coronary artery disease who are at risk for sudden death. Multicenter Unsustained Tachycardia Trial Investigators. *N Engl J Med.* 2000;342(26):1937-1945.

24. Yokokawa M, Kim HM, Baser K, et al. Predictive value of programmed ventricular stimulation after catheter ablation of post-infarction ventricular tachycardia. *J Am Coll Cardiol.* 2015;65(18):1954-1959.

25. Zaman S, Narayan A, Thiagalingam A, et al. Long-term arrhythmia-free survival in patients with severe left ventricular dysfunction and no inducible ventricular tachycardia after myocardial infarction. *Circulation.* 2014;129(8):848-854.

26. Buxton AE, Lee KL, Hafley GE, et al. Relation of ejection fraction and inducible ventricular tachycardia to mode of death in patients with coronary artery disease: an analysis of patients enrolled in the multicenter unsustained tachycardia trial. *Circulation.* 2002;106(19):2466-2472.

27. Zaman S, Kumar S, Sullivan J, et al. Significance of inducible very fast ventricular tachycardia (cycle length 200-230 ms) after early reperfusion for ST-segment-elevation myocardial infarction. *Circ Arrhythm Electrophysiol.* 2013;6(5):884-890.

28. Kumar S, Sivagangabalan G, Choi MC, Eipper V, Thiagalingam A, Kovoor P. Long-term outcomes of inducible very fast ventricular tachycardia (cycle length 200-250 ms) in patients with ischemic cardiomyopathy. *J Cardiovasc Electrophysiol.* 2010;21(3):262-269.

29. Zaman S, Kumar S, Narayan A, et al. Induction of ventricular tachycardia with the fourth extrastimulus and its relationship to risk of arrhythmic events in patients

with post-myocardial infarct left ventricular dysfunction. *Europace.* 2012;14(12): 1771-1777.

30. Piccini JP, Hafley GE, Lee KL, et al. Mode of induction of ventricular tachycardia and prognosis in patients with coronary disease: the Multicenter UnSustained Tachycardia Trial (MUSTT). *J Cardiovasc Electrophysiol.* 2009;20(8):850-855.

31. Bourke JP, Richards DA, Ross DL, McGuire MA, Uther JB. Does the induction of ventricular flutter or fibrillation at electrophysiologic testing after myocardial infarction have any prognostic significance? *Am J Cardiol.* 1995;75(7):431-435.

32. Daubert JP, Zareba W, Hall WJ, et al. Predictive value of ventricular arrhythmia inducibility for subsequent ventricular tachycardia or ventricular fibrillation in Multicenter Automatic Defibrillator Implantation Trial (MADIT) II patients. *J Am Coll Cardiol.* 2006;47(1):98-107.

33. Mittal S, Hao SC, Iwai S, et al. Significance of inducible ventricular fibrillation in patients with coronary artery disease and unexplained syncope. *J Am Coll Cardiol.* 2001;38(2):371-376.

34. Monahan KM, Hadjis T, Hallett N, Casavant D, Josephson ME. Relation of induced to spontaneous ventricular tachycardia from analysis of stored far-field implantable defibrillator electrograms. *Am J Cardiol.* 1999;83(3):349-353.

35. Zaman S, Sivagangabalan G, Narayan A, Thiagalingam A, Ross DL, Kovoor P. Outcomes of early risk stratification and targeted implantable cardioverter-defibrillator implantation after ST-elevation myocardial infarction treated with primary percutaneous coronary intervention. *Circulation.* 2009;120(3):194-200.

36. Gatzoulis KA, Tsiachris D, Arsenos P, et al. Arrhythmic risk stratification in post-myocardial infarction patients with preserved ejection fraction: the PRESERVE EF study. *Eur Heart J.* 2019;40(35):2940-2949.

37. Brilakis ES, Shen WK, Hammill SC, et al. Role of programmed ventricular stimulation and implantable cardioverter defibrillators in patients with idiopathic dilated cardiomyopathy and syncope. *Pacing Clin Electrophysiol.* 2001;24(11): 1623-1630.

38. Grimm W, Hoffmann J, Menz V, Luck K, Maisch B. Programmed ventricular stimulation for arrhythmia risk prediction in patients with idiopathic dilated cardiomyopathy and nonsustained ventricular tachycardia. *J Am Coll Cardiol.* 1998;32(3): 739-745.

39. Daubert JP, Winters SL, Subacius H, et al. Ventricular arrhythmia inducibility predicts subsequent ICD activation in nonischemic cardiomyopathy patients: a DEFINITE substudy. *Pacing Clin Electrophysiol.* 2009;32(6):755-761.

40. Rolf S, Haverkamp W, Borggrefe M, Breithardt G, Bocker D. Induction of ventricular fibrillation rather than ventricular tachycardia predicts tachyarrhythmia recurrences in patients with idiopathic dilated cardiomyopathy and implantable cardioverter defibrillator for secondary prophylaxis. *Europace.* 2009;11(3):289-296.

41. Khairy P, Landzberg MJ, Gatzoulis MA, et al. Value of programmed ventricular stimulation after tetralogy of fallot repair: a multicenter study. *Circulation.* 2004;109(16):1994-2000.

42. Mehta D, Mori N, Goldbarg SH, Lubitz S, Wisnivesky JP, Teirstein A. Primary prevention of sudden cardiac death in silent cardiac sarcoidosis: role of programmed ventricular stimulation. *Circ Arrhythm Electrophysiol.* 2011;4(1):43-48.

43. Shivkumar K. Catheter ablation of ventricular arrhythmias. *N Engl J Med.* 2019;380(16):1555-1564.

44. Guandalini GS, Liang JJ, Marchlinski FE. Ventricular tachycardia ablation: past, present, and future perspectives. *JACC Clin Electrophysiol.* 2019;5(12):1363-1383.

45. Sweeney MO. The contradiction of appropriate shocks in primary prevention ICDs: increasing and decreasing the risk of death. *Circulation.* 2010;122(25): 2638-2641.

46. Pacifico A, Ferlic LL, Cedillo-Salazar FR, Nasir Jr N, Doyle TK, Henry PD. Shocks as predictors of survival in patients with implantable cardioverter-defibrillators. *J Am Coll Cardiol.* 1999;34(1):204-210.

47. Bardy GH, Lee KL, Mark DB, et al. Amiodarone or an implantable cardioverter-defibrillator for congestive heart failure. *N Engl J Med.* 2005;352(3):225-237.

48. Connolly SJ, Dorian P, Roberts RS, et al. Comparison of beta-blockers, amiodarone plus beta-blockers, or sotalol for prevention of shocks from implantable cardioverter defibrillators: the OPTIC Study: a randomized trial. *JAMA.* 2006;295(2):165-171.

49. Kheiri B, Barbarawi M, Zayed Y, et al. Antiarrhythmic drugs or catheter ablation in the management of ventricular tachyarrhythmias in patients with implantable cardioverter-defibrillators: a systematic review and meta-analysis of randomized controlled trials. *Circ Arrhythm Electrophysiol.* 2019;12(11):e007600.

50. Santangeli P, Muser D, Maeda S, et al. Comparative effectiveness of antiarrhythmic drugs and catheter ablation for the prevention of recurrent ventricular tachycardia in patients with implantable cardioverter-defibrillators: a systematic review and meta-analysis of randomized controlled trials. *Heart Rhythm.* 2016;13(7): 1552-1559.

51. Li J, Saba S, Wang NC. Ventricular tachycardia ablation versus antiarrhythmic-drug escalation. *N Engl J Med.* 2016;375(15):1498-1500.

52. Tanawuttiwat T, Nazarian S, Calkins H. The role of catheter ablation in the management of ventricular tachycardia. *Eur Heart J.* 2016;37(7):594-609.

53. Komatsu Y, Hocini M, Nogami A, et al. Catheter ablation of refractory ventricular fibrillation storm after myocardial infarction. *Circulation.* 2019;139(20):2315-2325.

54. Kuck KH, Schaumann A, Eckardt L, et al. Catheter ablation of stable ventricular tachycardia before defibrillator implantation in patients with coronary heart disease (VTACH): a multicentre randomised controlled trial. *Lancet.* 2010;375(9708):31-40.

55. Reddy VY, Reynolds MR, Neuzil P, et al. Prophylactic catheter ablation for the prevention of defibrillator therapy. *N Engl J Med.* 2007;357(26):2657-2665.

56. Dukkipati SR, Koruth JS, Choudry S, Miller MA, Whang W, Reddy VY. Catheter ablation of ventricular tachycardia in structural heart disease: indications, strategies, and outcomes-Part II. *J Am Coll Cardiol.* 2017;70(23):2924-2941.

57. Willems S, Tilz RR, Steven D, et al. Preventive or deferred ablation of ventricular tachycardia in patients with ischemic cardiomyopathy and implantable defibrillator (BERLIN VT): a multicenter randomized trial. *Circulation.* 2020;141(13):1057-1067.

58. Vergara P, Tzou WS, Tung R, et al. Predictive score for identifying survival and recurrence risk profiles in patients undergoing ventricular tachycardia ablation. *Circ Arrhythm Electrophysiol.* 2018;11(12):e006730.

59. Konig S, Ueberham L, Muller-Rothing R, et al. Catheter ablation of ventricular arrhythmias and in-hospital mortality: insights from the German-wide Helios hospital network of 5052 cases. *Europace*. 2020;22(1):100-108.

60. Cheung JW, Yeo I, Ip JE, et al. Outcomes, costs, and 30-day readmissions after catheter ablation of myocardial infarct-associated ventricular tachycardia in the real world. *Circ Arrhythm Electrophysiol*. 2018;11(11):e006754.

61. Tung R, Vaseghi M, Frankel DS, et al. Freedom from recurrent ventricular tachycardia after catheter ablation is associated with improved survival in patients with structural heart disease: An International VT Ablation Center Collaborative Group study. *Heart Rhythm*. 2015;12(9):1997-2007.

62. Ghanbari H, Baser K, Yokokawa M, et al. Noninducibility in postinfarction ventricular tachycardia as an end point for ventricular tachycardia ablation and its effects on outcomes: a meta-analysis. *Circ Arrhythm Electrophysiol*. 2014;7(4):677-683.

63. Dinov B, Arya A, Schratter A, et al. Catheter ablation of ventricular tachycardia and mortality in patients with nonischemic dilated cardiomyopathy: can noninducibility after ablation be a predictor for reduced mortality? *Circ Arrhythm Electrophysiol*. 2015;8(3):598-605.

64. Cronin EM, Bogun FM, Maury P, et al. 2019 HRS/EHRA/APHRS/LAHRS expert consensus statement on catheter ablation of ventricular arrhythmias: executive summary. *Heart Rhythm*. 2020;17(1):e155-e205.

65. Page SP, Duncan ER, Thomas G, et al. Epicardial catheter ablation for ventricular tachycardia in heparinized patients. *Europace*. 2013;15(2):284-289.

66. Sawhney V, Breitenstein A, Ullah W, et al. Epicardial catheter ablation for ventricular tachycardia on uninterrupted warfarin: a safe approach for those with a strong indication for peri-procedural anticoagulation? *Int J Cardiol*. 2016;222:57-61.

67. Santangeli P, Muser D, Zado ES, et al. Acute hemodynamic decompensation during catheter ablation of scar-related ventricular tachycardia: incidence, predictors, and impact on mortality. *Circ Arrhythm Electrophysiol*. 2015;8(1):68-75.

68. Nof E, Stevenson WG, John RM. Catheter ablation for ventricular arrhythmias. *Arrhythm Electrophysiol Rev*. 2013;2(1):45-52.

69. Tschabrunn CM, Roujol S, Dorman NC, Nezafat R, Josephson ME, Anter E. High-resolution mapping of ventricular scar: comparison between single and multi-electrode catheters. *Circ Arrhythm Electrophysiol*. 2016;9(6):e003841.

70. Zhang J, Cooper DH, Desouza KA, et al. Electrophysiologic scar substrate in relation to vt: noninvasive high-resolution mapping and risk assessment with ECGI. *Pacing Clin Electrophysiol*. 2016;39(8):781-791.

71. Sapp JL, Dawoud F, Clements JC, Horacek BM. Inverse solution mapping of epicardial potentials: quantitative comparison with epicardial contact mapping. *Circ Arrhythm Electrophysiol*. 2012;5(5):1001-1009.

72. Mountantonakis SE, Park RE, Frankel DS, et al. Relationship between voltage map "channels" and the location of critical isthmus sites in patients with post-infarction cardiomyopathy and ventricular tachycardia. *J Am Coll Cardiol*. 2013;61(20):2088-2095.

73. Nayyar S, Wilson L, Ganesan AN, et al. High-density mapping of ventricular scar: a comparison of ventricular tachycardia (VT) supporting channels with channels that do not support VT. *Circ Arrhythm Electrophysiol*. 2014;7(1):90-98.

74. Irie T, Yu R, Bradfield JS, et al. Relationship between sinus rhythm late activation zones and critical sites for scar-related ventricular tachycardia: systematic analysis of isochronal late activation mapping. *Circ Arrhythm Electrophysiol.* 2015;8(2):390-399.

75. Stevenson WG, Friedman PL, Sager PT, et al. Exploring postinfarction reentrant ventricular tachycardia with entrainment mapping. *J Am Coll Cardiol.* 1997;29(6):1180-1189.

76. Morady F, Kadish A, Rosenheck S, et al. Concealed entrainment as a guide for catheter ablation of ventricular tachycardia in patients with prior myocardial infarction. *J Am Coll Cardiol.* 1991;17(3):678-689.

77. Bogun F, Kim HM, Han J, et al. Comparison of mapping criteria for hemodynami-cally tolerated, postinfarction ventricular tachycardia. *Heart Rhythm.* 2006;3(1):20-26.

78. Tung S, Soejima K, Maisel WH, Suzuki M, Epstein L, Stevenson WG. Recognition of far-field electrograms during entrainment mapping of ventricular tachycardia. *J Am Coll Cardiol.* 2003;42(1):110-115.

79. El-Shalakany A, Hadjis T, Papageorgiou P, Monahan K, Epstein L, Josephson ME. Entrainment/mapping criteria for the prediction of termination of ventricular tachycardia by single radiofrequency lesion in patients with coronary artery disease. *Circulation.* 1999;99(17):2283-2289.

80. Stevenson WG, Wilber DJ, Natale A, et al. Irrigated radiofrequency catheter abla-tion guided by electroanatomic mapping for recurrent ventricular tachycardia after myocardial infarction: the multicenter thermocool ventricular tachycardia ablation trial. *Circulation.* 2008;118(25):2773-2782.

81. Bogun F, Good E, Reich S, et al. Isolated potentials during sinus rhythm and pace-mapping within scars as guides for ablation of post-infarction ventricular tachycardia. *J Am Coll Cardiol.* 2006;47(10):2013-2019.

82. Jais P, Maury P, Khairy P, et al. Elimination of local abnormal ventricular activi-ties: a new end point for substrate modification in patients with scar-related ventricular tachycardia. *Circulation.* 2012;125(18):2184-2196.

83. Arenal A, Glez-Torrecilla E, Ortiz M, et al. Ablation of electrograms with an iso-lated, delayed component as treatment of unmappable monomorphic ventricu-lar tachycardias in patients with structural heart disease. *J Am Coll Cardiol.* 2003;41(1):81-92.

84. Takigawa M, Relan J, Martin R, et al. Effect of bipolar electrode orientation on local electrogram properties. *Heart Rhythm.* 2018;15(12):1853-1861.

85. Marchlinski FE, Callans DJ, Gottlieb CD, Zado E. Linear ablation lesions for control of unmappable ventricular tachycardia in patients with ischemic and nonischemic cardiomyopathy. *Circulation.* 2000;101(11):1288-1296.

86. Glashan CA, Androulakis AFA, Tao Q, et al. Whole human heart histology to vali-date electroanatomical voltage mapping in patients with non-ischaemic cardio-myopathy and ventricular tachycardia. *Eur Heart J.* 2018;39(31):2867-2875.

87. de Chillou C, Groben L, Magnin-Poull I, et al. Localizing the critical isthmus of postinfarct ventricular tachycardia: the value of pace-mapping during sinus rhythm. *Heart Rhythm.* 2014;11(2):175-181.

88. Calkins H, Kalbfleisch SJ, el-Atassi R, Langberg JJ, Morady F. Relation between efficacy of radiofrequency catheter ablation and site of origin of idiopathic ventricular tachycardia. *Am J Cardiol.* 1993;71(10):827-833.

89. Stevenson WG, Sager PT, Natterson PD, Saxon LA, Middlekauff HR, Wiener I. Relation of pace mapping QRS configuration and conduction delay to ventricular tachycardia reentry circuits in human infarct scars. *J Am Coll Cardiol*. 1995;26(2):481-488.

90. Brunckhorst CB, Delacretaz E, Soejima K, Maisel WH, Friedman PL, Stevenson WG. Identification of the ventricular tachycardia isthmus after infarction by pace mapping. *Circulation*. 2004;110(6):652-659.

91. Bogun F, Taj M, Ting M, et al. Spatial resolution of pace mapping of idiopathic ventricular tachycardia/ectopy originating in the right ventricular outflow tract. *Heart Rhythm*. 2008;5(3):339-344.

92. Azegami K, Wilber DJ, Arruda M, Lin AC, Denman RA. Spatial resolution of pace-mapping and activation mapping in patients with idiopathic right ventricular outflow tract tachycardia. *J Cardiovasc Electrophysiol*. 2005;16(8):823-829.

93. Goyal R, Harvey M, Daoud EG, et al. Effect of coupling interval and pacing cycle length on morphology of paced ventricular complexes. Implications for pace mapping. *Circulation*. 1996;94(11):2843-2849.

94. Tilz RR, Makimoto H, Lin T, et al. Electrical isolation of a substrate after myocardial infarction: a novel ablation strategy for unmappable ventricular tachycardias—feasibility and clinical outcome. *Europace*. 2014;16(7):1040-1052.

95. Di Biase L, Santangeli P, Burkhardt DJ, et al. Endo-epicardial homogenization of the scar versus limited substrate ablation for the treatment of electrical storms in patients with ischemic cardiomyopathy. *J Am Coll Cardiol*. 2012;60(2):132-141.

96. Aziz Z, Shatz D, Raiman M, et al. Targeted ablation of ventricular tachycardia guided by wavefront discontinuities during sinus rhythm: a new functional substrate mapping strategy. *Circulation*. 2019;140(17):1383-1397.

97. Volkmer M, Ouyang F, Deger F, et al. Substrate mapping vs. tachycardia mapping using CARTO in patients with coronary artery disease and ventricular tachycardia: impact on outcome of catheter ablation. *Europace*. 2006;8(11):968-976.

98. Berruezo A, Fernandez-Armenta J, Andreu D, et al. Scar dechanneling: new method for scar-related left ventricular tachycardia substrate ablation. *Circ Arrhythm Electrophysiol*. 2015;8(2):326-336.

99. Komatsu Y, Maury P, Sacher F, et al. Impact of substrate-based ablation of ventricular tachycardia on cardiac mortality in patients with implantable cardioverter-defibrillators. *J Cardiovasc Electrophysiol*. 2015;26(11):1230-1238.

100. Silberbauer J, Oloriz T, Maccabelli G, et al. Noninducibility and late potential abolition: a novel combined prognostic procedural end point for catheter ablation of postinfarction ventricular tachycardia. *Circ Arrhythm Electrophysiol*. 2014;7(3):424-435.

101. Arenal A, Hernández J, Calvo D, et al. Safety, long-term results, and predictors of recurrence after complete endocardial ventricular tachycardia substrate ablation in patients with previous myocardial infarction. *Am J Cardiol*. 2013;111:499-505.

102. Vergara P, Trevisi N, Ricco A, et al. Late potentials abolition as an additional technique for reduction of arrhythmia recurrence in scar related ventricular tachycardia ablation. *J Cardiovasc Electrophysiol*. 2012;23(6):621-627.

103. Kumar S, Baldinger SH, Romero J, et al. Substrate-based ablation versus ablation guided by activation and entrainment mapping for ventricular tachycardia: a systematic review and meta-analysis. *J Cardiovasc Electrophysiol*. 2016;27(12):1437-1447.

104. Di Biase L, Burkhardt JD, Lakkireddy D, et al. Ablation of Stable VTs versus substrate ablation in ischemic cardiomyopathy: The VISTA Randomized Multicenter Trial. *J Am Coll Cardiol.* 2015;66(25):2872-2882.
105. Bogun FM, Desjardins B, Good E, et al. Delayed-enhanced magnetic resonance imaging in nonischemic cardiomyopathy: utility for identifying the ventricular arrhythmia substrate. *J Am Coll Cardiol.* 2009;53(13):1138-1145.
106. Valles E, Bazan V, Marchlinski FE. ECG criteria to identify epicardial ventricular tachycardia in nonischemic cardiomyopathy. *Circ Arrhythm Electrophysiol.* 2010;3(1):63-71.
107. Berruezo A, Mont L, Nava S, Chueca E, Bartholomay E, Brugada J. Electrocardiographic recognition of the epicardial origin of ventricular tachycardias. *Circulation.* 2004;109(15):1842-1847.
108. Martinek M, Stevenson WG, Inada K, Tokuda M, Tedrow UB. QRS characteristics fail to reliably identify ventricular tachycardias that require epicardial ablation in ischemic heart disease. *J Cardiovasc Electrophysiol.* 2012;23(2):188-193.
109. Piers SR, Silva Mde R, Kapel GF, Trines SA, Schalij MJ, Zeppenfeld K. Endocardial or epicardial ventricular tachycardia in nonischemic cardiomyopathy? The role of 12-lead ECG criteria in clinical practice. *Heart Rhythm.* 2014;11(6):1031-1039.
110. Bottoni N, Quartieri F, Lolli G, Iori M, Manari A, Menozzi C. Sudden death in a patient with idiopathic right ventricular outflow tract arrhythmia. *J Cardiovasc Med (Hagerstown).* 2009;10(10):801-803.
111. Noda T, Shimizu W, Taguchi A, et al. Malignant entity of idiopathic ventricular fibrillation and polymorphic ventricular tachycardia initiated by premature extrasystoles originating from the right ventricular outflow tract. *J Am Coll Cardiol.* 2005;46(7):1288-1294.
112. Viskin S, Rosso R, Rogowski O, Belhassen B. The "short-coupled" variant of right ventricular outflow ventricular tachycardia: a not-so-benign form of benign ventricular tachycardia? *J Cardiovasc Electrophysiol.* 2005;16(8):912-916.
113. Marine JE. Nonsustained ventricular tachycardia in the normal heart: risk stratification and management. *Card Electrophysiol Clin.* 2016;8(3):525-543.
114. Katritsis DG, Zareba W, Camm AJ. Nonsustained ventricular tachycardia. *J Am Coll Cardiol.* 2012;60(20):1993-2004.
115. Boukens BJ, Christoffels VM, Coronel R, Moorman AF. Developmental basis for electrophysiological heterogeneity in the ventricular and outflow tract myocardium as a substrate for life-threatening ventricular arrhythmias. *Circ Res.* 2009;104(1):19-31.
116. Dixit S, Gerstenfeld EP, Callans DJ, Marchlinski FE. Electrocardiographic patterns of superior right ventricular outflow tract tachycardias: distinguishing septal and free-wall sites of origin. *J Cardiovasc Electrophysiol.* 2003;14(1):1-7.
117. Prystowsky EN, Padanilam BJ, Joshi S, Fogel RI. Ventricular arrhythmias in the absence of structural heart disease. *J Am Coll Cardiol.* 2012;59(20):1733-1744.
118. Betensky BP, Park RE, Marchlinski FE, et al. The V(2) transition ratio: a new electrocardiographic criterion for distinguishing left from right ventricular outflow tract tachycardia origin. *J Am Coll Cardiol.* 2011;57(22):2255-2262.
119. Ouyang F, Mathew S, Wu S, et al. Ventricular arrhythmias arising from the left ventricular outflow tract below the aortic sinus cusps: mapping and catheter

ablation via transseptal approach and electrocardiographic characteristics. *Circ Arrhythm Electrophysiol*. 2014;7(3):445-455.

120. Liao Z, Zhan X, Wu S, et al. Idiopathic ventricular arrhythmias originating from the pulmonary sinus cusp: prevalence, electrocardiographic/electrophysiological characteristics, and catheter ablation. *J Am Coll Cardiol*. 2015;66(23): 2633-2644.

121. Dukkipati SR, Choudry S, Koruth JS, Miller MA, Whang W, Reddy VY. Catheter ablation of ventricular tachycardia in structurally normal hearts: indications, strategies, and outcomes-Part I. *J Am Coll Cardiol*. 2017;70(23):2909-2923.

122. Suleiman M, Asirvatham SJ. Ablation above the semilunar valves: when, why, and how? Part I. *Heart Rhythm*. 2008;5(10):1485-1492.

123. Chen S, Lu X, Peng S, et al. Ablation at right coronary cusp as an alternative and favorable approach to eliminate premature ventricular complexes originating from the proximal left anterior fascicle. *Circ Arrhythm Electrophysiol*. 2020;13(5):e008173.

124. Liu Y, Fang Z, Yang B, et al. Catheter Ablation of Fascicular Ventricular Tachycardia: Long-Term Clinical Outcomes and Mechanisms of Recurrence. *Circ Arrhythm Electrophysiol*. 2015;8(6):1443-1451.

125. Ip JE, Liu CF, Thomas G, Cheung JW, Markowitz SM, Lerman BB. Unifying mechanism of sustained idiopathic atrial and ventricular annular tachycardia. *Circ Arrhythm Electrophysiol*. 2014;7(3):436-444.

126. Al'Aref SJ, Ip JE, Markowitz SM, et al. Differentiation of papillary muscle from fascicular and mitral annular ventricular arrhythmias in patients with and without structural heart disease. *Circ Arrhythm Electrophysiol*. 2015;8(3):616-624.

127. Briceno DF, Santangeli P, Frankel DS, et al. QRS morphology in lead V1 for the rapid localization of idiopathic ventricular arrhythmias originating from the left ventricular papillary muscles: A novel electrocardiographic criterion. *Heart Rhythm*. 2020;17(10):1711-1718.

128. Yokokawa M, Good E, Chugh A, et al. Intramural idiopathic ventricular arrhythmias originating in the intraventricular septum: mapping and ablation. *Circ Arrhythm Electrophysiol*. 2012;5(2):258-263.

129. Nucifora G, Muser D, Masci PG, et al. Prevalence and prognostic value of concealed structural abnormalities in patients with apparently idiopathic ventricular arrhythmias of left versus right ventricular origin: a magnetic resonance imaging study. *Circ Arrhythm Electrophysiol*. 2014;7(3):456-462.

130. Saffitz JE. Arrhythmogenic cardiomyopathy: advances in diagnosis and disease pathogenesis. *Circulation*. 2011;124(15):e390-e392.

131. Hoffmayer KS, Machado ON, Marcus GM, et al. Electrocardiographic comparison of ventricular arrhythmias in patients with arrhythmogenic right ventricular cardiomyopathy and right ventricular outflow tract tachycardia. *J Am Coll Cardiol*. 2011;58(8):831-838.

132. Bastiaenen R, Pantazis A, Gonna H, et al. The ventricular ectopic QRS interval (VEQSI): Diagnosis of arrhythmogenic right ventricular cardiomyopathy in patients with incomplete disease expression. *Heart Rhythm*. 2016;13(7):1504-1512.

133. Philips B, Madhavan S, James CA, et al. Arrhythmogenic right ventricular dysplasia/cardiomyopathy and cardiac sarcoidosis: distinguishing features when the diagnosis is unclear. *Circ Arrhythm Electrophysiol*. 2014;7(2):230-236.

134. Naruse Y, Sekiguchi Y, Nogami A, et al. Systematic treatment approach to ventricular tachycardia in cardiac sarcoidosis. *Circ Arrhythm Electrophysiol.* 2014;7(3):407-413.

135. Bohnen M, Stevenson WG, Tedrow UB, et al. Incidence and predictors of major complications from contemporary catheter ablation to treat cardiac arrhythmias. *Heart Rhythm.* 2011;8(11):1661-1666.

136. Peichl P, Wichterle D, Pavlu L, Cihak R, Aldhoon B, Kautzner J. Complications of catheter ablation of ventricular tachycardia: a single-center experience. *Circ Arrhythm Electrophysiol.* 2014;7(4):684-690.

137. Bloch Thomsen PE, Jons C, Raatikainen MJ, et al. Long-term recording of cardiac arrhythmias with an implantable cardiac monitor in patients with reduced ejection fraction after acute myocardial infarction: the Cardiac Arrhythmias and Risk Stratification After Acute Myocardial Infarction (CARISMA) study. *Circulation.* 2010;122(13):1258-1264.

138. Scirica BM, Braunwald E, Belardinelli L, et al. Relationship between nonsustained ventricular tachycardia after non-ST-elevation acute coronary syndrome and sudden cardiac death: observations from the metabolic efficiency with ranolazine for less ischemia in non-ST-elevation acute coronary syndrome-thrombolysis in myocardial infarction 36 (MERLIN-TIMI 36) randomized controlled trial. *Circulation.* 2010;122(5):455-462.

139. Cheema AN, Sheu K, Parker M, Kadish AH, Goldberger JJ. Nonsustained ventricular tachycardia in the setting of acute myocardial infarction: tachycardia characteristics and their prognostic implications. *Circulation.* 1998;98(19):2030-2036.

140. Heidbuchel H, Tack J, Vanneste L, Ballet A, Ector H, Van de Werf F. Significance of arrhythmias during the first 24 hours of acute myocardial infarction treated with alteplase and effect of early administration of a beta-blocker or a bradycardiac agent on their incidence. *Circulation.* 1994;89(3):1051-1059.

141. Makikallio TH, Barthel P, Schneider R, et al. Prediction of sudden cardiac death after acute myocardial infarction: role of Holter monitoring in the modern treatment era. *Eur Heart J.* 2005;26(8):762-769.

142. Yokokawa M, Liu TY, Yoshida K, et al. Automated analysis of the 12-lead electrocardiogram to identify the exit site of postinfarction ventricular tachycardia. *Heart Rhythm.* 2012;9(3):330-334.

143. de Riva M, Watanabe M, Zeppenfeld K. Twelve-lead ECG of ventricular tachycardia in structural heart disease. *Circ Arrhythm Electrophysiol.* 2015;8(4):951-962.

144. Andreu D, Fernandez-Armenta J, Acosta J, et al. A QRS axis-based algorithm to identify the origin of scar-related ventricular tachycardia in the 17-segment American Heart Association model. *Heart Rhythm.* 2018;15(10):1491-1497.

145. Myerburg RJ, Kessler KM, Castellanos A. Sudden cardiac death. Structure, function, and time-dependence of risk. *Circulation.* 1992;85(suppl 1):I2-I10.

146. Wolfe CL, Nibley C, Bhandari A, Chatterjee K, Scheinman M. Polymorphous ventricular tachycardia associated with acute myocardial infarction. *Circulation.* 1991;84(4):1543-1551.

147. Nayyar S, Ganesan AN, Brooks AG, Sullivan T, Roberts-Thomson KC, Sanders P. Venturing into ventricular arrhythmia storm: a systematic review and meta-analysis. *Eur Heart J.* 2013;34(8):560-571.

148. Marchlinski FE, Haffajee CI, Beshai JF, et al. Long-term success of irrigated radiofrequency catheter ablation of sustained ventricular tachycardia: post-approval THERMOCOOL VT Trial. *J Am Coll Cardiol.* 2016;67(6):674-683.

149. Santangeli P, Frankel DS, Tung R, et al. Early mortality after catheter ablation of ventricular tachycardia in patients with structural heart disease. *J Am Coll Cardiol.* 2017;96:2105-2101.

150. Marchlinski FE, Haffajee CI, Beshai JF, et al. Long-term success of irrigated radiofrequency catheter ablation of sustained ventricular tachycardia: post-approval THERMOCOOL VT Trial. *J Am Coll Cardiol.* 2016;67(6):674-683.

151. Frankel DS, Mountantonakis SE, Robinson MR, Zado ES, Callans DJ, Marchlinski FE. Ventricular tachycardia ablation remains treatment of last resort in structural heart disease: argument for earlier intervention. *J Cardiovasc Electrophysiol.* 2011;22(10):1123-1128.

152. Sapp JL, Wells GA, Parkash R, et al. Ventricular tachycardia ablation versus escalation of antiarrhythmic drugs. *N Engl J Med.* 2016;375(2):111-121.

153. Santangeli P, Rame JE, Birati EY, Marchlinski FE. Management of ventricular arrhythmias in patients with advanced heart failure. *J Am Coll Cardiol.* 2017;69(14):1842-1860.

154. Doval HC, Nul DR, Grancelli HO, et al. Nonsustained ventricular tachycardia in severe heart failure. Independent marker of increased mortality due to sudden death. GESICA-GEMA Investigators. *Circulation.* 1996;94(12):3198-3203.

155. Singh SN, Fisher SG, Carson PE, Fletcher RD. Prevalence and significance of nonsustained ventricular tachycardia in patients with premature ventricular contractions and heart failure treated with vasodilator therapy. Department of Veterans Affairs CHF STAT Investigators. *J Am Coll Cardiol.* 1998;32(4):942-947.

156. Teerlink JR, Jalaluddin M, Anderson S, et al. Ambulatory ventricular arrhythmias in patients with heart failure do not specifically predict an increased risk of sudden death. PROMISE (Prospective Randomized Milrinone Survival Evaluation) Investigators. *Circulation.* 2000;101(1):40-46.

157. O'Neill JO, Young JB, Pothier CE, Lauer MS. Severe frequent ventricular ectopy after exercise as a predictor of death in patients with heart failure. *J Am Coll Cardiol.* 2004;44(4):820-826.

158. Chen J, Johnson G, Hellkamp AS, et al. Rapid-rate nonsustained ventricular tachycardia found on implantable cardioverter-defibrillator interrogation: relationship to outcomes in the SCD-HeFT (Sudden Cardiac Death in Heart Failure Trial). *J Am Coll Cardiol.* 2013;61(21):2161-2168.

159. Iacoviello M, Forleo C, Guida P, et al. Ventricular repolarization dynamicity provides independent prognostic information toward major arrhythmic events in patients with idiopathic dilated cardiomyopathy. *J Am Coll Cardiol.* 2007;50(3):225-231.

160. Zecchin M, Di Lenarda A, Gregori D, et al. Are nonsustained ventricular tachycardias predictive of major arrhythmias in patients with dilated cardiomyopathy on optimal medical treatment? *Pacing Clin Electrophysiol.* 2008;31(3):290-299.

161. Grimm W, Christ M, Bach J, Muller HH, Maisch B. Noninvasive arrhythmia risk stratification in idiopathic dilated cardiomyopathy: results of the Marburg Cardiomyopathy Study. *Circulation.* 2003;108(23):2883-2891.

162. Delacretaz E, Stevenson WG, Ellison KE, Maisel WH, Friedman PL. Mapping and radiofrequency catheter ablation of the three types of sustained monomorphic ventricular tachycardia in nonischemic heart disease. *J Cardiovasc Electrophysiol.* 2000;11(1):11-17.

163. Oloriz T, Silberbauer J, Maccabelli G, et al. Catheter ablation of ventricular arrhythmia in nonischemic cardiomyopathy: anteroseptal versus inferolateral scar sub-types. *Circ Arrhythm Electrophysiol.* 2014;7(3):414-423.

164. Halliday BP, Cleland JGF, Goldberger JJ, Prasad SK. Personalizing risk stratification for sudden death in dilated cardiomyopathy: the past, present, and future. *Circulation.* 2017;136(2):215-231.

165. Andreu D, Ortiz-Perez JT, Boussy T, et al. Usefulness of contrast-enhanced cardiac magnetic resonance in identifying the ventricular arrhythmia substrate and the approach needed for ablation. *Eur Heart J.* 2014;35(20):1316-1326.

166. Kanagasundram A, John RM, Stevenson WG. Sustained monomorphic ventricular tachycardia in nonischemic heart disease: arrhythmia-substrate correlations that inform the approach to ablation. *Circ Arrhythm Electrophysiol.* 2019;12(11):e007312.

167. Groh WJ. Arrhythmias in the muscular dystrophies. *Heart Rhythm.* 2012;9(11):1890-1895.

168. Katritsis D. Progressive cardiac conduction disease. In: Zipes DP, Jalife J, eds. *Cardiac Electrophysiology: From Cell to Bedside.* 7th ed. Elsevier, Philadelphia, PA, USA. 2017.

169. van Rijsingen IA, Arbustini E, Elliott PM, et al. Risk factors for malignant ventricular arrhythmias in lamin a/c mutation carriers a European cohort study. *J Am Coll Cardiol.* 2012;59(5):493-500.

170. Gopinathannair R, Etheridge SP, Marchlinski FE, Spinale FG, Lakkireddy D, Olshansky B. Arrhythmia-induced cardiomyopathies: mechanisms, recognition, and management. *J Am Coll Cardiol.* 2015;66(15):1714-1728.

171. Ellis ER, Josephson ME. What about tachycardia-induced cardiomyopathy? *Arrhythm Electrophysiol Rev.* 2013;2(2):82-90.

172. Huizar JF, Ellenbogen KA, Tan AY, Kaszala K. Arrhythmia-induced cardiomyopathy. *JACC.* 2019;73(18):2328-2344.

173. Shinbane JS, Wood MA, Jensen DN, Ellenbogen KA, Fitzpatrick AP, Scheinman MM. Tachycardia-induced cardiomyopathy: a review of animal models and clinical studies. *J Am Coll Cardiol.* 1997;29(4):709-715.

174. Lishmanov A, Chockalingam P, Senthilkumar A, Chockalingam A. Tachycardia-induced cardiomyopathy: evaluation and therapeutic options. *Congest Heart Fail.* 2010;16(3):122-126.

175. Dinov B, Fiedler L, Schonbauer R, et al. Outcomes in catheter ablation of ventricular tachycardia in dilated nonischemic cardiomyopathy compared with ischemic cardiomyopathy: results from the Prospective Heart Centre of Leipzig VT (HELP-VT) Study. *Circulation.* 2014;129(7):728-736.

176. Muser D, Santangeli P, Castro SA, et al. Long-term outcome after catheter ablation of ventricular tachycardia in patients with nonischemic dilated cardiomyopathy. *Circ Arrhythm Electrophysiol.* 2016;9(10):e004328.

177. Gokoglan Y, Mohanty S, Gianni C, et al. Scar homogenization versus limited-substrate ablation in patients with nonischemic cardiomyopathy and ventricular tachycardia. *J Am Coll Cardiol.* 2016;68(18):1990-1998.

178. Tokuda M, Tedrow UB, Kojodjojo P, et al. Catheter ablation of ventricular tachycardia in nonischemic heart disease. *Circ Arrhythm Electrophysiol.* 2012;5(5):992-1000.

179. Bai R, Di Biase L, Shivkumar K, et al. Ablation of ventricular arrhythmias in arrhythmogenic right ventricular dysplasia/cardiomyopathy: arrhythmia-free survival after endo-epicardial substrate based mapping and ablation. *Circ Arrhythm Electrophysiol.* 2011;4(4):478-485.
180. Dalal D, Jain R, Tandri H, et al. Long-term efficacy of catheter ablation of ventricular tachycardia in patients with arrhythmogenic right ventricular dysplasia/cardiomyopathy. *J Am Coll Cardiol.* 2007;50(5):432-440.
181. Philips B, Madhavan S, James C, et al. Outcomes of catheter ablation of ventricular tachycardia in arrhythmogenic right ventricular dysplasia/cardiomyopathy. *Circ Arrhythm Electrophysiol.* 2012;5(3):499-505.
182. Santangeli P, Zado ES, Supple GE, et al. Long-term outcome with catheter ablation of ventricular tachycardia in patients with arrhythmogenic right ventricular cardiomyopathy. *Circ Arrhythm Electrophysiol.* 2015;8(6):1413-1421.
183. Monserrat L, Elliott PM, Gimeno JR, Sharma S, Penas-Lado M, McKenna WJ. Non-sustained ventricular tachycardia in hypertrophic cardiomyopathy: an independent marker of sudden death risk in young patients. *J Am Coll Cardiol.* 2003;42(5):873-879.
184. Dukkipati SR, d'Avila A, Soejima K, et al. Long-term outcomes of combined epicardial and endocardial ablation of monomorphic ventricular tachycardia related to hypertrophic cardiomyopathy. *Circ Arrhythm Electrophysiol.* 2011;4(2):185-194.
185. Santangeli P, Di Biase L, Lakkireddy D, et al. Radiofrequency catheter ablation of ventricular arrhythmias in patients with hypertrophic cardiomyopathy: safety and feasibility. *Heart Rhythm.* 2010;7(8):1036-1042.
186. Inada K, Seiler J, Roberts-Thomson KC, et al. Substrate characterization and catheter ablation for monomorphic ventricular tachycardia in patients with apical hypertrophic cardiomyopathy. *J Cardiovasc Electrophysiol.* 2011;22(1):41-48.
187. Kumar S, Barbhaiya C, Nagashima K, et al. Ventricular tachycardia in cardiac sarcoidosis: characterization of ventricular substrate and outcomes of catheter ablation. *Circ Arrhythm Electrophysiol.* 2015;8(1):87-93.
188. Muser D, Santangeli P, Pathak RK, et al. Long-term outcomes of catheter ablation of ventricular tachycardia in patients with cardiac sarcoidosis. *Circ Arrhythm Electrophysiol.* 2016;9(8):e004333.
189. Papageorgiou N, Providencia R, Bronis K, et al. Catheter ablation for ventricular tachycardia in patients with cardiac sarcoidosis: a systematic review. *Europace.* 2018;20(4):682-691.
190. Nademanee K, Veerakul G, Chandanamattha P, et al. Prevention of ventricular fibrillation episodes in Brugada syndrome by catheter ablation over the anterior right ventricular outflow tract epicardium. *Circulation.* 2011;123(12):1270-1279.
191. Miller MA, al. e. Arrhythmic Mitral Valve Prolapse. *JACC.* 2018.
192. Sriram CS, Syed FF, Ferguson ME, et al. Malignant bileaflet mitral valve prolapse syndrome in patients with otherwise idiopathic out-of-hospital cardiac arrest. *J Am Coll Cardiol.* 2013;62(3):222-230.
193. Basso C, Perazzolo Marra M, Rizzo S, et al. Arrhythmic Mitral Valve Prolapse and Sudden Cardiac Death. *Circulation.* 2015;132(7):556-566.
194. Dejgaard LA, al. e. The Mitral Annulus Disjunction Arrhythmic Syndrome. *JACC.* 2018.

195. Essayagh B, Sabbag A, Antoine C, et al. Presentation and Outcome of Arrhythmic Mitral Valve Prolapse. *J Am Coll Cardiol.* 2020;76(6):637-649.

196. Nademanee K, Veerakul G, Chandanamattha P, et al. Prevention of ventricular fibrillation episodes in Brugada syndrome by catheter ablation over the anterior right ventricular outflow tract epicardium. *Circulation.* 2011;123(12):1270-1279.

197. Zhang P, Tung R, Zhang Z, et al. Characterization of the epicardial substrate for catheter ablation of Brugada syndrome. *Heart Rhythm.* 2016;13(11):2151-2158.

198. Pappone C, Brugada J, Vicedomini G, et al. Electrical substrate elimination in 135 consecutive patients with brugada syndrome. *Circ Arrhythm Electrophysiol.* 2017;10(5):e005053.

199. Fernandes GC, Fernandes A, Cardoso R, et al. Ablation strategies for the management of symptomatic Brugada syndrome: a systematic review. *Heart Rhythm.* 2018;15(8):1140-1147.

200. Nademanee K, Haissaguerre M, Hocini M, et al. Mapping and ablation of ventricular fibrillation associated with early repolarization syndrome. *Circulation.* 2019;140(18):1477-1490.

201. Kapel GF, Reichlin T, Wijnmaalen AP, et al. Left-sided ablation of ventricular tachycardia in adults with repaired tetralogy of Fallot: a case series. *Circ Arrhythm Electrophysiol.* 2014;7(5):889-897.

202. Laredo M, Frank R, Waintraub X, et al. Ten-year outcomes of monomorphic ventricular tachycardia catheter ablation in repaired tetralogy of Fallot. *Arch Cardiovasc Dis.* 2017;110(5):292-302.

203. Kapel GF, Sacher F, Dekkers OM, et al. Arrhythmogenic anatomical isthmuses identified by electroanatomical mapping are the substrate for ventricular tachycardia in repaired Tetralogy of Fallot. *Eur Heart J.* 2017;38(4):268-276.

204. von Rotz M, Aeschbacher S, Bossard M, et al. Risk factors for premature ventricular contractions in young and healthy adults. *Heart.* 2017;103(9):702-707.

205. Agarwal SK, Simpson Jr RJ, Rautaharju P, et al. Relation of ventricular premature complexes to heart failure (from the Atherosclerosis Risk In Communities [ARIC] Study). *Am J Cardiol.* 2012;109(1):105-109.

206. Marcus GM. Evaluation and management of premature ventricular complexes. *Circulation.* 2020;141(17):1404-1418.

207. Morshedi-Meibodi A, Evans JC, Levy D, Larson MG, Vasan RS. Clinical correlates and prognostic significance of exercise-induced ventricular premature beats in the community: the Framingham Heart Study. *Circulation.* 2004;109(20):2417-2422.

208. Cheriyath P, He F, Peters I, et al. Relation of atrial and/or ventricular premature complexes on a two-minute rhythm strip to the risk of sudden cardiac death (the Atherosclerosis Risk in Communities [ARIC] study). *Am J Cardiol.* 2011;107(2):151-155.

209. Dukes JW, Dewland TA, Vittinghoff E, et al. Ventricular ectopy as a predictor of heart failure and death. *J Am Coll Cardiol.* 2015;66(2):101-109.

210. Agarwal V, Vittinghoff E, Whitman IR, Dewland TA, Dukes JW, Marcus GM. Relation between ventricular premature complexes and incident heart failure. *Am J Cardiol.* 2017;119(8):1238-1242.

211. Qureshi W, Shah AJ, Salahuddin T, Soliman EZ. Long-term mortality risk in individuals with atrial or ventricular premature complexes (results from the Third National Health and Nutrition Examination Survey). *Am J Cardiol.* 2014;114(1):59-64.

212. Frolkis JP, Pothier CE, Blackstone EH, Lauer MS. Frequent ventricular ectopy after exercise as a predictor of death. *N Engl J Med.* 2003;348(9):781-790.

213. Jouven X, Zureik M, Desnos M, Courbon D, Ducimetiere P. Long-term outcome in asymptomatic men with exercise-induced premature ventricular depolarizations. *N Engl J Med.* 2000;343(12):826-833.

214. Marine JE, Shetty V, Chow GV, et al. Prevalence and prognostic significance of exercise-induced nonsustained ventricular tachycardia in asymptomatic volunteers: BLSA (Baltimore Longitudinal Study of Aging). *J Am Coll Cardiol.* 2013;62(7):595-600.

215. Baldesberger S, Bauersfeld U, Candinas R, et al. Sinus node disease and arrhythmias in the long-term follow-up of former professional cyclists. *Eur Heart J.* 2008;29(1):71-78.

216. Verdile L, Maron BJ, Pelliccia A, Spataro A, Santini M, Biffi A. Clinical significance of exercise-induced ventricular tachyarrhythmias in trained athletes without cardiovascular abnormalities. *Heart Rhythm.* 2015;12(1):78-85.

217. Biffi A, Maron BJ, Culasso F, et al. Patterns of ventricular tachyarrhythmias associated with training, deconditioning and retraining in elite athletes without cardiovascular abnormalities. *Am J Cardiol.* 2011;107(5):697-703.

218. Dello Russo A, Pieroni M, Santangeli P, et al. Concealed cardiomyopathies in competitive athletes with ventricular arrhythmias and an apparently normal heart: role of cardiac electroanatomical mapping and biopsy. *Heart Rhythm.* 2011;8(12):1915-1922.

219. Willems S, Hoffmann BA, Schaeffer B, et al. Mapping and ablation of ventricular fibrillation-how and for whom? *J Interv Card Electrophysiol.* 2014;40(3):229-235.

220. Haissaguerre M, Shoda M, Jais P, et al. Mapping and ablation of idiopathic ventricular fibrillation. *Circulation.* 2002;106(8):962-967.

221. Haissaguerre M, Shah DC, Jais P, et al. Role of Purkinje conducting system in triggering of idiopathic ventricular fibrillation. *Lancet.* 2002;359(9307):677-678.

222. Shimizu W. Arrhythmias originating from the right ventricular outflow tract: how to distinguish "malignant" from "benign"? *Heart Rhythm.* 2009;6(10):1507-1511.

223. Kim YR, Nam GB, Kwon CH, et al. Second coupling interval of nonsustained ventricular tachycardia to distinguish malignant from benign outflow tract ventricular tachycardias. *Heart Rhythm.* 2014;11(12):2222-2230.

224. Bansch D, Oyang F, Antz M, et al. Successful catheter ablation of electrical storm after myocardial infarction. *Circulation.* 2003;108(24):3011-3016.

225. Haissaguerre M, Extramiana F, Hocini M, et al. Mapping and ablation of ventricular fibrillation associated with long-QT and Brugada syndromes. *Circulation.* 2003;108(8):925-928.

226. Birati EY, Belhassen B, Bardai A, Wilde AA, Viskin S. The site of origin of torsade de pointes. *Heart.* 2011;97(20):1650-1654.

227. Santoro F, Di Biase L, Hranitzky P, et al. Ventricular fibrillation triggered by PVCs from papillary muscles: clinical features and ablation. *J Cardiovasc Electrophysiol.* 2014;25(11):1158-1164.

228. Sadek MM, Benhayon D, Sureddi R, et al. Idiopathic ventricular arrhythmias originating from the moderator band: Electrocardiographic characteristics and treatment by catheter ablation. *Heart Rhythm.* 2015;12(1):67-75.

229. Walters TE, Rahmutula D, Szilagyi J, et al. Left ventricular dyssynchrony predicts the cardiomyopathy associated with premature ventricular contractions. *JACC.* 2018;72(23 Pt A):2870-2882.
230. Latchamsetty R, Bogun F. Premature ventricular complex-induced cardiomyopathy. *JACC Clin Electrophysiol.* 2019;5(5):537-550.
231. Walters TE, Rahmutula D, Szilagyi J, et al. Left Ventricular dyssynchrony predicts the cardiomyopathy associated with premature ventricular contractions. *J Am Coll Cardiol.* 2018;72(23 Pt A):2870-2882.
232. Baman TS, Lange DC, Ilg KJ, et al. Relationship between burden of premature ventricular complexes and left ventricular function. *Heart Rhythm.* 2010;7(7):865-869.
233. Sadron Blaye-Felice M, Hamon D, Sacher F, et al. Premature ventricular contraction-induced cardiomyopathy: related clinical and electrophysiologic parameters. *Heart Rhythm.* 2016;13(1):103-110.
234. Yarlagadda RK, Iwai S, Stein KM, et al. Reversal of cardiomyopathy in patients with repetitive monomorphic ventricular ectopy originating from the right ventricular outflow tract. *Circulation.* 2005;112(8):1092-1097.
235. Niwano S, Wakisaka Y, Niwano H, et al. Prognostic significance of frequent premature ventricular contractions originating from the ventricular outflow tract in patients with normal left ventricular function. *Heart.* 2009;95(15):1230-1237.
236. Olgun H, Yokokawa M, Baman T, et al. The role of interpolation in PVC-induced cardiomyopathy. *Heart Rhythm.* 2011;8(7):1046-1049.
237. Carballeira Pol L, Deyell MW, Frankel DS, et al. Ventricular premature depolarization QRS duration as a new marker of risk for the development of ventricular premature depolarization-induced cardiomyopathy. *Heart Rhythm.* 2014;11(2):299-306.
238. Latchamsetty R, Yokokawa M, Morady F, et al. Multicenter outcomes for catheter ablation of idiopathic premature ventricular complexes. *JACC Clin Electrophysiol.* 2015;1(3):116-123.
239. Ling Z, Liu Z, Su L, et al. Radiofrequency ablation versus antiarrhythmic medication for treatment of ventricular premature beats from the right ventricular outflow tract: prospective randomized study. *Circ Arrhythm Electrophysiol.* 2014;7(2):237-243.

Index

Page numbers followed by "b," "f," and "t," indicate boxes, figures, and tables, respectively.